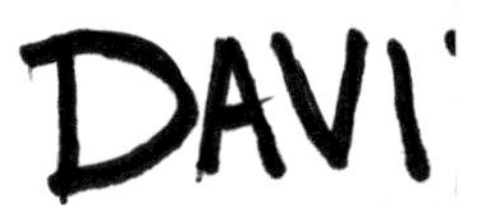
DAVI

MW00712101

DAVID SUH

CONGENITAL HEART DISEASE IN THE ADULT

CONGENITAL HEART DISEASE IN THE ADULT

Welton M. Gersony, MD
Alexander S. Nadas Professor of Pediatrics
College of Physicians and Surgeons
Columbia University
Professor of Pediatrics
Cornell University
Director, Columbia-Cornell
Pediatric Cardiovascular Center
New York Presbyterian Hospital
New York, New York

AND

Marlon S. Rosenbaum, MD
Assistant Professor of Clinical Medicine
and Clinical Pediatrics
College of Physicians & Surgeons
Columbia University
Director, Adult Congenital Heart Disease
New York Presbyterian Hospital
New York, New York

FOREWORD BY

Myron L. Weisfeldt, MD
Bard Professor of Medicine
College of Physicians & Surgeons
Columbia University
Chairman, Department of Medicine
New York Presbyterian Hospital
New York, New York

ILLUSTRATIONS BY

Richard A. Gersony, MD
Gersony Medical Media
New York, New York

CONTRIBUTOR

Kwame Anyane-Yeboa, MD
Associate Professor of Clinical Pediatrics
College of Physicians and Surgeons
Columbia University
New York, New York

McGRAW-HILL
Medical Publishing Division

New York / Chicago / San Francisco / Lisbon / London / Madrid / Mexico City
Milan / New Delhi / San Juan / Seoul / Singapore / Sydney / Toronto

McGraw-Hill

A Division of The ***McGraw-Hill*** *Companies*

CONGENITAL HEART DISEASE IN THE ADULT

1234567890 IMP/IMP 0987654321

ISBN: 0-07-032909-5

This book was set in Times Roman by Matrix Publishing Services.
Photo preparation was done by Jay's Publishing Services.
The editors were Darlene Cooke, Kathleen McCullough, and Scott Kurtz.
The production supervisor was Philip Galea.
The cover designer was Aimee Nordin.
The interior designer was Marsha Cohen/Parallelogram Graphics.
The index was prepared by Edwin Durbin.

The printer and binder was Imago (U.S.A.), Inc., in China.

This book is printed on acid-free paper.

Library of Congress Cataloging-in-Publication Data
Cataloging-in-Publication Data is on file with the Library of Congress.

CONTENTS

Welton M. Gersony and Marlon S. Rosenbaum have written a valuable and insightful introduction to the sparse cardiological literature depicting our current understanding of the life-long history of congenital heart disease in the modern era. Reflecting their years of experience, these authors characterize congenital heart disease as initially diagnosed and manifested in the adult and as modified by surgical interventions at variable points in the natural history. They challenge themselves to portray the long-term consequences of palliative operations (as performed in the early era of surgical intervention) and modern "corrective" procedures. They identify the needs and approaches to further surgical intervention in the former group. Their experience allows them to elucidate those aspects of "corrective" surgery that are not fully corrective. Finally, the consequences and options for further medical and/or surgical management emerge from their experience base.

If only a book such as this had been present and available during my own cardiology fellowship, my areas of personal interest might have changed significantly! Because of my own fascination with congenital heart disease and my inadequate understanding of the details of complex disease, I spent one month during a cardiology fellowship in Chicago, in the clinical laboratories of Morris Lev. He was arguably the most sophisticated pathologist and the most creative pioneer in understanding the detailed anatomy of congenital heart disease. Morris Lev accumulated hearts at various stages in development and correction from all over the world. These collections of hearts have been displayed by him and his disciples over the years in extraordinary fashion at national cardiology meetings.

What Lev understood and portrayed was a deep understanding of the basic anatomy of congenital heart disease. Then, the further evolution of the specialty resulted from the elucidation of the hemodynamic consequences of the various defects and their combinations in the cardiac catheterization laboratory. Enlargement, dilation, secondary hypertrophy, and ultimately hemodynamic failure and intolerance of the hemodynamic burden were cardinal principles. We are beginning to understand the molecular stimuli that result in remodeling and hypertrophy in the presence of hemodynamic stress and the response to neurohormonal stimuli. But we have yet to truly understand the ultimate molecular basis for the transition from hemodynamic compensation to progressive cardiac muscle dysfunction, though such an understanding will almost certainly emerge soon. The building blocks of the clinical, observational, and pathophysiological principles as presented by Gersony and Rosenbaum will be the reference core for such knowledge in the area of congenital heart disease.

The present monograph is organized categorically, depicting each important congenital heart disease lesion as acyanotic or cyanotic, from the common and simple to the complex and unusual. With each of these disorders there is a presentation of the classic findings and natural history for earlier and later identification of the congenital lesion. There is a presentation of the surgical approach as modified over the past fifty years to correct or palliate the lesion, and there is a wonderful presentation of the secondary consequences and the natural history of each lesion itself, and the problems and consequences related to the types of surgical interventions used, the partial corrections, and any later, more complete correction of these lesions. Finally, there is a presentation of end-stage medical and surgical management. The book relies heavily on echocardiographic, noninvasive assessment of the lesions and their natural history and the parameters of importance in the echocardiographic-Doppler characterization of the condition and the stage and adaptation.

The presentation is straightforward and assumes little in the way of sophisticated knowledge on the part of the reader. There are many thoughtful comments on management and strategies, both medical and surgical. There are clear statements where specific approaches improve the clinical state and natural history of the condition. Where there is doubt, the authors, on the basis of experience and knowledge, allow themselves to speculate or conjecture about the potential approaches and value of a variety of therapeutic options.

Dr. Welton M. Gersony was a fellow at the Children's Hospital Medical Center of Harvard Medical School in Boston. He has been the director of the Division of Pediatric Cardiology at the Columbia-Presbyterian Medical Center for the past thirty years. He is currently the Alexander S. Nadas Professor of Pediatrics and has been in every sense a major leader of the field of congenital heart disease at an international level, in part through creating an extraordinarily renowned clinical program. Similarly, Dr. Marlon S. Rosenbaum received advanced cardiology training at the Massachusetts General Hospital. He has been a member of the Columbia-Presbyterian Medical Center for nearly fifteen years. His focus is on adult congenital heart disease, and particularly the electrophysiological aspects of congenital heart disease, and the long-term care of patients with difficult-to-manage congenital heart disease. He is the director of the program of Adult Congenital Heart Disease within the Department of Medicine for the College of Physicians and Surgeons and heads an endowed program.

This monograph should be of considerable value to large groups of physicians and students at various stages in their own careers, with variable relationships to congenital heart disease in the adult: (1) to the consulting cardiologist who, like myself, sees acquired heart disease routinely but yet occasionally has responsibility for identification or management of congenital heart disease at many different stages; (2) to the cardiology fellow in pursuing the kind of deep understanding and conceptual formulation of these diseases and lesions that is essential to his/her education; and, similarly, to trainees in pediatric cardiology who are concentrating their attention on congenital heart disease in the infant and child but who need to understand the longer-term manifestations; (3) to the general internist, who from time to time is faced with the diagnostic challenge of eliminating or considering congenital heart disease along with acquired disease; and (4) to the trainee in internal medicine, who is often bewildered by a host of information sources, none of which provide a real diagnosis-by-diagnosis presentation of the origin and the natural-history consequences and options for patients they encounter on an occasional basis. Unquestionably, medical housestaff who have this monograph available will breathe easier when they encounter and must present or discuss the next patient with adult congenital heart disease, an unusual cardiac examination, or a difficult-to-interpret electrocardiogram.

Myron L. Weisfeldt, M.D.
Bard Professor of Medicine
College of Physicians and Surgeons
Columbia University
Chairman, Department of Medicine
New York Presbyterian Hospital

The prognosis for children with congenital heart disease has improved remarkably over the past two decades as a result of increasingly successful reparative cardiac surgery. This has created an expanding population of young adults who have had corrective or palliative cardiac operations early in life. It has been estimated that there are over one million adults with congenital cardiac abnormalities in the United States. These patients present a unique challenge to the internist/cardiologist, who must care for them but may not be fully informed regarding the natural history, potential complications, and decision-making issues. At times, this can result in patients developing myocardial or pulmonary vascular complications that could have been prevented; whereas undue concern for minor lesions can result in unnecessary patient anxiety and "over testing." The pediatric cardiologist does not have expertise in adult medicine and cannot assume total responsibility for an individual adult patient. A partnership should evolve between the pediatric cardiologist and his counterpart in adult medicine. This is especially important for the twenty- to thirty-year-old, who must give up a long-standing confident relationship with a pediatric specialist. The number of cardiologists specializing in congenital heart disease must grow, since for optimal care of the adult with congenital heart disease, the transition to a knowledgeable adult physician must be seamless.

The purpose of this book is to familiarize physicians with the broad spectrum of congenital heart defects, including both unoperated-upon and operated-upon patients. Each chapter focuses on a specific lesion, reviewing the anatomy, physiology, clinical presentation, surgical repair, and potential long-term problems encountered in adulthood. Particular emphasis has been placed on the optimal evaluation and follow-up care of these patients. Included are physical and laboratory findings, indications for invasive assessment, and management planning. Special sections on pregnancy and the genetics of congenital heart disease are provided.

For each chapter, a summary section is provided that reviews the most important information regarding each congenital heart lesion, allowing a patient's status to be better categorized when the patient is first referred to an internist/cardiologist for evaluation. The critical issues are identified in shortened form, and an algorithm is included, which illustrates a clinical practice plan for management of each defect and its variations, based on the patient's current status. Guidelines related to frequency of visits, appropriate testing, and criteria for intervention are outlined.

We would like to acknowledge the valuable assistance of David Brick, David Crowe, and Donna Heller in the preparation of this textbook.

Welton M. Gersony, M.D.
Marlon S. Rosenbaum, M.D.

CONGENITAL HEART DISEASE IN THE ADULT

PART I

ACYANOTIC HEART DISEASE

CHAPTER 1

ATRIAL SEPTAL DEFECT

Atrial septal defect (ASD) is a common congenital cardiac defect that accounts for 7% of all cardiac anomalies. There are three types of these defects: secundum, primum, and sinus venosus. The secundum defect is the most common and is located in the middle portion of the atrial septum (Fig. 1-1). Primum defects occur in the inferior atrial septum just superior to the inflow portion of both atrioventricular (AV) valves (Fig. 1-2). The defect almost always is associated with a cleft in the anterior leaflets of the mitral and tricuspid AV valve. Sinus venosus defects are located at the posterosuperior atrial border adjacent to the superior vena cava and usually are associated with anomalous drainage of the right upper or middle lobe pulmonary vein (Fig. 1-3).

Secundum and sinus venosus ASDs cause a left-to-right shunting at the atrial level that results in right ventricular volume overload and enlargement of the right atrium (RA), right ventricle (RV), and pulmonary artery (PA). Clinically detectable defects have little or no pressure gradient between the left atrium and right atrium. Since the flow across an ASD occurs in diastole when the AV valves are open, the degree of shunting is related to the relative compliance of the right and left ventricles as well as the size of the defect. As a result, a newborn infant who has a hypertrophied RV with compliance similar to that in the LV does not develop significant left-to-right shunting until physiologic right ventricular hypertrophy resolves during the first year of life. Once left-to-right shunting occurs, progressive dilatation of the right side of the heart ensues.

CLINICAL FEATURES

Despite substantial pulmonary blood flow, children and adolescents with ASDs are usually asymptomatic. Symptoms are more common in adults, who may experience palpitations, exertional dyspnea, and fatigue. Older adults with an ASD may present with congestive heart failure, often as a result of the development of atrial tachyarrhythmias. The incidence of atrial fibrillation or flutter increases progressively after the age of 40. The late presentation of patients with an ASD also may be due to the development of coronary artery disease, systemic hypertension, or natural aging. These processes result in decreased left ventricular compliance, increasing left-to-right shunting, and worsening

FIGURE 1-1*A*

Subcostal view in a patient with a moderate-size secundum atrial septal defect. Arrow points to the ASD. LA, left atrium; RA, right atrium.

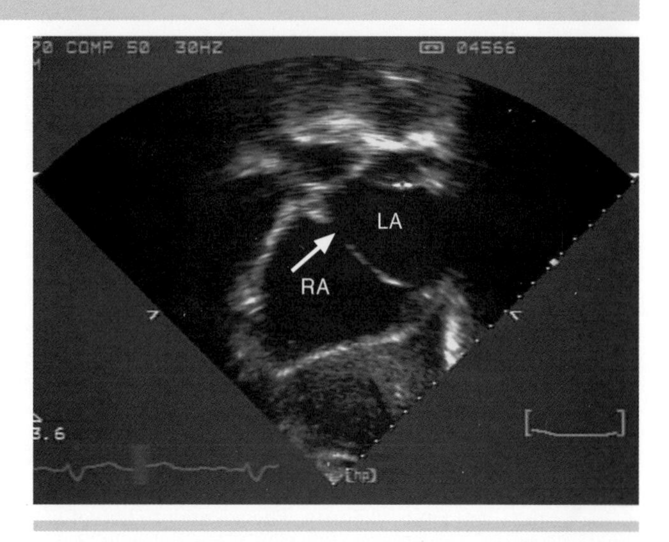

FIGURE 1-1*B*

Color Doppler from the subcostal view in the same patient showing left-to-right shunting across the ASD.

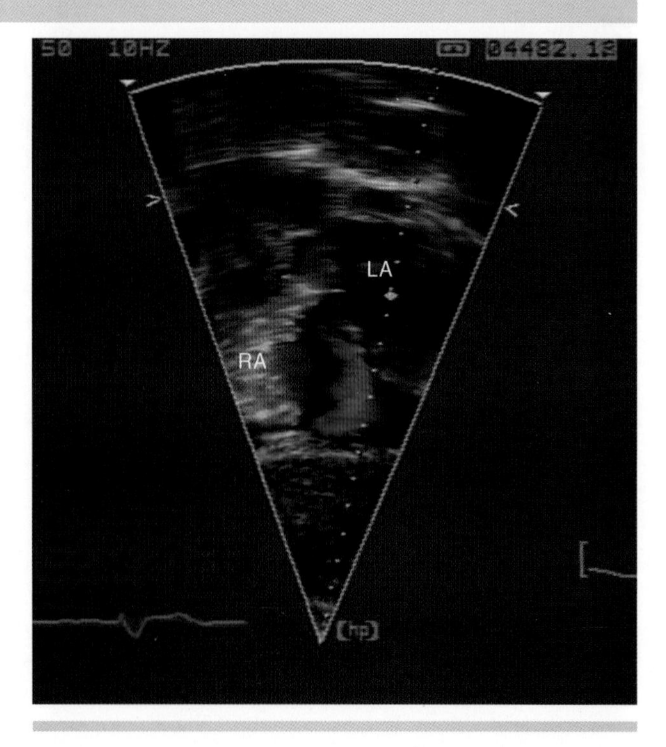

FIGURE 1-2

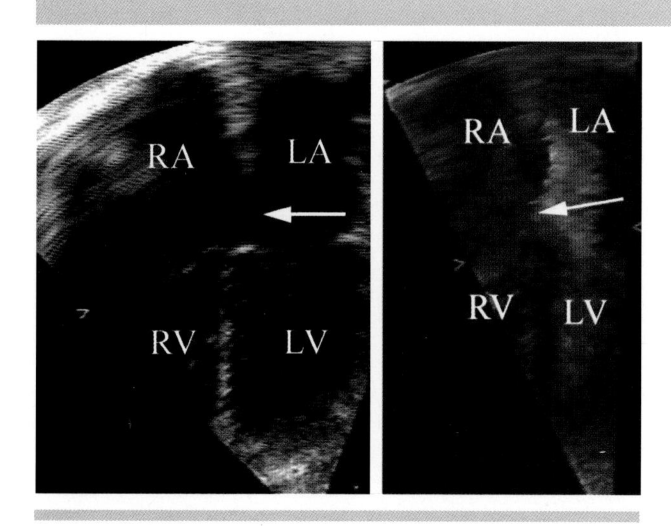

(Left) Apical 4-chamber view in a patient with a large primum atrial septal defect (ASD). The right heart is dilated. The arrow points to the deficiency in the atrial septum adjacent to the atrioventricular valve. (Right) Color Doppler from the same patient showing a left-to-right shunt across the defect. RA, right atrium; LA, left atrium; RV, right ventricle; LV, left ventricle.

symptoms. Patients with a primum ASD and mitral regurgitation will be symptomatic earlier than will individuals with an uncomplicated secundum ASD.

On occasion, an ASD is discovered during pregnancy when the increase in circulating blood volume calls attention to a prominent systolic murmur or results in symptoms of dyspnea. An unoperated patient also may be at increased risk for paradoxical embolism during pregnancy because of the increased incidence of pelvic thrombophlebitis during this period.

Pulmonary hypertension develops in a significant number of unoperated patients beyond age 40. In a series of 123 patients with secundum or sinus venosus ASD, pulmonary artery systolic pressure averaged 47 mm Hg in the patients operated on after age 41. Severe pulmonary hypertension with progressive pulmonary vascular obstructive disease develops in only 5 to 10% of patients with ASD but is a serious complication. As vascular disease evolves in later life, there is initially a decrease in left-to-right atrial shunting, followed by varying degrees of bidirectional shunting. Once long-standing pulmonary hypertension is present, tricuspid regurgitation and right-sided heart failure may develop and dominate the clinical picture. It is not possible to predict which patients will develop pulmonary vascular obstruction, but the disease appears to predominate in women.

Patients with a primum ASD may be diagnosed earlier, when mitral regurgitation is also present. Mitral regurgitation results from the cleft formed between the left superior and inferior AV valve leaflets. As is the case for all forms of endocardial cushion defects, the degree of AV valve regurgitation varies considerably from patient to patient. Mitral valve prolapse is present in 20% of patients with secundum ASD; however, significant mitral regurgitation is unusual.

FIGURE 1-3

A, Subcostal short-axis view showing a sinus venosus atrial septal defect (ASD). The broken arrow points to the defect, which is located in a superior and posterior portion of the atrial septum. *B*, Color Doppler from the same patient, which shows left-to-right shunting across the defect. RA, right atrium; LA, left atrium; SVC, superior vena cava; IVC, inferior vena cava; RPA, right pulmonary artery.

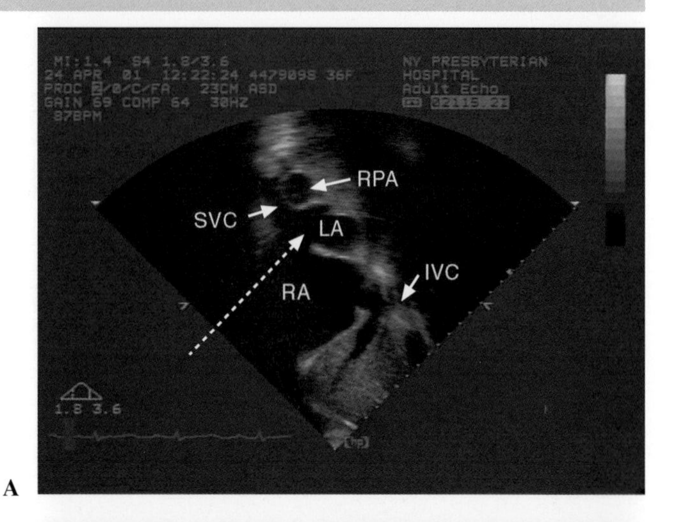

A

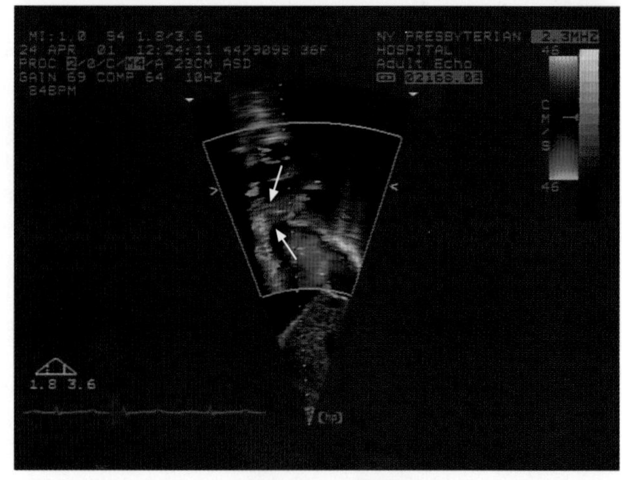

B

Physical Examination

The typical findings in a patient with an uncomplicated ASD may include a prominent right ventricular impulse along the left sternal border that reflects right ventricular volume overload. A systolic ejection murmur is frequently audible along the left upper sternal border because of increased flow across the right ventricular outflow tract. The murmur may be transmitted over the lungs secondary to turbulence in the pulmonary arteries. The second heart sound usually is widely split and fixed and may be an important finding in establishing a clinical diagnosis. When pulmonary blood flow is high, an early diastolic murmur may be audible at the lower left sternal border, reflecting increased flow across the tricuspid valve. Although these findings are indicative of a hemodynamically significant ASD, it is not uncommon to encounter adults with large left-to-right shunts who have more subtle examination findings. This is probably the cause for late discovery of ASD in some adults.

If pulmonary hypertension secondary to elevated pulmonary vascular resistance has developed, the widely split second heart sound is replaced by a narrowly split S_2 with an accentuated P_2. The tricuspid flow murmur disappears, and the systolic ejection murmur becomes shorter. A variable ejection click may be heard during expiration at the left upper to midsternal border because of right ventricular ejection into a dilated pulmonary trunk. Tricuspid insufficiency and pulmonary regurgitation may develop subsequently, and a medium-pitched protodiastolic murmur at the left midsternal border and/or a pansystolic murmur at the left lower sternal border become audible.

Noninvasive Evaluation

The *electrocardiogram* in a patient with a secundum ASD typically reveals sinus rhythm with an axis between 0 and +120 degrees. An RSR′ in V_1 is present in almost all hemodynamically significant lesions. Primum defects will show a characteristic left superior axis, as is found in patients with an AV canal (Fig. 1-4). The P-wave axis may be abnormal in sinus venosus defects, indicating a nonsinus atrial rhythm.

The *chest x-ray* in a patient with uncomplicated ASD may show enlargement of the right ventricle, best seen in the lateral view, and pulmonary artery dilatation with evidence of pulmonary overcirculation. However, it is not uncommon for the cardiac silhouette and pulmonary vascularity to be normal; this does not exclude the presence of a hemodynamically significant ASD. If the pulmonary vascular resistance is elevated, right ventricular volume overload disappears and cardiac size may decrease. In the most severe cases, there is a marked discrepancy between the dilated proximal pulmonary arteries and the diminished vascularity of the peripheral vessels.

Echocardiography has replaced cardiac catheterization for most children and most young adults with ASDs. A properly performed study is usually sufficient to visualize and size the defect, delineate a cleft mitral valve with a primum ASD (Fig. 1-5*A*,*B*), and estimate the amount of left-to-right atrial shunting on the basis of RA and RV enlargement, and determine the location of at least three of the four pulmonary veins. This is important because of the association with anomalous pulmonary venous drainage in ASDs, which occurs rarely in secundum defects but is present in 90% of sinus venosus communications. Doppler echocardiography is also helpful in estimating right ventricular pressure when tricuspid regurgitation is present or, when there is significant pulmonary hypertension, by the configuration of the ventricular septum during systole.

In adults, transthoracic echocardiography may be suboptional if imaging problems prevent adequate visualization of the ASD and pulmonary veins; subcostal long and short axis views and parasternal short axis imaging are most useful. Echo "dropout" in the region of the atrial septum or difficulty in visualizing the defect or locating the pulmonary veins may necessitate a transesophageal echocardiogram. Sinus venosus defects are particularly difficult to image in adults by transthoracic echo because of their superoposterior location and require adequate subcostal imaging. In this group, transesophageal echocardiography has been most useful.

FIGURE 1-4

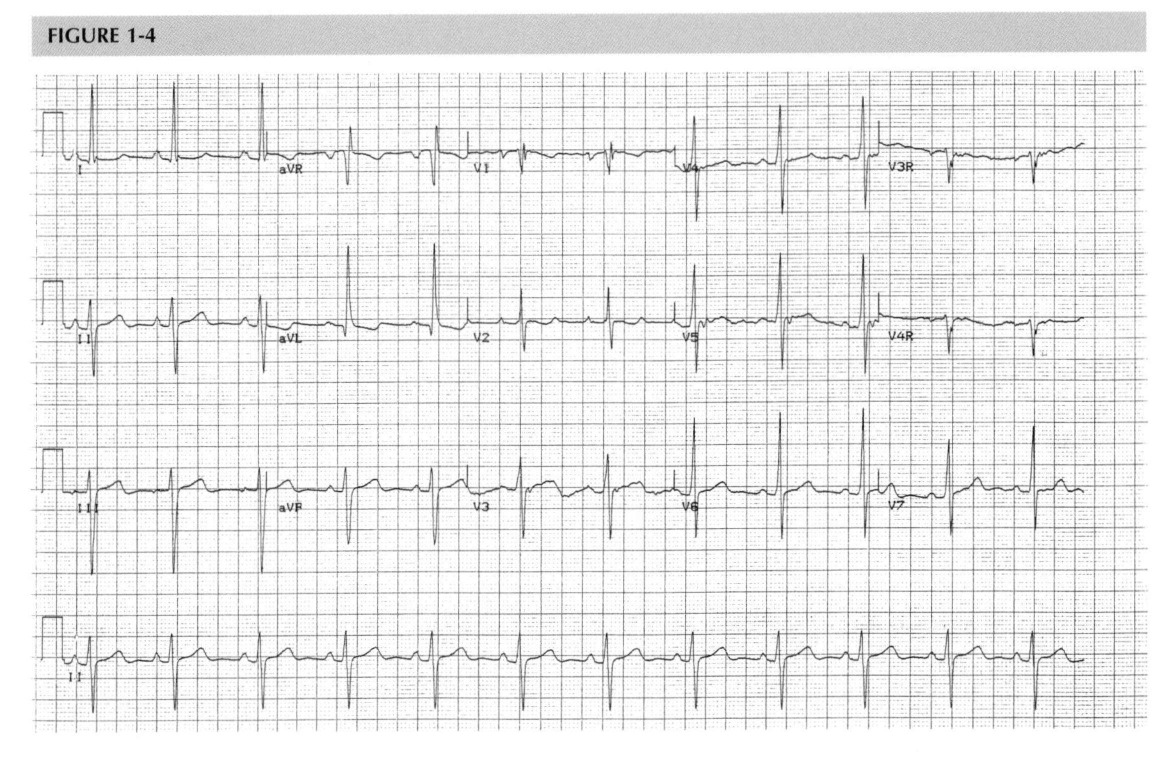

A 12-lead electrocardiogram from an adult with a primum atrial septal defect, which shows left axis deviation and a right-sided conduction delay, typical of an endocardial cushion defect.

Although echocardiography can resolve most of the pertinent issues, cardiac MRI can be a valuable resource in visualizing pulmonary or systemic venous anomalies as well as the ASD.

Cardiac Catheterization

The rationale for preoperative cardiac catheterization varies between institutions, but it is almost never required in children and young adults with an uncomplicated ASD. In older patients, cardiac catheterization is sometimes performed to address specific issues that cannot be assessed by echocardiography. These issues include the possibility of elevated pulmonary vascular resistance (PVR), the presence of anomalous pulmonary venous connections, and the assessment for possible associated mitral regurgitation. Coronary angiography may be required in patients over 40 years of age to determine whether coronary revascularization also is required.

When cardiac catheterization is performed, the femoral approach should be used to facilitate crossing of the ASD and measure the left and right atrial pressures. Sinus venosus defects may be difficult to cross because of their posterosuperior location. A series of oxygen saturations should be obtained in the superior vena cava (SVC), inferior vena cava (IVC), RA, RV, PA, and left atrium (LA) to calculate the PVR and Q_p/Q_s. A 10% step-up in the RA during a single series is usually indicative of a significant left-to-right shunt at the atrial level. However, it is important to recognize that there are potential pitfalls in the calculation of Q_p/Q_s by oximetry, including errors in the measurement of the saturation and in determining a true mixed venous saturation, both of which can change the calculations significantly. Some laboratories use a weighted average of SVC and IVC saturation for the mixed venous calculation. Others use only the SVC as the mixed venous site. Since the calculations are subject to error, it is important to recognize that right-sided heart dilatation and volume overload are the most important findings in determining whether an ASD is hemodynamically significant. Mild arterial desaturation (O_2 saturation 92 to 94%) may be present because of streaming of blood into the LA from the IVC through a secundum defect or from the SVC through a sinus venosus defect. Direct drainage of a left SVC into the LA is an unusual cause of arterial desaturation and is distinctly different from the more common anomaly, in which the left SVC enters the coronary sinus and does not cause desaturation.

Other causes of an O_2 step-up in the RA include a ventricular septal defect (VSD) with tricuspid insufficiency, a common AV valve with an endocardial cushion defect, anomalous pulmonary venous connections, a VSD with an LV-to-RA shunt, a sinus of Valsalva communication into the right atrium, a coronary artery fistula into the RA, and an unroofed coronary sinus. The RA saturation also will be elevated if a systemic AV fistula is present, but this also would be associated with an O_2 increase in the vena cava which drains the fistula. The presence of a markedly increased O_2 saturation in the SVC most often is due to an anomalous pulmonary venous connection. If the atrial septum cannot be crossed or if the location of the pulmonary veins is uncertain, left and right pulmonary angiograms can be done to visualize the pulmonary venous return. A left ventriculogram is performed when mitral regurgitation is suspected, most commonly in patients with primum defects that are associated with abnormalities of the left AV valve. An unroofed coronary sinus is a defect in the coronary sinus as it runs along the left AV groove, permitting fully saturated left atrial blood to enter the coronary sinus and right atrium.

MANAGEMENT

All hemodynamically significant ASDs should be closed. When the diagnosis is made in childhood, elective surgical repair or device closure is performed during the preschool years. Older patients should undergo ASD closure once the diagnosis has been established. Age does not appear to be a contraindication to repair of ASDs. Even patients with significant left-to-right shunts operated on after age 60 have shown significant symptomatic improvement and improved survival compared with patients treated medically.

Early closure of an ASD is recommended to prevent the sequelae of right-sided heart dilatation and pulmonary hypertension, which often lead to the development of supraventricular arrhythmias, pulmonary vascular obstructive disease, congestive heart failure, and, rarely, paradoxical embolism. Once supraventricular arrhythmias develop, they often do not improve after the defect is closed.

FIGURE 1-5*A*

Parasternal short-axis view in a patient with a cleft mitral valve. The arrow points to the cleft. LV, left ventricle; RV, right ventricle.

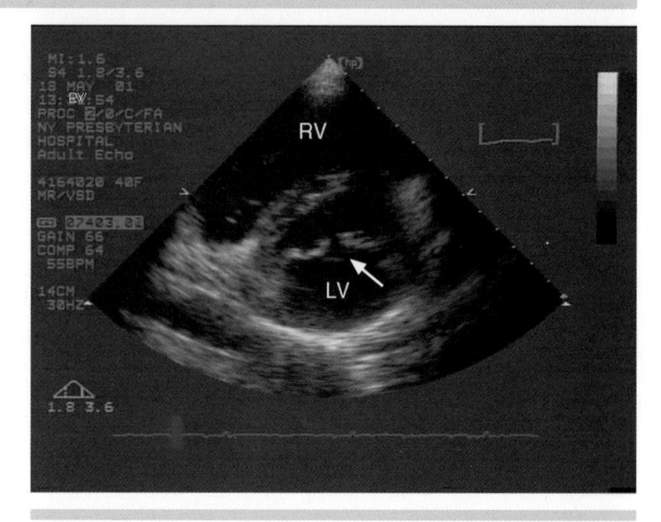

FIGURE 1-5*B*

Color Doppler from the same patient showing the origin of AV valve regurgitation from the cleft (arrow).

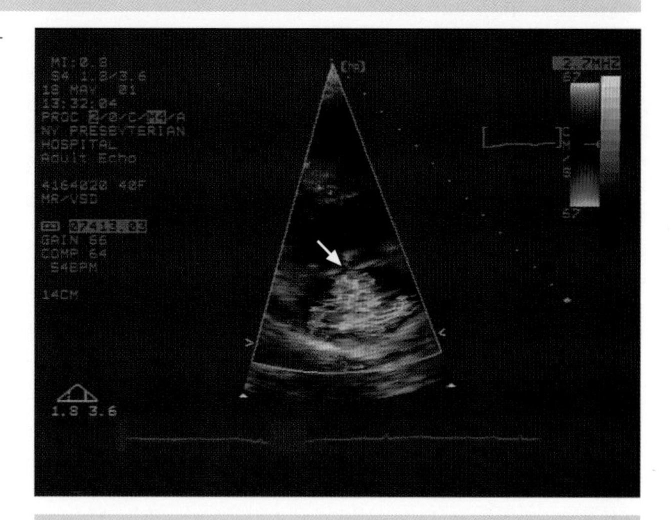

"Echo" Atrial Septal Defect

Technical advances in cardiac imaging, along with the widespread use of echocardiography, have resulted in the occasional detection of a small ASD that would not have been recognized clinically. Although ASD closure is not usually recommended for these defects if the right heart dimensions are normal, it is now appreciated that a significant percentage of adults with cryptogenic stroke have a patent foramen ovale or small ASD with provocable right-to-left shunting during a Valsalva maneuver. Treatment of patients who have had neurologic events with a small atrial communication is controversial. Management options include chronic anticoagulation, antiplatelet agents, and closure of the defect by surgery or with a device inserted during cardiac catheterization.

Pulmonary Hypertension

Although most patients with an ASD have a $Q_p/Q_s > 2.0$ and normal pulmonary vascular resistance, older patients may present for evaluation with an elevated pulmonary vascular resistance and a relatively small left-to-right shunt. If the left-to-right shunt is nevertheless significant, the ASD can be closed with the expectation that preexisting pulmonary hypertension will be improved or at least stabilized by the reduction in pulmonary blood flow.

If moderate to severe elevation of PVR is present and the Q_p/Q_s is <2.0, the decision regarding surgery may be difficult, as it is in any patient with increased PVR. In these patients, the issue is whether elimination of the small left-to-right shunt will reduce pulmonary artery pressure and decrease or halt the progression of pulmonary vascular obstructive disease. In borderline situations, it may be useful to evaluate the response to oxygen and other pulmonary vasodilators, such as nitric oxide or prostacyclin, and/or temporary occlusion of the defect during cardiac catheterization to assess the reactivity of the pulmonary vascular bed and assess whether permanent closure will be tolerated. Experience with such patients is limited. In a large reported series of secundum or sinus venosus ASD patients, pulmonary vascular obstructive disease was present in 6% of the patients. Patients with PVR <15 U/m^2 appeared to benefit from surgery with functional improvement, whereas those with PVR >15 U/m^2 were managed medically and had a short life expectancy.

Patients with PVR and right-to-left shunting are inoperable. Closure of the ASD will worsen the symptoms by eliminating the right-to-left shunt, which is important in maintaining systemic output at the expense of desaturation. Aggressive pulmonary vasodilator therapy may be helpful in some of these patients. Heart-lung transplantation and lung transplantation with intracardiac repair are the final treatment options for severely symptomatic patients with inoperable pulmonary vascular disease.

Surgical Repair

Secundum defects may be repaired primarily in most instances or with a pericardial patch for large defects. Ostium primum defects are repaired with a pericardial patch. Suture repair of the mitral valve cleft is almost always required. If mitral regurgitation persists after repair of the left AV valve, further attempts at repair may not be successful and valve replacement may be necessary. The use of transesophageal echocardiography in the operating room may help guide the surgeons in assessing the adequacy of mitral valve repair. Repair of a sinus venosus defect is affected by the presence of a right anomalous pulmonary venous connection. The patch is placed to the right of the anomalous vein to divert flow directly into the LA. Anomalous drainage of the right upper pulmonary vein high in the SVC makes the ASD closure more difficult.

Complications

In the past, repair of a primum defect was associated with a 5% risk of complete heart block. This complication is rarely encountered today because of a better understanding of the location of the AV node and the bundle of His. The development of a "Waring blender" syndrome is rare and refers to the development of hemolysis from a residual jet of AV valve regurgitation against a Dacron patch. Superior vena cava obstruction has been described after repair of the anomalous right pulmonary vein in association with a sinus venosus ASD. The proximity of the sinus venosus defect to the sinus node may result in sinus node dysfunction if it is damaged during the repair.

Device Atrial Septal Defect Closure

Percutaneous ASD closure devices are now available that obviate the need for surgical correction of selected patients with a secundum ASD. These devices permit percutaneous closure of an ASD or patent foramen ovale during cardiac catheterization (see Fig. 1-6). Two of these devices are currently being used. The largest experience has been with small and medium-size secundum defects, although larger devices have been developed to close the large defects. Although the complication rate has been very low, the main issues concern the potential for thromboembolic complication, acute embolization of the device and incomplete closure with a residual shunt. It is expected that the use of these devices will increase and eventually replace surgery for many patients with secundum defects.

LONG-TERM FOLLOW-UP

The long-term survival of patients who have undergone repair of secundum and sinus venosus ASDs appears to be related to the age at operation. Reported actuarial 27-year survival rates indicate no difference in survival between age- and sex-matched controls when surgery was carried out before age 24. In contrast, survival rates are significantly lower than those in controls in the group of patients operated on between ages 25 and 41 and after age 41. Cardiac failure, stroke, and atrial fibrillation occurred significantly more frequently in older patients.

Supraventricular arrhythmias may persist after surgery in older patients and also may develop over time in patients in whom rhythm abnormalities were not present preoperatively. A recent study of postoperative adults with ASDs found an increased incidence of late supraventricular tachycardia when repair was performed after age 40. Sick sinus syndrome may develop occasionally after the repair of a sinus venosus defect. A permanent pacemaker is required for the rare patient with sick sinus syndrome and symptomatic bradycardia. Left AV valve regurgitation in patients with primum defects may require late medical and/or surgical management. Subacute bacterial endocarditis (SBE) prophylaxis should be continued in patients with postoperative primum defects because of abnormalities of the left AV valve. This prophylaxis is not recommended for secundum and sinus venosus defects beyond 6 months after surgery unless there are associated valvar abnormalities.

FIGURE 1-6

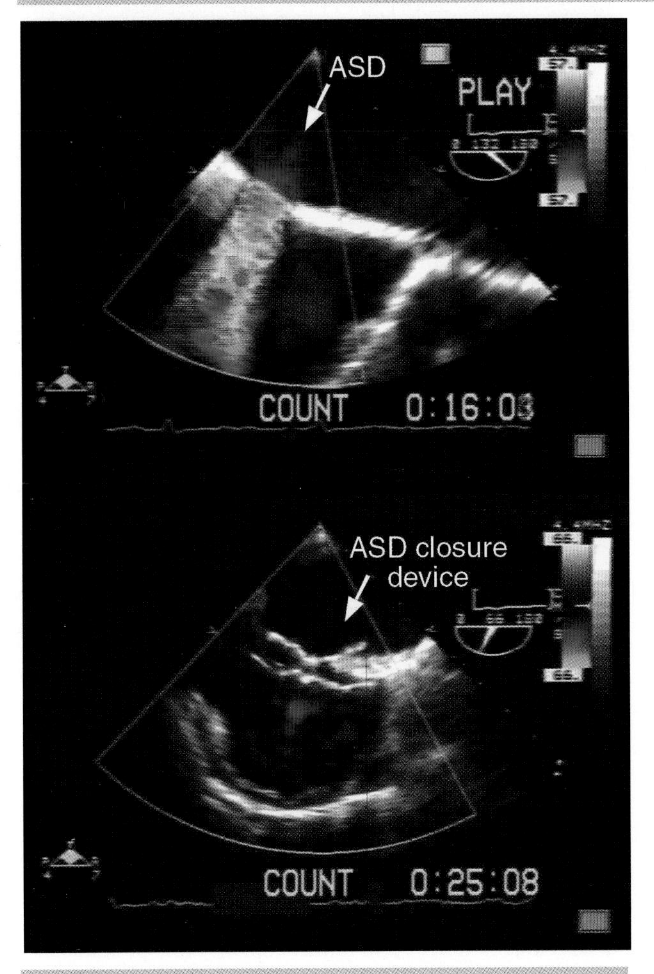

(Top) Color Doppler from a transesophageal echocardiogram in a patient with a secundum atrial septal defect (ASD). A left-to-right shunt is present across the ASD. (Bottom) The ASD has been closed using an ASD closure device. There is no residual shunt across the defect.

PARTIAL ANOMALOUS PULMONARY VENOUS CONNECTIONS

Partial anomalous pulmonary venous connections occasionally may be mistaken for an ASD. This lesion can result in right ventricular volume overload if a significant left-to-right shunt is present. Anomalous pulmonary venous connections may arise from either the right lung or the left lung. They may drain directly into the RA or via the vena cavae, innominate vein, or coronary sinus. The most frequently encountered anomalous connections are, in descending order, right upper or middle lobe pulmonary vein into the right atrium or SVC, left pulmonary vein into the innominate vein, and right pulmonary vein into the IVC. When the left pulmonary vein is anomalous, it usually drains into the innominate vein via a vertical vein. Bilateral partial anomalous connections are rare but have been reported.

In the "scimitar syndrome," pulmonary venous drainage from the right lung drains into the IVC. In some of these cases, there is dextroposition of the heart into the right side of the chest with hypoplasia of the right lung and pulmonary artery. Pulmonary sequestration and bronchial artery collateral to the right lung may also be present in some cases.

Although a single anomalous pulmonary vein represents only one-quarter of the anatomic pulmonary blood flow from the lungs, the actual left-to-right shunt may be larger because venous return into the lower-pressure right atrium may promote more blood flow through the corresponding lung segment. Nevertheless, anomalous drainage of a single pulmonary vein without an associated ASD usually does not require surgical correction in asymptomatic adults because the left-to-right shunt is generally not substantial enough to cause right-sided heart dilatation. However, in a rare symptomatic patient, partial anomalous pulmonary venous return with a large left-to-right shunt requires surgical intervention.

SUMMARY

Large Left-to-Right Shunt

Patients with a significant left-to-right shunt should undergo closure of the defect. Percutaneous closure may replace surgery for appropriately sized ASDs. When present, anomalous pulmonary veins are incorporated into the left atrium. Mitral valve insufficiency may require repair; tricuspid valve surgery rarely is needed.

Tiny Defect (Echo Diagnosis)

An extremely small ASD or patent foramen ovale discovered in a patient with no symptoms or physical findings of an ASD should be followed, since there is no evidence that prophylactic closure provides an advantage. Long-term follow-up of such patients has shown no clinical manifestations. Borderline cases are encountered in which small but nevertheless well-defined left-to-right shunts are noted through ASDs that are well delineated by imaging techniques. These patients must be dealt with on an individual basis, depending on the age, sex, and overall clinical status of the patient. The optimal treatment of patients with patent foramen ovale (PFO) and cryptogenic stroke has not been determined. Chronic anticoagulation, aspirin, and closure have been utilized.

Atrial Septal Defect with Pulmonary Vascular Obstructive Disease

Patients who have mild elevation of pulmonary vascular resistance but still have a significant left-to-right shunt may benefit from surgery. Pulmonary pressure will fall in keeping with the decrease in flow, and progressive disease may be prevented. Patients with severe pulmonary vascular disease should not undergo ASD closure. Pulmonary vasodilator therapy may be useful. Lung and heart-lung transplantations are options for severely symptomatic patients.

Postoperative Atrial Septal Defect

Adults who have an ASD repaired should be followed for late arrhythmias, usually supraventricular or sick sinus syndrome. If residual mitral insufficiency was originally present, this lesion should be reevaluated at reasonably frequent intervals since progressive AV valve disease can occur even after the original ASD was successfully repaired and whether or not an original valvuloplasty was done.

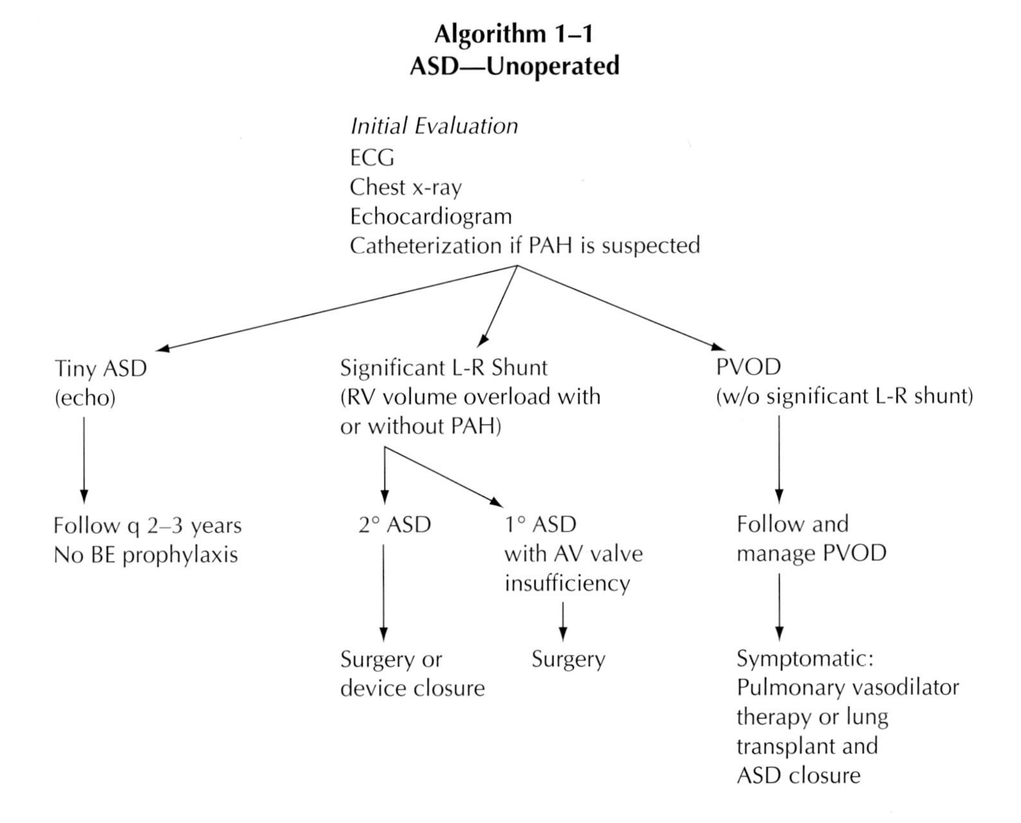

KEY: ASD, atrial septal defect; A-V, atrioventricular; ECG, electrocardiogram; PAH, pulmonary artery hypertrophy; PVOD, pulmonary vascular obstructive disease; RV, right ventricle; SBE, subacute bacterial endocarditis; w/o, without; 2°, secundum; 1°, primum.

Algorithm 1–2
ASD—Operated

Initial Evaluation
ECG
Chest x-ray
Echocardiogram
Holter

↓

Follow q 2 years
(more often for 1° ASD
re A-V valve regurgitation
or subvalvular AS)

No BE prophylaxis for repaired
secundum or sinus venosus

BE prophylaxis for primum

KEY: AS, aortic stenosis; ASD, atrial septal defect; A-V, atrium-ventricle; BE, bacterial endocarditis; ECG; electrocardiogram

BIBLIOGRAPHY

Anderson M, Moller I, Lyngborg K, et al: The natural history of small atrial septal defect: Long-term follow-up with serial heart catheterization. *Am Heart J* 92:302, 1976.

Berger F, Ewert P, Bjkornstad PG, et al: Transcatheter closure as standard treatment for most interatrial defects: Experience in 200 patients treated with the Amplatzer Septal Occluder. *Cardiol Young* 9(5):468, 1999.

Berger F, Vogel M, Kramer A, et al: Incidence of atrial flutter/fibrillation in adults with atrial septal defect before and after surgery. *Ann Thorac Surg* 68:75, 1999.

Brassard M, Fouron JC, van Doesburg NH, et al: Outcome of children with atrial septal defect considered too small for surgical closure. *Am J Cardiol* 83(11):1552, 1999.

Burke RP, Horvath K, Landzberg M, et al: Long-term follow-up after surgical repair of ostium primum atrial septal defect in adults. *J Am Coll Cardiol* 27(3):696, 1996.

Campbell M: Natural history of atrial septal defect. *Br Heart J* 32:820, 1970.

Cherian G, Uthaman CB, Durairaj M, et al: Pulmonary hypertension in isolated secundum atrial septal defect: High frequency in young patients. *Am Heart J* 105:952, 1983.

Craig RJ, Selzer A: Natural history and prognosis of atrial septal defect. *Circulation* 37:805, 1968.

Di Tullio M, Sacco RL, Gopal A, et al: Patent foramen ovale as a risk factor for cryptogenic stroke. *Ann Intern Med* 117:461, 1992.

Gatzoulis MA, Freeman MA, Siu SC, et al: Atrial arrhythmia after surgical closure of atrial septal defects in adults. *N Engl J Med* 18(11):839, 1999.

Gatzoulis MA, Hechter S, Webb GD, Williams WG: Surgery for partial atrioventricular septal defect in the adult. *Ann Thorac Surg* 67(2):504, 1999.

Gatzoulis MA, Redington AN, Somerville J, Shore DF: Should atrial septal defects in adults be closed? *Ann Thorac Surg* 61(2):657, 1996.

Hagen PT, Scholz DG, Edwards WD: Incidence and size of patent foramen ovale during the first 10 decades of life: An autopsy of 965 normal hearts. *Mayo Clin Proc* 59:17, 1984.

Helber U, Baumann R, Seboldt H, et al: Atrial septal defect in adults: Cardiopulmonary exercise capacity before and 4 months and 10 years after defect closure. *J Am Coll Cardiol* 29(6):1345, 1997.

Horvath KA, Burke RP, Collins JJ Jr, Cohn LH: Surgical treatment of adult atrial septal defect: Early and long-term results. *J Am Coll Cardiol* 20:1156, 1992.

King RM, Puga FJ, Danielson GK, et al: Prognostic factors and surgical treatment of partial atrioventricular canal. *Circulation* 74:142, 1986.

King TD, Mills NL: Non-operative closure of atrial septal defects. *Surgery* 75:383, 1974.

Konstantinides S, Geibel A, Olschewski M, et al: A comparison of surgical and medical therapy for atrial septal defect in adults. *N Engl J Med* 333(8):469, 1995.

Kyger ER, Frazier OH, Cooley DA, et al: Sinus venosus atrial septal defect: Early and late results following closure in 109 patients. *Ann Thorac Surg* 25:44, 1978.

Latson LA, Benson LN, Hellenbrand WE, et al: Early results of multicenter trial of the Bard Clamshell Septal Occluder. *Circulation* 84:2161a, 1991.

Lock JE, Rome JJ, David R, et al: Transcatheter closure of atrial septal defects: Experimental studies. *Circulation* 79:1091, 1989.

Markman P, Howitt G, Wade EG: Atrial septal defect in the middle aged and elderly. *Q J Med* 34:409, 1965.

Mattila S, Merikallio E, Tala P: ASD in patients over 40 years of age. *Scand J Thorac Cardiovasc Surg* 13:21, 1979.

Meijboom F, Hess J, Szatmari A, et al: Long-term follow-up (9 to 20 years) after surgical closure of atrial septal defect at a young age. *Am J Cardiol* 72:431, 1993.

Murphy JG, Gersh BJ, McGoon MD, et al: Long-term outcome after surgical repair of isolated atrial septal defect: Follow-up at 27 to 32 years. *N Engl J Med* 323(24):1645, 1990.

O'Toole JD, Reddy PS, Curtiss EL, Shaver JA: The mechanism of splitting of the second heart sound in atrial septal defect. *Circulation* 56:105, 1977.

Reid JM, Stevenson JC: Cardiac arrhythmias following successful surgical closure of atrial septal defect. *Br Heart J* 29:742, 1967.

Rome JJ, Keane JF, Perry SB, et al: Double-umbrella closure of atrial defects: Initial clinical applications. *Circulation* 82:751, 1990.

St. John Sutton MG, Tajik AJ, McGoon DC: Atrial septal defect in patients ages 60 years or older: Operative results and long-term postoperative follow-up. *Circulation* 64:402, 1981.

Schenck MH, Sterba R, Foreman CK, et al: Improvement in noninvasive electrophysiologic findings in children after transcatheter atrial septal defect closure. *Am J Cardiol* 76:695, 1995.

Shah D, Azhar M, Oakley CM, et al: Natural history of secundum atrial septal defect in adults after medical or surgical treatment: A historical prospective study. *Br Heart J* 71:224, 1994.

Steele PM, Fuster V, Cohen M, et al: Isolated atrial septal defect with pulmonary vascular obstructive disease—long-term follow-up and prediction of outcome after surgical correction. *Circulation* 76(5):1037, 1987.

CHAPTER 2

ATRIOVENTRICULAR CANAL

An atrioventricular (AV) canal defect, also known as an atrioventricular septal defect, is defined as a deficiency of septal tissue immediately above and below the AV valve in conjunction with abnormalities of the atrioventricular valves. This results in a primum atrial septal defect (ASD), abnormalities of the right and left AV valves, and a deficiency in the inlet portion of the ventricular septum. The AV valve abnormalities may be severe; the valves are distinctly different anatomically from the normal mitral and tricuspid valves. The left-sided valve consists of left lateral, left superior, and left inferior leaflets. The right-sided AV valve consists of right lateral, right superior, and right inferior leaflets. In addition to these abnormalities, the aorta is elevated and anteriorly deviated, producing a different relationship than the mitral-aortic continuity observed in normal hearts. In AV canal defects, the LV inflow tract is shortened and the LVOT is narrowed, producing a so-called "gooseneck" deformity of the outflow tract.

AV canal defects can be broadly characterized as complete, partial, and intermediate. Much of the distinction between complete and partial AV canal defects lies in the morphology and attachments of the left superior leaflet. In the complete form of AV canal defect, there are both a primum ASD and inlet-type VSD, and there are no connections between the left superior and left inferior AV valve leaflets. In the milder form of atrioventricular septal defect, known as partial AV canal defect, a primum ASD is present, the ventricular septal defect is small, and the common AV valve is replaced by two separate AV valves, which are connected at the border of the left superior and left inferior leaflets. Variations between these two extremes are referred to as intermediate forms of AV canal defect.

In addition to the anatomic classification, a complete AV canal defect can be defined hemodynamically by the nonrestrictive large VSD that is present regardless of the specific details of the anatomy of the AV valve. In a complete AV canal defect, there is always right ventricular and pulmonary artery hypertension based on the large ventricular communication, whereas in the other forms, the VSD may be small and pulmonary artery pressures may be relatively normal. In a complete AV canal defect, shunting occurs at both the atrial level and ventricular level, and there are varying degrees of AV valve insufficiency. The hemodynamic distinctions make decision making about repair of these entities easier (see Figs. 2-1*A* and *B* and 2-2*A* and *B*).

Complete AV canal defect is further classified into three types (Rastelli type A, B, C), which relate to the extent to which the left superior leaflet extends across the crest of

FIGURE 2-1

A. Apical four-chamber view during diastole in a patient with a complete atrioventricular (AV) canal defect demonstrating the large atrial and ventricular communication and bridging leaflets that traverse the interventricular septum. *B*. AV canal systole. Apical four-chamber view during systole in the same patient with a complete AV canal defect. There is a large inlet-type ventricular septal defect and a primum atrial septal defect. The AV valve is closed. The arrow points to the chordal attachments that insert on the crest of the ventricular septum. ASD, atrial septal defect; VSD, ventricular septal defect; RV, right ventricle; left ventricle.

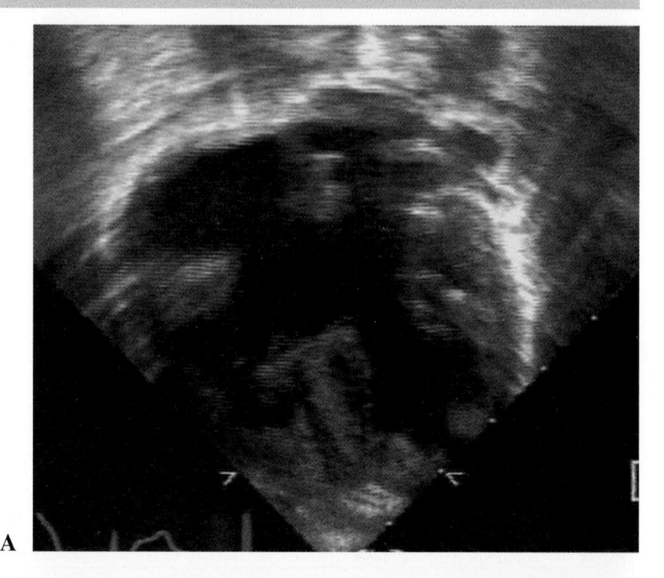

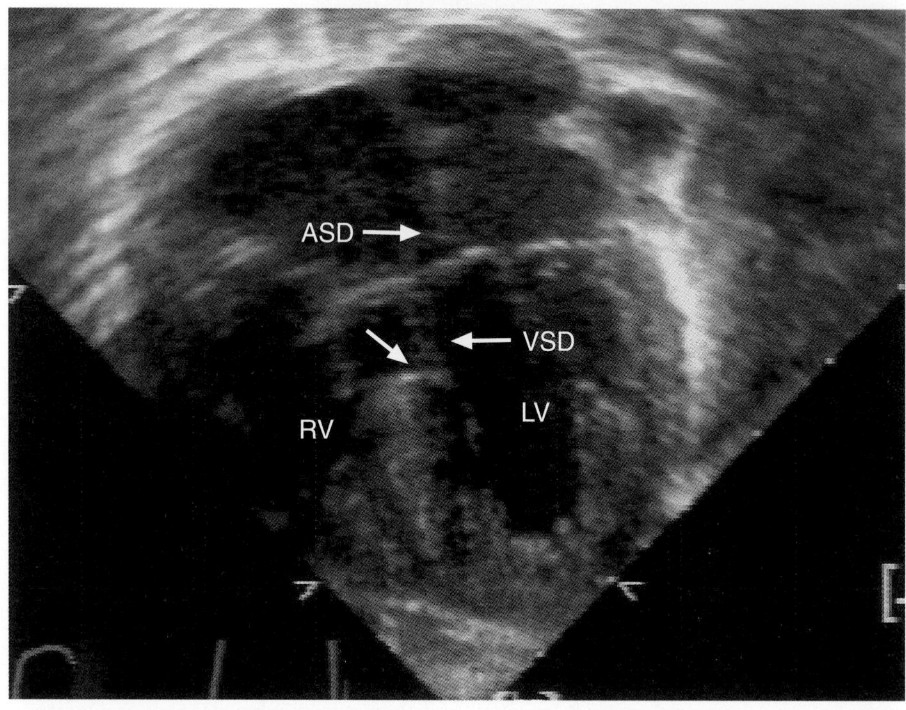

FIGURE 2-2

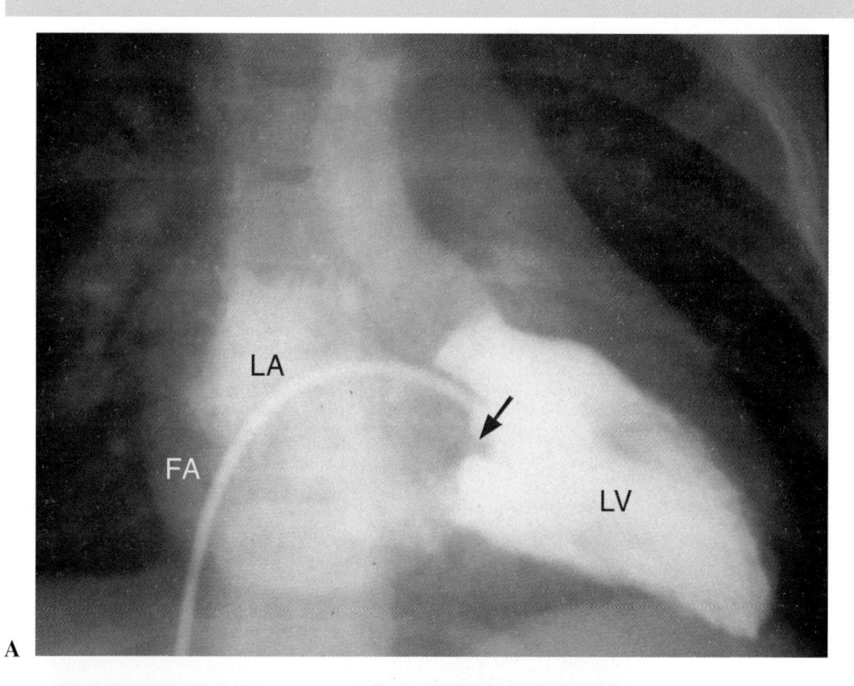

A

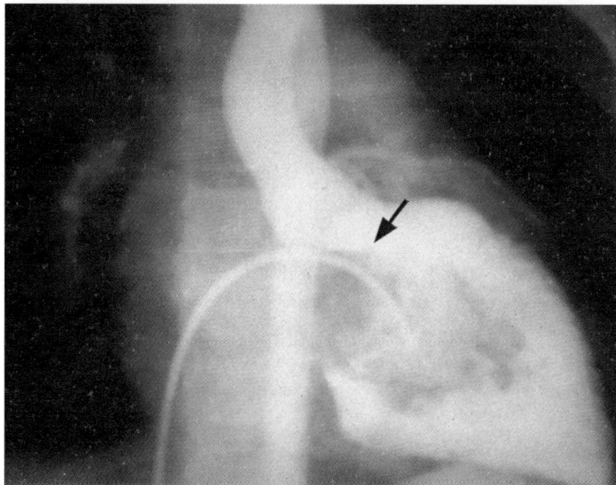

B

Left ventricular angiogram in systole in a patient with a cleft mitral valve (arrow). Significant AV valve insufficiency is present with filling of both the left atrium and the right atrium. LV = left ventricle; LA = left atrium; RA = right atrium. *B.* Cineangiogram frame taken in diastole shows the gooseneck deformity of the left ventricular outflow tract (arrow).

the ventricular septum into the right ventricle. In all cases, a primum ASD and a VSD are present. In type A, the chordal attachments are to the crest of the ventricular septum. In type B, which is extremely rare, there is mild bridging of the left superior leaflet with chordal attachments to the medial papillary muscle in the right ventricle. In type C, there is marked bridging of the left superior leaflet into the right ventricle. The leaflet freely floats over the crest of the ventricular septum without chordal attachments to the crest of the septum.

In the classic form of complete AV canal defect, the sizes of the ventricles are similar. However, right or left ventricular chamber dominance may occur, and one ventricle or the other may be sufficiently underdeveloped to preclude a four-chamber surgical repair (unbalanced AV canal). In such cases, the condition must be treated surgically as a form of single ventricle (Chap. 12).

CLINICAL FEATURES IN INFANCY AND CHILDHOOD

Patients with a complete AV canal present to the pediatric cardiologist in early infancy with various combinations of large left-to-right shunts and AV valve insufficiency. As with other large communications between the left-sided and right-sided heart circulations (e.g., VSD, patent ductus arteriosus, truncus arteriosus), symptoms usually begin after a few weeks of life; increased pulmonary vascular resistance at birth limits the left-to-right shunt during the early neonatal period. However, once heart failure ensues, these patients often are difficult to manage medically, and early surgical intervention is required to prevent chronic heart failure and failure to thrive.

Surgical results have improved markedly over the last decade; left-to-right shunts can be eliminated, and valvuloplasty decreases the degree of regurgitation, significantly if not completely. Even if patients can be managed successfully medically, surgery should be carried out within the first 4 to 5 months of life to prevent pulmonary vascular obstructive disease. This complication occurs more frequently and earlier in these patients than do other large left-to-right shunts, such as an isolated large VSD. Patients with Down syndrome are especially susceptible to upper airway and pulmonary complications and to early pulmonary vascular obstructive disease. Although partial and intermediate forms may occasionally produce early symptoms, this usually is based on left AV valve insufficiency with a large primum ASD. If AV valve insufficiency is not severe in an asymptomatic patient and pulmonary artery pressure is relatively normal, surgery can be delayed.

Unoperated patients with complete AV canal defects who survive into adult life almost invariably have pulmonary vascular obstructive disease and no more than moderate AV valve insufficiency. Down syndrome is present in 75% of patients with complete AV canal, but is much less frequently seen in patients with partial AV canal defects.

MANAGEMENT

Surgical Repair

Surgery for complete AV canal defect consists of closure of the intraventricular communication with a patch, partitioning of the common AV valve into separate right and left components, and patch closure of the primum ASD. It is important to avoid sutures in the region of the AV node and bundle of His, and in recent years the incidence of postoperative complete heart block has diminished significantly. Some surgeons perform the repair with a single patch and attach the AV valve leaflets at the appropriate level within the patch. Others use a two-patch method.

In the partial form of AV canal defect, only a single patch is required. Repair of left AV valve regurgitation is performed when there is at least moderate regurgitation. In patients with a primum ASD and little or no AV valve regurgitation, there is a debate concerning the benefits of valvuloplasty on the left AV valve. As with complete AV canal defect, it is important that the orifices of the left and right AV valves remain relatively equal in size and unobstructed. It is rare that right AV valvuloplasty is required, and tricuspid insufficiency is not usually a clinical problem.

Tetralogy of Fallot is an associated defect in 10% of patients with AV canal defect. The presence of significant RV outflow tract obstruction limits left-to-right shunting and prevents heart failure and late pulmonary vascular obstructive disease. The physiology is that of tetralogy of Fallot, often with progressive obstruction leading to severe cyanosis, resulting in the need for surgical intervention. Surgical repairs are complex, but in recent years, successful repair has been achieved in the great majority of these patients.

Among postoperative patients with AV canal, the major concern is the degree of residual left AV valve insufficiency. This insufficiency varies from trivial to severe, and management ranges from early to late reoperation or replacement to decades of observation without the necessity for AV valve reintervention. Residual right AV valve insufficiency is rarely clinically significant enough to require surgical reintervention.

Patients with postoperative AV canal also are prone to the development of subvalvar aortic stenosis. This complication occurs in approximately 10% of these patients, and has multiple etiologies. LVOT obstruction may be due to: (1) narrowing of the junction between the aortic valve and the left superior leaflet, (2) discrete subaortic stenosis, (3) excess AV valve tissue in the LVOT, and (4) the result of an abnormally positioned papillary muscle. Reoperation for subvalvar aortic stenosis is not unusual; fibrous tissue usually can be removed, allowing relief of the obstruction. However, some patients may be prone to recurrent outflow tract obstruction and may require more extensive surgery in the LVOT, such as a modified Konno procedure. This consists of a right ventriculotomy with incision and patch enlargement of the ventricular septum just below the aortic valve.

CLINICAL FEATURES IN ADULTS

An adult with complete AV canal defect most often has a history of cardiac surgery during infancy, and some of these patients may have had reoperation for left AV valve insufficiency or subaortic stenosis. Reoperation for residual left-to-right shunts is not common. Unoperated patients almost invariably have pulmonary vascular obstructive disease, and if surgical repair was done late, postoperative patients also may have elevated pulmonary artery pressure because of persistent or progressive pulmonary vascular obstructive disease. Patients who have been operated on for AV canal defect and pulmonary stenosis may have residual pulmonary stenosis and/or insufficiency as well as the other complications associated with AV canal surgery. Surgically acquired complete heart block requiring a pacemaker occasionally is encountered.

Physical Examination

An adult with a repaired form of AV canal defect who is doing well clinically usually has only a murmur of mild left AV valve insufficiency. Some patients may have advanced AV valve insufficiency, and the clinical findings will be consistent with that diagnosis. A diastolic rumble frequently accompanies the murmur of AV valve regurgitation, but true AV valve stenosis is rare. Clinically important right AV valve insufficiency is encountered rarely. When a harsh systolic ejection murmur is audible along the left middle and upper sternal border radiating to the base, subaortic obstruction should be considered. Patients who have had surgery for associated pulmonary stenosis will have the typical to-and-fro murmurs of pulmonary stenosis and/or insufficiency audible at the left middle and upper sternal border as well as the other findings associated with a postsurgical AV canal. Murmurs suggesting residual ASDs or VSDs are not expected. Pulmonary hypertension should be suspected in the presence of a loud single second heart sound and a right ventricular heave.

Noninvasive Evaluation

The chest x-ray may show a normal cardiac silhouette when left AV valve insufficiency is only mild. Pulmonary hypertension may be suspected on the basis of large main and central pulmonary arteries. Cardiomegaly may suggest a residual left-to-right shunt and/or significant AV valve regurgitation. The *electrocardiogram* reveals the classic pattern of left axis and right ventricular conduction delay. Complete right bundle branch block is common after surgical intervention. *Echocardiography* delineates the location and severity of residual AV valve regurgitation and determines whether significant left ventricular outflow tract obstruction exists. Assessment of ventricular function and RV pressure by tricuspid regurgitation jet are important components of the echocardiographic examination.

Cardiac Catheterization

Cardiac catheterization may be required in patients with significant residual abnormalities after initial surgical repair in infancy or childhood. The presence of a residual shunt at the atrial or ventricular level is documented and quantitated. Pulmonary artery pressure and resistance are measured, and ventricular function is assessed. If left ventricular outflow tract obstruction is suspected, hemodynamics and angiography will indicate the severity. A left ventricular angiogram also will demonstrate the presence of left AV valve insufficiency and show the typical "gooseneck" deformity of the left ventricular outflow tract.

LONG-TERM FOLLOW-UP

Patients who have had AV canal defect repair during childhood should be followed closely for late manifestations, including (1) left AV valve insufficiency or, rarely, stenosis, (2) subaortic obstruction, and (3) development of atrial and occasionally ventricular arrhythmias. Patients who had repair of AV canal defect with right ventricular outflow obstruction may have progressive pulmonary valve insufficiency, which, in conjunction with tricuspid valve incompetence, can result in severe dilatation of the right ventricle. The status of the right ventricle should be monitored closely as in postoperative adults with tetralogy of Fallot. Late pulmonary valve replacement may ultimately be considered in some cases. Patients with pulmonary hypertension as a result of early vascular obstruction disease should be followed closely (see Chap. 16). Surgical reintervention should be considered for patients with severe residual or recurrent structural abnormalities such as left AV valve regurgitation, subaortic stenosis, and residual shunts.

SUMMARY

Atrioventricular canal defect is a lesion characterized by a primum ASD, AV valve abnormalities, and an inlet VSD. In complete AV canal defect, there is a large contiguous atrial and ventricular defect with a common AV valve entering both ventricles. Some patients have right ventricular outflow tract obstruction (tetralogy of Fallot) associated with this lesion. Down syndrome is present in the majority of cases of complete AV canal defect.

Most infants with complete AV canal defect do not survive childhood without surgical repair. Exceptions include a rare unoperated patient with pulmonary stenosis, in whom the pulmonary vascular bed is protected from high pressure and a large left-to-right shunt, and individuals with pulmonary vascular obstructive disease, which prevents progressive heart failure from large left-to-right shunts. No more than moderate left AV valve insufficiency is noted in such patients. Patients with pulmonary vascular disease have limited life expectancy but may reach adulthood.

A patient with AV canal defect after surgical repair in infancy will have a clinical course dependent on the effectiveness of the original surgery, which includes elimination of the left-to-right shunt, and reduction of left AV valve insufficiency to no more than mild to moderate. Since the development of subaortic stenosis is not unusual, postoperative patients must be monitored for this possibility. Late surgical management of AV canal

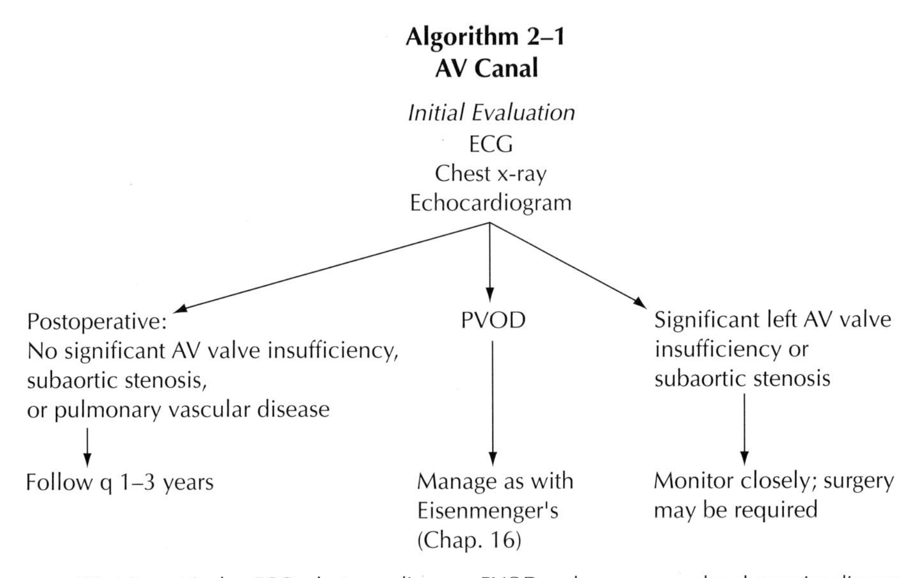

KEY: AV, atrioventricular; ECG, electrocardiogram; PVOD, pulmonary vascular obstructive disease.

defect includes repeat left AV valve repair or replacement and relief of subaortic obstruction. Assessment of the right ventricular outflow tract in terms of residual pulmonary stenosis and/or insufficiency is required in patients whose original lesion was AV canal defect with tetralogy of Fallot. Individuals with pulmonary vascular obstructive disease are managed similarly to any patient with Eisenmenger's syndrome (Chap. 16).

BIBLIOGRAPHY

Anderson RH, Baker EJ, Ho SY, et al: The morphology and diagnosis of AVSDs. *Cardiol Young* 1:290, 1991.

Bergin ML, Warnes CA, Tajik AJ, Danielson GK: Partial AV canal defect: Long-term follow-up after initial repair in patients ≥40 years old. *J Am Coll Cardiol* 25:1189, 1995.

Burke RP, Horvath K, Landzberg M, et al: Long-term follow-up after surgical repair of ostium primum atrial septal defect in adults. *J Am Coll Cardiol* 27:696, 1996.

Fyler DC: Endocardial cushion defects, in *Nadas' Pediatric Cardiology*, DC Fyler, ed. Philadelphia, Hanley & Belfus, 1992, p 577.

Goldfaden DM, Jones M, Morrow AG: Long-term results of repair of incomplete persistent AV canal. *J Thorac Cariovasc Surg* 82:69, 1981.

King RM, Puga FJ, Danielson GK, et al: Prognostic factors and surgical treatment of partial atrioventricular canal. *Circulation* 74:142, 1986.

Kirklin JW, Barratt-Boyes BG: AV canal defect, in *Cardiac Surgery,* 2d ed., JW Kirklin, BG Barratt-Boyes, eds. New York, Churchill Livingstone, 1993, p 693.

Lukacs L, Szanto G, Kassai I, Lengyel M: Late results after repair of partial AVSD. *Tex Heart Inst J* 19:265, 1992.

Meehan JJ, Delius RE, Behrendt DM, et al: Long term outcome following repair of incomplete AVSDs. *Circulation* 94(Suppl 1):117, 1996.

Najm HK, Coles JG, Endo M, et al: Complete atrioventricular septal defects: Results of repair, risk factors, and freedom from reoperation. *Circulation* 96:II-311, 1997.

Rastelli GC, Kirklin JW, Titus JL: Anatomic observations on complete form of persistent common AV canal with special reference to AV valves. *Mayo Clin Proc* 41:296, 1966.

Roberson DA, Muhiudeen KA, Silverman NH, et al: Intraoperative transesophageal echocardiography of AVSD. *J Am Coll Cardiol* 18:357, 1991.

Smallhorn JF, Perrin D, Musewe N, et al: The role of transesophageal echocardiography in the evaluation of patients with AVSD. *Cardiol Young* 1:324, 1991.

Somerville J: Ostium primum defect: Factors causing deterioration in the natural history. *Br Heart J* 27:413, 1965.

Studer M, Blackstone EH, Kirklin JW, et al: Determinants of early and late results of repair of atrioventricular septal (canal) defects. *J Thorac Cardiovasc Surg* 84:523, 1982.

Van Mierop LHS, Alley RD, Kausel HW, et al: The anatomy and embryology of endocardial cushion defects. *J Thorac Cardiovasc Surg* 43:71, 1962.

CHAPTER 3

VENTRICULAR SEPTAL DEFECT

Ventricular septal defect (VSD) is the most common congenital cardiac defect that is present at birth, accounting for 25% of congenital cardiac lesions and occurring in 1.5 to 2.5 per 1000 live births. These defects are classified anatomically as perimembranous, supracristal, muscular, and inlet (endocardial cushion) (Fig. 3-1).

Perimembranous defects account for 80% of all VSD (Figs. 3-2 and 3-3). The defect lies adjacent to the tricuspid annulus in the region of the anteroseptal commissure immediately inferior to the infundibular septum, involving the membranous ventricular septum. When viewed from the left ventricle, the defect lies in the posterior region of the left ventricular outflow tract beneath the commissure between the right and noncoronary cusps of the aortic valve. This defect often is referred to as a subaortic VSD.

Five to 20% of VSDs are muscular (Fig. 3-4*A* and *B*). Although they may be located anywhere within the muscular septum, the majority are found in the midmuscular region. Anterior defects are frequently multiple. Multiple defects occasionally produce a so-called Swiss cheese defect. A small but significant number are at the apex of the right ventricle (apical VSD).

Supracristal (subpulmonary) defects account for 5 to 10% of VSDs (Fig. 3-5). The defect lies immediately beneath the pulmonary and aortic valves, which are separated by a thin rim of fibrous tissue. From the left ventricular side, the defect is in the outflow portion of the ventricular septum, immediately beneath the right coronary cusp or in the commissure between the right and left cusps. The right aortic cusp or noncoronary cusp may prolapse into the defect and produce aortic regurgitation. Supracristal defects are reported more frequently in Japan and China than in western countries.

A small percentage of isolated VSDs are located beneath the septal leaflet of the tricuspid valve and are known as an atrioventricular (AV) canal defect or an endocardial cushion defect. This defect nearly always is associated with abnormalities of the AV valves, but if there is an associated primum ASD, they are classified as a form of AV canal (Chap. 2).

CLINICAL PRESENTATION

The diagnosis of a VSD typically is made within the first few weeks of life after the discovery of a systolic murmur. The timing coincides with the fall in pulmonary vascular re-

FIGURE 3-1

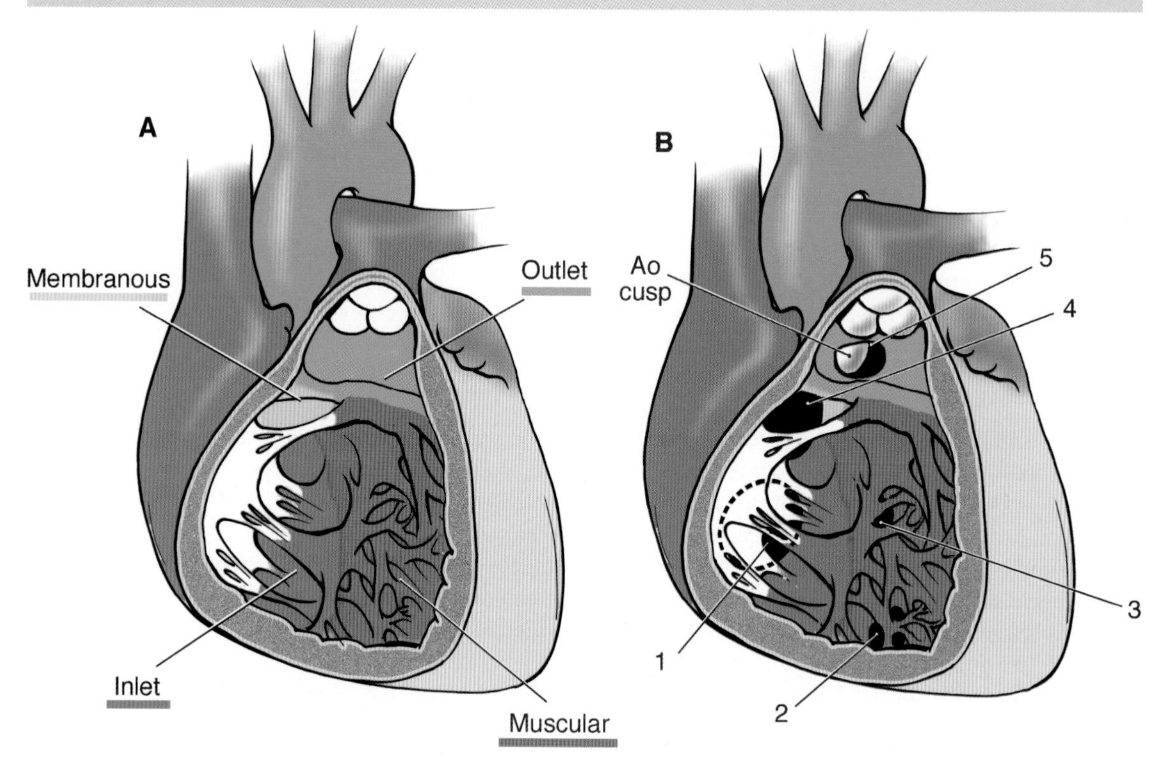

Ventricular septal defect. Panel *A* shows the segments of the ventricular septum. Ventricular septal defects may occur in the outlet (Conal) septum, membranous septum, inlet septum, or muscular septum. Panel *B* indicates various types of ventricular septal defects. 1 = inlet VSD, 2 = muscular apical septal defect, 3 = midmuscular defect, 4 = membranous ventricular septal defect, 5 = subpulmonary VSD. (Note prolapsing aortic cusp) into the defect.

sistance, which begins shortly after birth and results in progressive left-to-right shunting through the defect. The left-to-right shunt produces an increase in pulmonary blood flow that, if the shunt is large enough, results in volume overload of the left ventricle.

A small VSD produces only a modest left-to-right shunt (Q_p/Q_s <2.0) that does not cause symptoms, left ventricular dilatation, or pulmonary hypertension. Many of these defects close spontaneously, usually within the first year of life but sometimes later.

A moderate-size VSD results in enough left-to-right shunting to produce pulmonary overcirculation and volume overload of the left ventricle. The Q_p/Q_s is typically 2.0 to 3.0 with normal or slightly elevated pulmonary artery pressure. Mild congestive heart failure may develop after the second month of life, but these symptoms generally can be controlled with digoxin and diuretics. Most moderate-size VSDs become smaller within the first year of life, alleviating congestive failure and permitting normal growth and development.

FIGURE 3-2

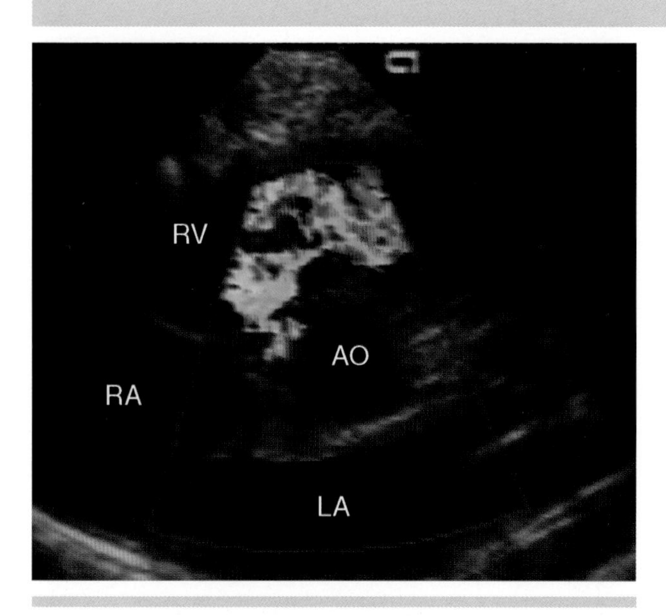

Color Doppler from a parasternal short-axis view in a patient with a perimembranous ventricular septal defect (VSD). There is a left-to-right shunt that arises at approximately 10 o'clock around the aortic orifice and communicates with the perimembranous portion of the right ventricle. RA, right atrium; LA, left atrium; Ao, aorta; RV, right ventricle.

Both small and moderate-size VSDs are termed restrictive because a pressure gradient is maintained between the left and right ventricles. The physiology and clinical manifestations of a large (nonrestrictive) VSD differ from those of a restrictive defect.

A large VSD results in systemic pressure in the right ventricle that is equal to or slightly lower than that in the left ventricle. Infants with a large VSD typically develop severe congestive heart failure by the end of the second month of life. The pulmonary vascular resistance is low, permitting massive left-to-right shunting with torrential pulmonary blood flow, systemic pulmonary artery pressure, left ventricular volume overload, and heart failure. These infants experience failure to thrive with feeding difficulties, inability to gain weight, and frequent respiratory infections. Anticongestive medications are used to control heart failure, and if adequate nutrition can be maintained to allow infant growth, regression in the size of the defect will result in an improvement in symptoms. Even large defects become smaller, either anatomically or relatively, and thus are restrictive. Those infants improve with medical management, and early surgical correction is not required. However, infants with intractable congestive heart failure and failure to thrive require early surgical repair. Although pulmonary artery banding was employed commonly in such patients in the 1960s and early 1970s to restrict pulmonary blood flow, in the present era of infant cardiac surgery, these defects can be repaired at very low surgical risk. Pulmonary artery banding for a VSD currently is reserved for the rare patient with multiple muscular VSDs (so called Swiss-cheese defects) or in the context of other complicated anatomy in which early closure of the defects is not feasible or would require a left ventriculotomy.

An infant with a large left-to-right shunt and severe pulmonary hypertension from an unrestricted VSD eventually may develop pulmonary vascular obstructive disease. If the

FIGURE 3-3

Apical four-chamber view in a patient with a perimembranous ventricular septal defect. Color Doppler shows a left-to-right shunt with a small jet (arrow) directed toward the right ventricular apex. RA, right atrium; LA, left atrium; LV, left ventricle; RV, right ventricle.

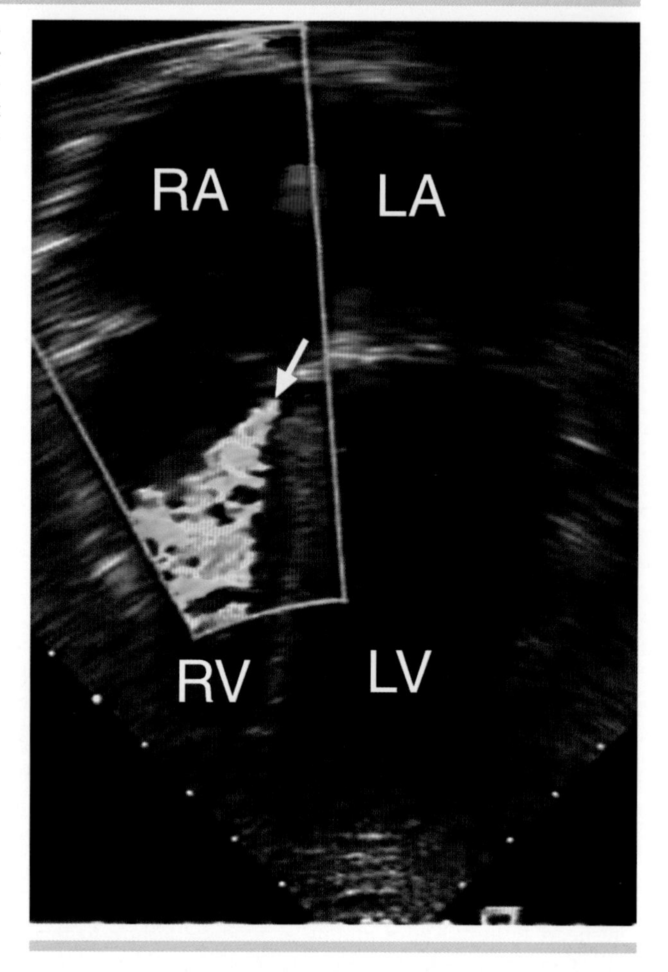

defect is not closed, shear stress damage to the pulmonary vascular bed results in pathologic changes in the pulmonary artery, including muscular hypertrophy and intimal hyperplasia. These changes in the pulmonary vascular bed are progressive if pulmonary hypertension is not eliminated. Patients who develop elevated pulmonary vascular resistance manifest diminished left-to-right shunting and pulmonary blood flow, and this decreases left ventricular volume overload and congestive failure. Thus, while these pathologic changes in the pulmonary circulation result in alleviation of congestive heart failure, the end result is fixed elevation of pulmonary vascular resistance, irreversible damage to the pulmonary vascular bed, and chronic severe pulmonary hypertension (Eisenmenger's syndrome). If an infant has VSD closure or a spontaneous decrease in the size of the communication before 2 years of age, this sequence of events will not occur.

Once pulmonary vascular obstructive disease is severe and pulmonary vascular resistance approaches systemic vascular resistance, bidirectional shunting is present.

FIGURE 3-4*A*

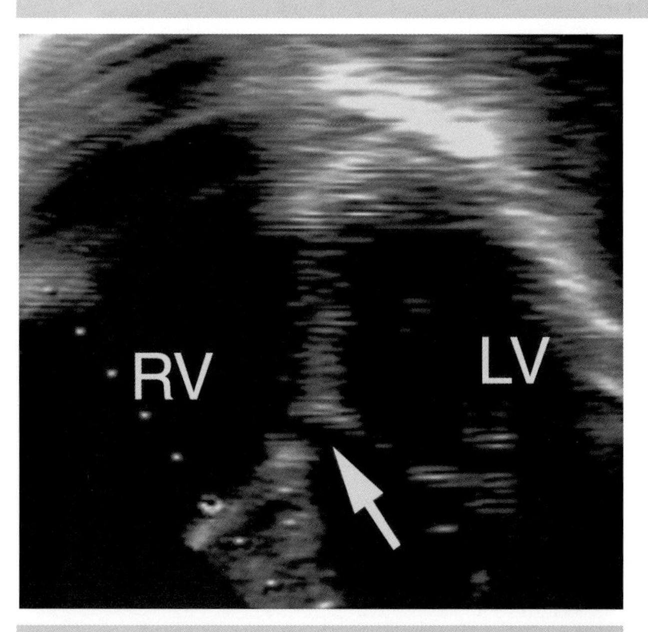

Apical four-chamber view in an adult with a muscular ventricular septal defect (VSD). The arrow points to a small VSD located in the muscular portion of the ventricular septum. RV, right ventricle; LV, left ventricle.

FIGURE 3-4*B*

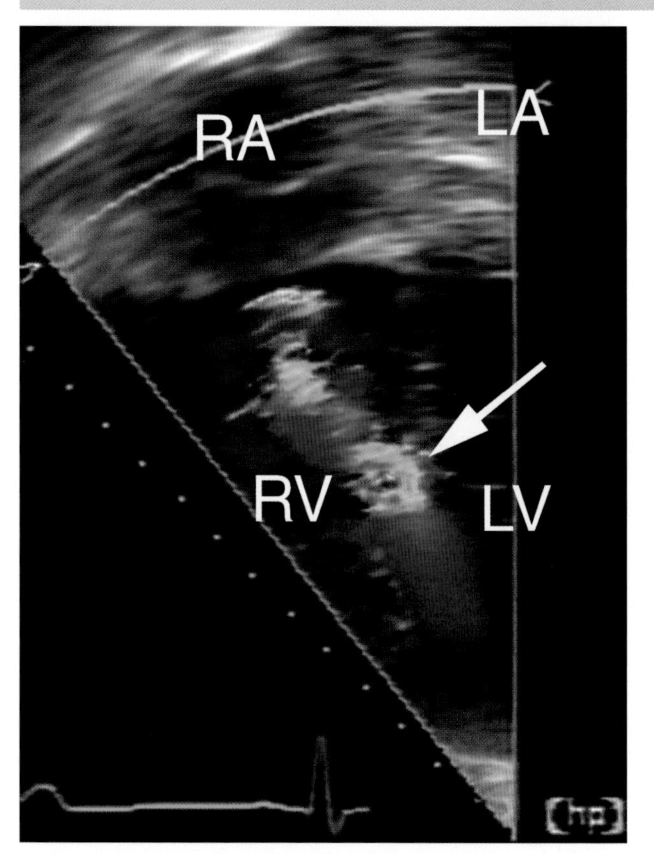

Color Doppler from an apical four-chamber view from the same patient. There is a left-to-right shunt through the ventricular septal defect, which is directed toward the right atrioventricular valve. RA, right atrium; LA, left atrium; RV, right ventricle; LV, left ventricle.

FIGURE 3-5

Color Doppler from a parasternal short-axis view in a patient with a supracristal (subpulmonary) ventricular septal defect (VSD). There is a left-to-right shunt from the left ventricle into the right ventricular outflow tract. Note that the VSD is visualized at approximately 1 o'-clock around the aortic orifice just below the pulmonary valve. This view is useful in distinguishing a subpulmonary VSD from a perimembranous defect that is located adjacent to the tricuspid valve. See also Fig. 3-3. Ao, aorta; RA, right atrium; LA, left atrium; RV, right ventricle.

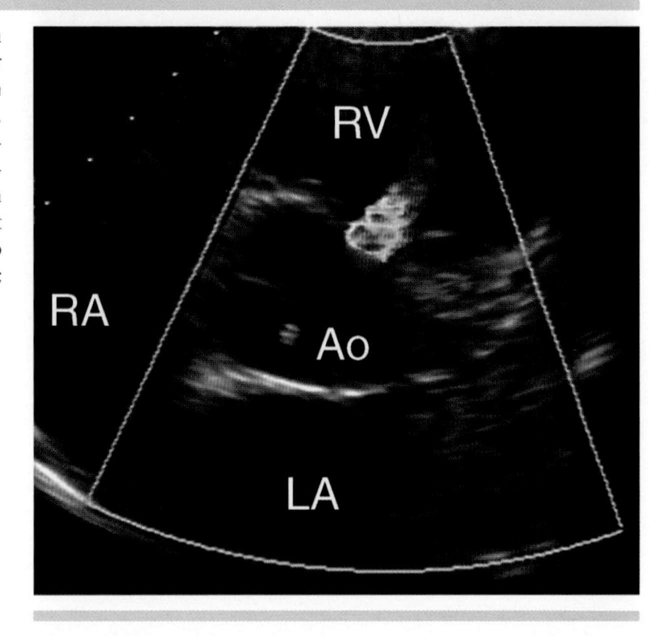

Ultimately, with further elevation of pulmonary vascular resistance, the shunt becomes predominantly right-to-left. At this stage, usually in adolescence or adulthood, there is overt cyanosis and polycythemia. Closure of the VSD is contraindicated when the pulmonary vascular resistance is severely elevated, since it would eliminate the portion of the systemic cardiac output that is dependent on right-to-left shunting through the VSD (Chap. 16).

NATURAL HISTORY

A substantial percentage of VSDs undergo spontaneous regression in size or complete closure over time. This has a favorable influence on the natural history of this defect. Small defects are more likely to close than are large ones, but even large VSDs may become small or moderate in size during infancy, either anatomically or relatively, as the child grows.

The mechanism of VSD closure is related to the location of the defect. Perimembranous defects become smaller or close by ingrowth of endocardial cushion tissue or adherence of the septal leaflet of the tricuspid valve to the defect, forming a membranous septal aneurysm that obstructs the VSD (Figs. 3-6 and 3-7). Rarely, VSD closure may result from prolapse of an aortic cusp into the defect, producing aortic regurgitation. Small trabecular defects in the muscular septum are the most likely to close as a result of endocardial proliferation and ventricular hypertrophy within the right ventricle.

FIGURE 3-6

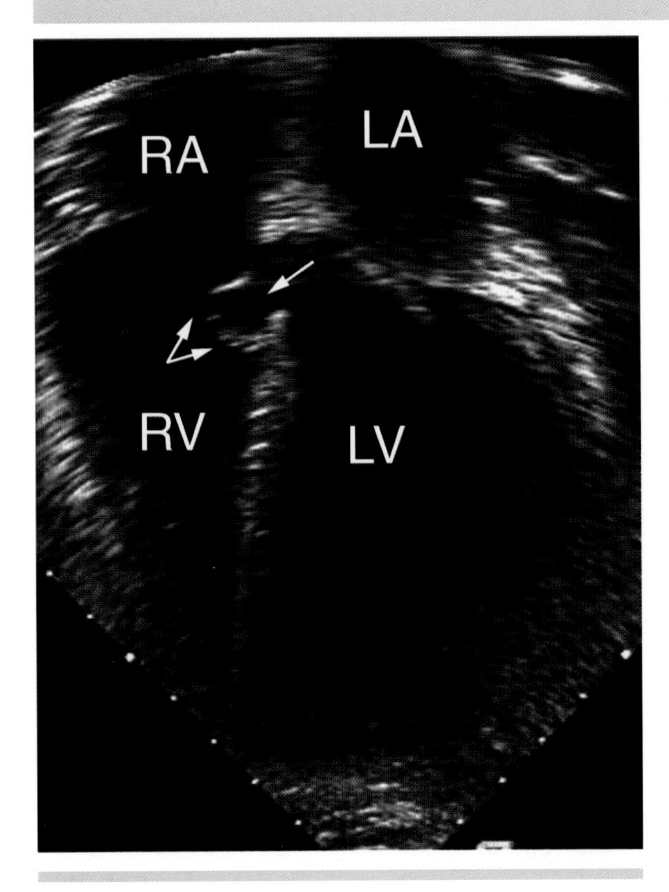

Apical four-chamber view in a patient with a perimembranous VSD, which has been partially closed by the development of aneurysmal tissue (double arrow). This restricts blood flow through the defect. The arrow points to the VSD. RA, right atrium; LA, left atrium; RV, right ventricle; LV, left ventricle.

Hypertrophy and scarring along the moderator band may divide the right ventricle into inflow and outflow chambers (double-chamber right ventricle). The VSD may be closed by proliferating tissue and produce significant right ventricular outflow obstruction. When patients with a large VSD develop infundibular pulmonary stenosis, the degree of obstruction may vary from mild to severe. When shunting is right-to-left and the anatomy of the right ventricular outflow tract is distinctive, the lesion is classified as tetralogy of Fallot. An occasional patient subsequently diagnosed as having tetralogy of Fallot will have a history of a large left-to-right shunt from a VSD during infancy (Chap. 10).

MANAGEMENT OF ADULTS

Adults with a history of a VSD include those with small, moderate, or large defects as well as postoperative patients. The history, physical examination, and noninvasive studies are generally adequate in determining the clinical status of the patient.

FIGURE 3-7

Membranous septal aneurysm in a patient with a ventricular septal defect. A left ventriculogram shows the aneurysm (arrow) bulging into the right ventricle. Dye is noted entering the right ventricle and pulmonary artery, demonstrating a small left-to-right shunt. LV = left ventricle, RV = right ventricle, MPA = main pulmonary artery.

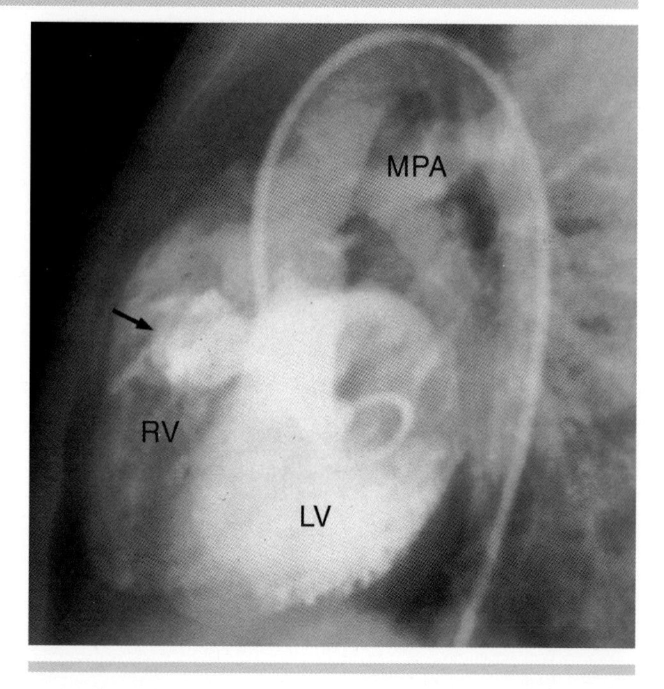

Small Ventricular Septal Defect

A small VSD is the most common form of the defect encountered in adults. Since the left-to-right shunt is small, the increase in pulmonary blood flow is insignificant and is not sufficient to cause left ventricular (LV) dilatation. Symptoms are not present.

Physical examination of a patient with a perimembranous defect characteristically reveals a thrill at the left middle to lower sternal border. The apical impulse is not displaced, and the second heart sound is normal. A prominent harsh pansystolic murmur is heard maximally at the left middle to lower sternal border. When the defect is muscular, the murmur may be well circumscribed at the lower border and occasionally may end before the second heart sound because of closure of the defect during late systole.

The *electrocardiogram* is most often within normal limits. The *chest x-ray* shows a normal cardiac silhouette without pulmonary overcirculation or pulmonary artery dilatation.

The *echocardiogram* shows normal right- and left-sided cardiac dimensions and normal ventricular function. The size of the defect may be assessed with two-dimensional imaging and color Doppler. When the VSD is small, a large gradient will be measured across the defect by continuous-wave Doppler, reflecting normal right ventricular (RV) pressure.

When the physical findings and noninvasive studies indicate the presence of a small VSD, no additional studies are required. Cardiac catheterization is not necessary and does not add to the noninvasive evaluation.

Small VSDs do not cause hemodynamic deterioration over time. However, periodic follow-up is recommended to detect the occasional patient who develops aortic insufficiency. Bacterial endocarditis (BE) prophylaxis is required.

Moderate Ventricular Septal Defect

Moderate VSD is defined as a defect that is restrictive in regard to pressure but nevertheless produces a large left-to-right shunt. A large VSD may become smaller but still remain moderate in terms of shunt size. The adult cardiologist is least likely to encounter an adult with a moderate-size VSD, since these defects either become smaller or have been repaired during early childhood.

Physical examination reflects the volume overload on the left side of the heart. The apical impulse may be displaced, and an LV heave may be present. A thrill is usually present at the left middle to lower sternal border along with a grade III to IV holosystolic murmur that is similar to the murmur of a small VSD. In addition, the increased blood flow across the mitral valve may produce a diastolic flow rumble.

The *electrocardiogram* may show a pattern of "diastolic overload" manifested by deep Q waves in leads V_5, V_6, I, and AV_L. The *chest x-ray* may reveal left ventricular enlargement with enlarged pulmonary arteries and pulmonary overcirculation.

Echocardiography delineates the size and location of the defect and its effect on the cardiac chambers. Although it may be difficult to quantitate VSD size as precisely as is done in a child, a patient with a moderate-size VSD can be recognized by cardiac chamber enlargement. Chronically elevated pulmonary blood flow produces dilatation of the pulmonary artery, left atrium, and left ventricle. The right ventricle is usually normal unless pulmonary hypertension is present. Right ventricular pressure usually can be estimated by a properly aligned continuous-wave Doppler across the VSD or by a tricuspid regurgitant jet. Since the defect is restrictive in terms of pressure, a large gradient will be predicted despite the large left-to-right shunt.

Adults suspected of having a moderate-size VSD may require cardiac catheterization to quantitate the left-to-right shunt and measure pulmonary artery pressure and pulmonary vascular resistance. The size and location of the VSD are best delineated by a steep left anterior oblique (LAO) projection with cranial angulation. An aortogram may be necessary if aortic regurgitation is suspected or to exclude an associated patent ductus arteriosus.

Adults with a moderate-size VSD typically have a $Q_p/Q_s > 2.0$ with normal or mildly elevated pulmonary artery pressure. A patient with a moderate-size defect and a large shunt who requires VSD closure occasionally may be encountered. Greater degrees of pulmonary hypertension may reflect the development of pulmonary vascular disease after decades of high pulmonary blood flow, as occurs in some older adults with an atrial septal defect. Decision making regarding surgical intervention for a moderate-size VSD may be difficult under these circumstances. Pulmonary vascular obstructive disease (Eisenmenger's syndrome) does not develop in patients with normal pulmonary artery pressure.

Large Ventricular Septal Defect

Only rarely is an adult encountered with a large VSD and a significant left-to-right shunt with normal or minimally elevated pulmonary vascular resistance, since most large VSDs are closed in infancy. Nonoperated late adult survivors with a large VSD almost always develop a progressive increase in pulmonary vascular resistance secondary to shear stress–induced damage to the pulmonary arteriolar media and intima. This limits the left-to-right shunt, but the final result is chronic pulmonary vascular obstructive disease. The typical history is that of congestive heart failure during infancy that gradually improved spontaneously during the first 2 years of life as pulmonary arteriolar constriction began to develop. However, some patients with Eisenmenger's syndrome do not have such a history and apparently have pulmonary vascular obstructive disease from birth.

As pulmonary vascular resistance increases during childhood and adolescence, cyanosis becomes apparent as a result of increasing right-to-left shunting (Eisenmenger's syndrome) (Ch. 15). Once cyanosis and polycythemia are established, patients may complain of dyspnea, exercise intolerance, and headache and, in the late stages, cerebral ischemia, hemoptysis, and chest pain. Brain abscess and endocarditis also are potential complications. Patients may ultimately develop RV failure with pulmonary and tricuspid regurgitation, ascites, and peripheral edema, but the most common terminal illness is severe hypoxemia as pulmonary blood flow decreases. Arrhythmias are common in the latter stages of the disease, and sudden death is not uncommon.

Physical examination of a patient with a VSD who has developed Eisenmenger's syndrome reveals varying degrees of cyanosis and clubbing. A left parasternal heave is typically present, indicative of right ventricular hypertension. The second heart sound is loud and single, and a pulmonary ejection click may be present at the left midsternal border. A left sternal border ejection murmur is most often audible, but the murmur of a VSD is no longer present. Late in the disease, the murmurs of tricuspid and pulmonary regurgitation may be heard. The holosystolic murmur of tricuspid regurgitation murmur may be maximal at the cardiac apex as a result of massive RV enlargement, mimicking mitral regurgitation. When tricuspid regurgitation is significant, it results in a prominent V wave in the jugular venous pulse and produces a pulsatile liver, sometimes with fluid retention.

The *electrocardiogram* typically shows right ventricular hypertrophy (RVH); the *chest x-ray* reveals RV enlargement, a prominent main pulmonary artery, and tapering distal pulmonary vessels.

Patients with Eisenmenger's syndrome can lead productive lives for many decades, although their activities are limited. An occasional patient will display rapid progression of the disease and early symptoms in adolescence or early adulthood. Chronic pulmonary vasodilator therapy, similar to the regimens for primary pulmonary hypertension, may be useful in severe cases, but the only surgical option is transplantation. If right ventricular dysfunction is advanced, heart-lung transplantation is the preferred approach, whereas in patients with preserved RV systolic function without severe tricuspid regurgitation, lung transplant with simultaneous closure of the VSD may be feasible.

Although it is clear that patients with severely elevated pulmonary vascular resistance are not candidates for VSD closure, it is important for the cardiologist to recognize an adult with a moderate VSD and pulmonary hypertension who still has a significant left-to-right shunt and may be a candidate for VSD repair. The physical examination and noninvasive studies may not be definitive in this situation. Cardiac catheterization is required to determine the magnitude of the shunt, pulmonary artery pressure, and pulmonary vascular resistance. The assessment of these patients requires careful study in the catheterization laboratory, since small errors in oximetry have a large effect on the calculation of pulmonary vascular resistance and the assessment of operability. Patients with pulmonary hypertension who have a Q_p/Q_s >1.8 on room air without arterial desaturation generally are considered surgical candidates.

Some adults with a moderate to large VSD and severe pulmonary hypertension have a bidirectional shunt with mild arterial desaturation on room air that after the administration of 100% oxygen becomes a significant left to right shunt. Although this implies some reactivity of the pulmonary vascular bed, it is only a rare patient with these findings who will derive significant benefit from VSD closure. VSD closure in patients with severe fixed elevation of pulmonary vascular resistance is contraindicated because, aside from increased surgical risk, the patient will lose the ability to augment cardiac output by increasing right-to-left shunting through the VSD. Inappropriate closure will result in an even poorer prognosis, similar to that in patients with primary pulmonary hypertension.

VENTRICULAR SEPTAL DEFECT WITH AORTIC INSUFFICIENCY

A subpulmonary (supracristal) VSD creates a communication in the region of the aortic sinuses and can result in prolapse of an aortic cusp into the defect. In some cases this can be severe, resulting in marked aortic insufficiency, and in some instances the aortic cusp can virtually close the VSD. Most often progressive prolapse occurs in childhood, but the degree of abnormality may increase over the years, becoming severe in adolescence or young adulthood.

Physical examination in an unoperated patient with significant prolapse and aortic insufficiency will reveal the classic harsh pansystolic of a VSD accompanied by the usual high-pitched protodiastolic murmur of aortic insufficiency. In severe cases, the other physical manifestations of aortic regurgitation will be present (left ventricular heave, bounding pulses, and wide pulse pressure). However, few patients would reach this stage without having had previous cardiac surgery. The *electrocardiogram* will show left ventricular hypertrophy, and some patients will have ST-T wave abnormalities. The *chest x-ray* reveals various degrees of left ventricular enlargement. The *echocardiogram* defines the supracristal defect and the degree of aortic insufficiency as well as the severity of ventricular dilatation and the state of ventricular function (Fig. 3-8*A* and *B*). Occasionally the aortic regurgitation will be directed into the right ventricle.

Surgical treatment is directed at closing the VSD and carrying out an aortic valvuloplasty. It is usually not necessary to replace the aortic valve, but in severe cases this may be required. The results of surgery are good, but mild residual aortic insufficiency is often present and can be expected in adult patients with a history of surgical repair of a VSD with aortic insufficiency (AI).

Management of a patient with trivial AI and a small VSD may vary among centers. Some advocate early surgical repair of the VSD to prevent progressive AI, whereas others may wait for evidence of progression before operating on a patient with minimal disease. At the present time, there is no clear evidence whether the outcome will be affected by early intervention. However, all agree that no patient should be allowed to progress beyond mild to moderate AI without surgical repair.

Some patients may be encountered in whom AI continues to worsen despite surgery at an earlier age. In such cases, aortic valve replacement should be considered on the same basis as in any patient with aortic valve disease.

FIGURE 3-8*A*

Apical four-chamber view in a patient with a moderate-size subaortic ventricular septal defect (VSD). There is also overriding of the aorta across the ventricular septum. The arrow points to the VSD. Ao, aorta; LA, left atrium; RV, right ventricle; LV, left ventricle.

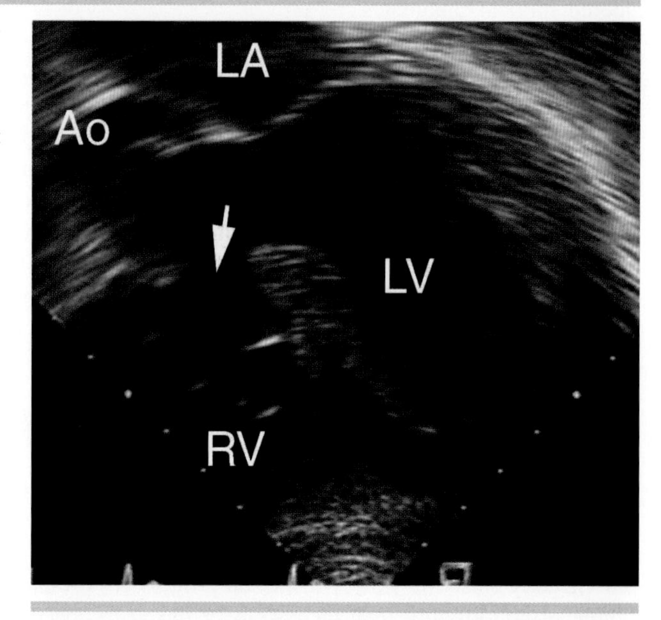

FIGURE 3-8*B*

VSD with aortic regurgitation. Color Doppler from an apical long-axis view in the same patient as Fig. 3-8*A*. The Doppler shows aortic regurgitation, which is directed across the VSD into the right ventricle. Ao, aorta; LA, left atrium; LV, left ventricle.

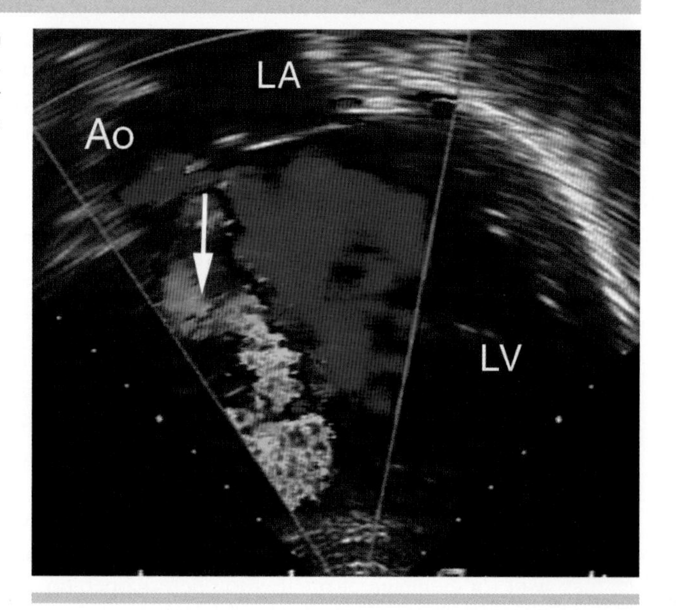

Surgical Repair

The surgical approach for VSD closure is related to the location of the VSD and the experience of the surgeon. Although the majority of perimembranous defects are now closed through the right atrium, a right ventriculotomy was used in many adults seen today who were operated on during childhood. When a right ventriculotomy has been performed, the postoperative electrocardiogram shows a right bundle branch block in most patients. A right bundle branch block also occurs in approximately a third of patients repaired via the right atrial approach. This presumably is related to sutures placed along the inferior border of the perimembranous VSD. On rare occasions, a right ventriculotomy results in right ventricular dysfunction and the late development of ventricular arrhythmias.

The surgical risk of VSD closure for perimembranous defects is extremely low. Rare complications include heart block from damage to the bundle of His (which runs inferior and posterior to the defect) and the inadvertent creation of aortic regurgitation. The method of closure of a muscular defect or defects varies with the location of the communication and surgical expertise. Most of these defects can be repaired via a right atrial or right ventricular approach. In rare instances of an apical VSD, a left ventriculotomy could be necessary, but this can be associated with postoperative left ventricular dysfunction and arrhythmias. Closure of muscular defects by catheter techniques is being carried out at some centers.

A subpulmonary VSD associated with aortic regurgitation is closed using a transverse incision in the infundibular portion of the right ventricle or through the pulmonary valve when the pulmonary artery is large. An aortic approach is used at some centers. The prolapsed aortic cusp is elevated and repaired.

LONG-TERM FOLLOW-UP

While VSD closure repair today is generally a low-risk operation at any age, it must be appreciated that today's adults may have undergone surgery during an era when myocardial preservation and surgical techniques were in the early stage of development. Consequently, it is not surprising that some postoperative adults have had complications such as ventricular dysfunction, arrhythmias, and heart block.

In the absence of these problems, one would expect a postoperative patient to be asymptomatic with normal cardiac function and chamber dimensions. The postoperative examination should be unremarkable. A significant cardiac murmur is not expected. The presence of a pansystolic murmur along the lower left sternal border may be indicative of a residual VSD or tricuspid regurgitation. If aortic regurgitation is present, it may be due to prolapse of an aortic cusp or result from a suture placed through one of the aortic cusps during closure of a perimembranous VSD. Patients who initially were treated with pulmonary artery banding before definitive repair and debanding of the pulmonary artery may have a murmur of pulmonary insufficiency along the left sternal border or a systolic murmur secondary to turbulence along the pulmonary artery and/or at the bifurcation.

Periodic follow-up of postoperative patients is recommended to observe for the development of ventricular arrhythmias, progression of conduction disease, ventricular dysfunction, or the development of aortic regurgitation. In addition, since a VSD may be associated with other cardiac defects, such as a bicuspid aortic valve, subaortic stenosis, a double-chambered right ventricle, and coarctation of the aorta, the development of a new or persistent murmur should prompt further assessment. Patients without a residual hemodynamic abnormality do not require antibiotic prophylaxis.

SUMMARY

With the exception of bicuspid aortic valve, VSD is the most common isolated congenital heart defect. Communications vary in position and size along the ventricular septum, and each has its own clinical profile in terms of associated abnormalities and natural history. Adults with an unoperated or previously repaired VSD come to the internist and adult cardiologist with varying presentations.

Small Restrictive Ventricular Septal Defect

Patients with small unoperated VSDs are asymptomatic and require no special management, with the exception of appropriate antibiotic prophylaxis to prevent endocarditis. On a risk-benefit basis, there is no evidence that surgical closure of these defects is warranted or that invasive diagnostic studies (cardiac catheterization) are required for further evaluation beyond history, physical examination, electrocardiography, chest x-ray, and echocardiography. These patients do not require limitation of physical activities, and there are no special issues for women who become pregnant.

Large Ventricular Septal Defect

Adult patients with large VSDs and a large left-to-right shunt associated with hyperkinetic pulmonary artery hypertension are almost never encountered. Virtually all such patients who have survived childhood with large communications have developed PVOD and must be managed accordingly. In recent years, the incidence of Eisenmenger's syndrome has decreased markedly since VSDs have been repaired during infancy, thus avoiding prolonged hyperkinetic pulmonary hypertension, resultant pulmonary vasoconstriction, and eventual pulmonary arteriolar anatomic obstructive changes. However, a few patients with PVOD may be encountered who have large VSDs and apparent high pulmonary vascular resistance from birth without a history of heart failure.

Patients with Eisenmenger's syndrome live for many years and with a prudent lifestyle can carry out most activities required for normal daily life. Close observation for severe polycythemia is required, and plasma exchange transfusions may be indicated in symptomatic patients with hematocrits in excess of 65%. Many patients will stabilize just below this level for many years. Iron deficiency must be avoided, since relative anemia can lead to symptoms of fatigue, and exercise dyspnea and may be associated with an increased risk of cerebrovascular events. Patients with the most advanced form of Eisenmenger's syndrome may be offered treatment with pulmonary vasodilator therapy, and for the most symptomatic, heart-lung transplantation or lung transplantation and VSD repair may be considered (Chap. 16).

Ventricular Septal Defect with Aortic Insufficiency

Patients with a restrictive subpulmonary (supracristal) VSD who have reached adulthood without surgery may continue to be followed if there is little or no aortic valve prolapse into the defect and no evidence of progressive aortic insufficiency. However, these patients have the potential to require operative intervention on the basis of aortic valve involvement.

Long-Term Follow-Up

Patients who have had successful repair of a VSD with no residual communication or associated lesions require minimal follow-up and have an excellent prognosis. Antibiotic prophylaxis is not necessary. As in most patients who have had open-heart surgery, these individuals require occasional follow-up regarding the possible development of late rhythm disturbances or myocardial dysfunction. A rare patient may develop discrete subvalvular aortic stenosis. Heart block with pacemaker insertion may be seen occasionally, but this complication is extremely rare in the modern era. Patients who have had concomitant repair of associated lesions must be evaluated for the status of the other defects. When VSD with aortic insufficiency has been repaired at least mild residual aortic insufficiency will often be present, and future decisions regarding reintervention are based on the status of the aortic valve.

Algorithm 3–1

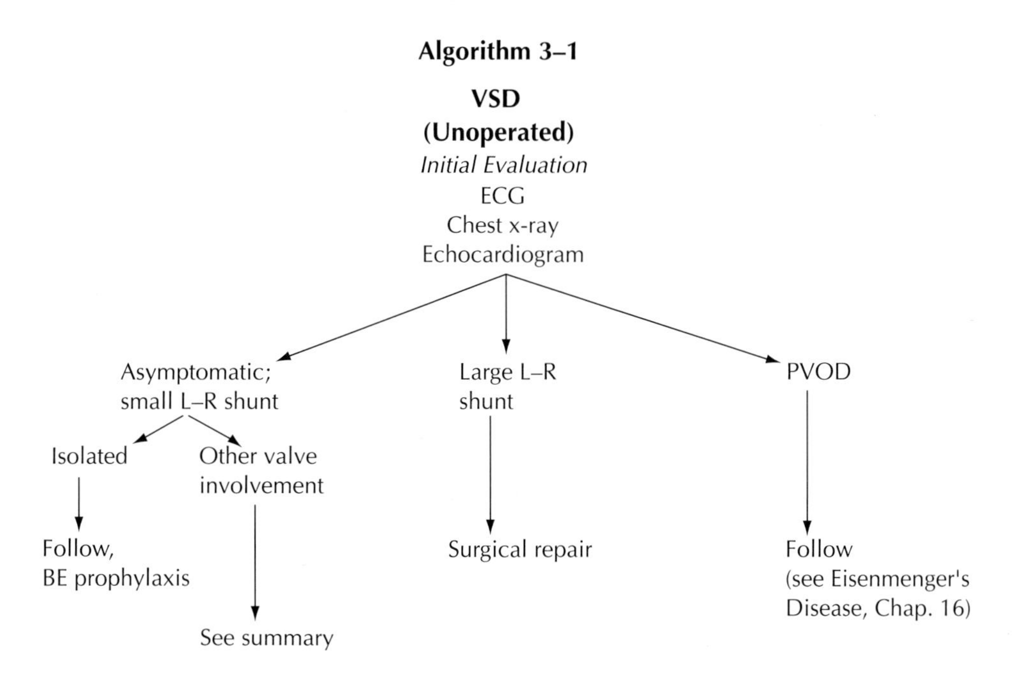

Algorithm 3–1 (Continued)

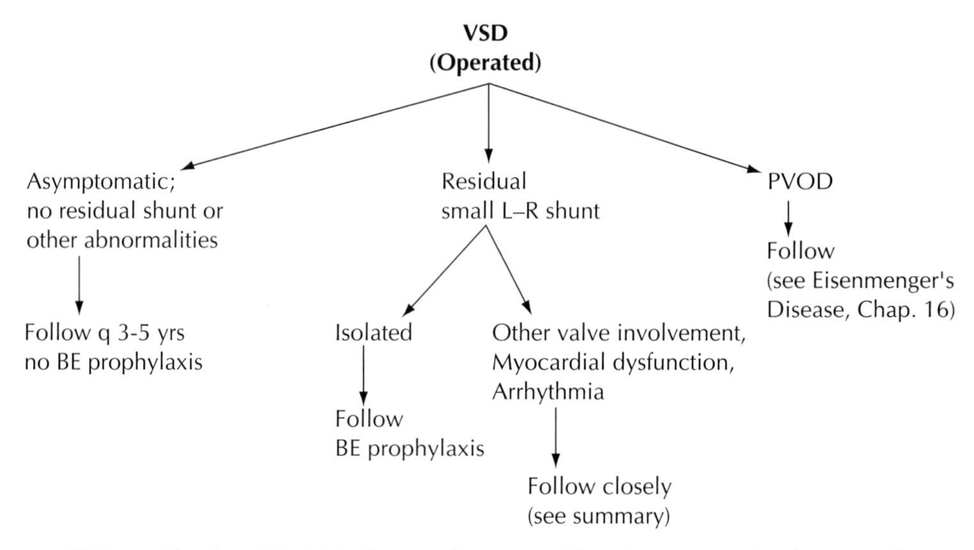

KEY: BE, bacterial endocarditis; ECG, electrocardiogram; PVOD, pulmonary vascular obstructive disease; VSD, ventricular septal defect; L–R, left to right.

BIBLIOGRAPHY

Anderson RH, Lenox CC, Zuberbuhler JR: Mechanisms of closure of perimembranous ventricular septal defect. *Am J Cardiol* 52:341, 1983.

Anderson RH, Wilcox BR: The surgical anatomy of ventricular septal defect (review). *J Cardiovasc Surg* 7:17, 1992.

Askenazi J, Ahnberg DS, Korngold E, et al: Quantitative radionuclide angiocardiography: Detection and quantitation of left to right shunts. *Am J Cardiol* 37:382, 1976.

Corone P, Doyan F, Gaudeau S, et al: Natural history of ventricular septal defect: A study involving 790 cases. *Circulation* 55:908, 1977.

Craig BG, Smallhorn JF, Burrows P, et al: Cross-sectional echocardiography in the evaluation of aortic valve prolapse associated with ventricular septal defect. *Am Heart J* 112:800, 1986.

Fishberger SB, Bridges ND, Keane JF, et al: Intraoperative device closure of ventricular septal defects. *Circulation* 88(Suppl):II-205, 1993.

Gasul BM, Dillon RF, Vrla V, Hait G: Ventricular septal defects: Their natural transformation into those with infundibular stenosis or into the cyanotic or non-cyanotic type of tetralogy of Fallot. *JAMA* 164:847, 1957.

Gersony WM, Hayes CJ, Driscoll DJ, et al: Bacterial endocarditis in patients with aortic stenosis, pulmonary stenosis, or ventricular septal defect. *Circulation* 87(Suppl I):I-121, 1993.

Kidd L, Driscoll DJ, Gersony WM, et al: Second natural history study of congenital heart defects: Results of treatment of patients with ventricular septal defects. *Circulation* 87(Suppl I):I-38, 1993.

Kirklin JW, DuShane JW: Indications for repair of ventricular septal defect. *Am J Cardiol* 12:75, 1963.

Lupi-Herrera E, Sandoval J, Seoane M, et al: The role of isoproterenol in the preoperative evaluation of high-pressure, high-resistance ventricular septal defect. *Chest* 81:42, 1982.

Moreno-Cabral RJ, Mamiya RT, Nakamura FF, et al: Ventricular septal defect and aortic insufficiency: Surgical treatment. *J Thorac Cardiovasc Surg* 73(3):358, 1977.

Muller WH Jr, Dammann JF Jr: The treatment of certain congenital malformations of the heart by the creation of pulmonic stenosis to reduce pulmonary hypertension and excessive pulmonary blood flow: A preliminary report. *Surg Gynecol Obstet* 95:213, 1952.

Neutze JM, Ishikawa T, Clarkson PM, et al: Assessment and follow-up of patients with ventricular septal defect and elevated pulmonary vascular resistance. *Am J Cardiol* 63:327, 1989.

Pieroni DR, Nishimura RA, Bierman FZ, et al: Second natural history study of congenital heart defects: Ventricular septal defect echocardiography. *Circulation* 87(Suppl I):I-80, 1993.

Ramaciotti C, Keren A, Silverman NH: Importance of (perimembranous) ventricular septal aneurysm in the natural history of isolated perimembranous ventricular septal defect. *Am J Cardiol* 57:268, 1986.

Rhodes LA, Keane JF, Keane JP, et al: Long follow-up (to 43 years) of ventricular septal defect with audible aortic regurgitation. *Am J Cardiol* 66:340, 1990.

Trusler GA, Williams WG, Smallhorn JS, Freedom RM: Late results after repair of aortic insufficiency associated with ventricular septal defect. *J Thorac Cardiovasc Surg* 103(2):276, 1992.

Weidman WH, DuShane JW, Ellison RC: Clinical course in adults with ventricular septal defect. *Circulation* 56(Suppl I):1-78, 1977.

Wu MH, Wu JM, Chang CI, et al: Implications of aneurysmal transformation in isolated perimembranous ventricular septal defect. *Am J Cardiol* 72:596, 1993.

CHAPTER 4

PATENT DUCTUS ARTERIOSUS

The ductus arteriosus is a unique structure that evolves from the sixth aortic arch and connects the pulmonary artery to the aorta during fetal life. This vessel, which is similar in size to the pulmonary artery and aorta in utero, has specific anatomic and physiologic characteristics that allow closure after birth. The ductal structure differs from that of other muscular arteries; there is a large amount of ground substance containing smooth muscle cells in a spiral arrangement with very few elastic fibers. After birth, the smooth muscle contracts, mucoid substance in the wall coalesces, and intimal cushions proliferate and protrude into the lumen. Over one or two days, blood flow stagnates and the ductus becomes sealed.

CLINICAL FEATURES

In the fetus, patency of the ductus arteriosus appears to be maintained by the combined relaxant effects of low oxygen tension and endogenously produced prostaglandins. At the time of birth in a full-term baby, prostaglandin levels abruptly fall and arterial Pao_2 increases. This stimulates the ductus to close physiologically and, soon afterward, anatomically. In a premature infant, prostaglandin levels continue to be elevated, and the ductus arteriosus remains patent. In the context of extreme prematurity, especially when associated with respiratory distress syndrome, the addition of a left-to-right shunt beyond the first few days of life may result in these infants being ventilator-dependent, and the ductus must be closed. This is carried out by the administration of indomethacin, which blocks prostaglandin, or, if necessary, surgical ligation. A smaller patent ductus arteriosus (PDA) that does not cause significant symptoms of impaired respiratory function and growth failure can be expected to close spontaneously in the first year of life in virtually all premature babies. However, when a term baby has a persistent PDA, this indicates that the internal structure of the ductus is abnormal and does not have the capacity to constrict after birth and close anatomically. If closure does not occur in the first weeks of life, continued patency can be expected.

During infancy, the ductus arteriosus in a term baby may require early surgical closure within the first months of life because of a large left-to-right shunt and congestive heart failure. Smaller defects are routinely closed somewhat later, and in the modern era, this often is done with coils or other closure devices during interventional cardiac catheterization. Surgical closure remains a safe option. A small ductus in an older child is closed to prevent the possibility of bacterial endocarditis (BE) rather than because of hemodynamic concerns about a trivial or small left-to-right shunt. An undiagnosed large PDA occasionally is encountered later in childhood.

An older child or adult can have a large PDA and pulmonary vascular obstructive disease. Although rarely encountered in the modern era, long-standing hyperkinetic pulmonary hypertension secondary to a large left-to-right shunt in an unoperated patient can result in medial and intimal proliferation in the pulmonary arteriolar bed, as occurs with large ventricular septal defects (Eisenmenger's syndrome). A rare patient living at high altitudes may have a form of primary pulmonary hypertension resulting from intrinsic vascular obstructive disease have an associated PDA.

A large PDA is rarely seen as a primary lesion in adulthood, although such patients are encountered occasionally in medically underserved regions. When an adult cardiologist discovers a patient with a PDA, it is usually a small communication that might have been overlooked in earlier years. Most of these patients are asymptomatic with small shunts, although an occasional patient with a moderate-size ductus may present in middle age in heart failure. A few cases are discovered in the context of bacterial endocarditis. Adults who have PDA and pulmonary vascular obstructive disease have varying degrees of right-to-left shunting and symptoms related to pulmonary hypertension.

PHYSICAL EXAMINATION

The physical examination of an adult patient with a small ductus arteriosus, either unoperated or with residual shunting after an earlier intervention, usually shows no signs of a hemodynamic abnormality. There are no obvious manifestations of a significant left-to-right shunt. The pulse pressure will be normal, the heart will not be hyperdynamic, and there will be no signs of congestive heart failure. The cardiac examination usually reveals a continuous "machinery" murmur at the left upper sternal border and the left infraclavicular area. The diagnosis may not be made in some patients until adulthood because the murmur may be soft and well localized to a small area at the left sternal border. Occasionally, it is difficult to recognize that the systolic murmur "spills over" into early diastole. With a moderate left-to-right shunt, the pulses may be prominent, and the pulse pressure may be increased with diastolic pressures as low as 30 to 50 mm Hg. Patients with these findings may complain of fatigue or shortness of breath. In patients with PDA and pulmonary hypertension secondary to pulmonary vascular disease, only a systolic ejection murmur is audible. If pulmonary hypertension is severe, a right ventricular impulse will be palpated in the substernal region and the early medium-pitched diastolic murmur of pulmonary insufficiency may be audible.

NONINVASIVE EVALUATION

The *electrocardiogram* either is normal or shows increased left ventricular voltage. Nonspecific ST-T wave changes may be observed. In the presence of pulmonary hypertension, right ventricular hypertrophy is noted. The *chest x-ray* may be normal or may show cardiomegaly and increased pulmonary vascular markings, depending on the size of the PDA. When a left-to-right shunt is present, the *echocardiogram* will demonstrate characteristic color Doppler flow from the aorta to the left pulmonary artery (Fig. 4-1). With small shunts, left ventricular volume will not be increased significantly. If the PDA can be imaged and proper alignment is achieved between the aorta and the left pulmonary artery, a gradient may be measured that can provide important information about pulmonary artery pressure. Delineation of a PDA can usually be made by transthoracic echocardiography using suprasternal views. Transesophageal echocardiography (TEE) may be required in difficult cases.

MANAGEMENT

In an adult with a recently discovered continuous murmur, it is essential to confirm that this abnormality is due to a PDA. Other causes of a continuous murmur include a coronary atrioventricular (AV) fistula, a ruptured sinus of Valsalva aneurysm into the right side

FIGURE 4-1

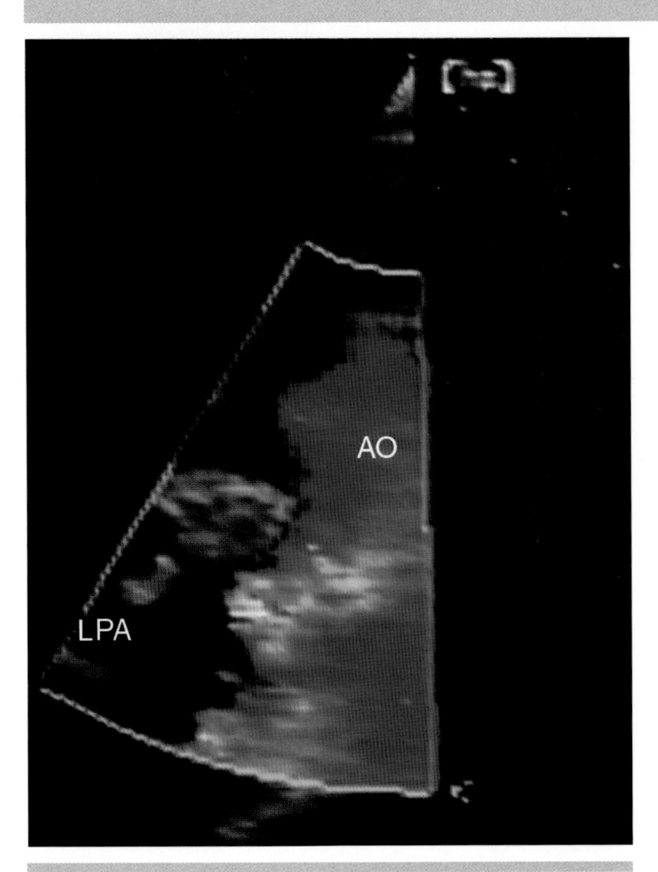

Color Doppler from a suprasternal view in a patient with a patent ductus arteriosus (PDA). Descending aortic blood flow is shown in blue, indicating flow away from the transducer. There is a red color jet in the left pulmonary artery, indicative of a left to right shunt through the PDA. Ao, aorta; LPA, left pulmonary artery.

of the heart or the left atrium, or a systemic AV fistula. A coronary AV fistula may be suspected on echocardiography because of the presence of a dilated proximal coronary artery, even when the insertion site of the fistula cannot be imaged. A communication between the sinus of Valsalva and the right ventricle usually can be visualized by echocardiography, although in adults the location of the shunt at the base of the aortic valve may be confused with a subaortic VSD. When the diagnosis is uncertain or when pulmonary hypertension is suspected, cardiac catheterization is indicated.

It generally is recommended that a small or moderate-sized PDA be closed by either interventional catheterization techniques, most often coil closure (Figs. 4-2 and 4-3*A* and *B*), or surgical ligation. The usual rationale for intervention with a small PDA is

FIGURE 4-2

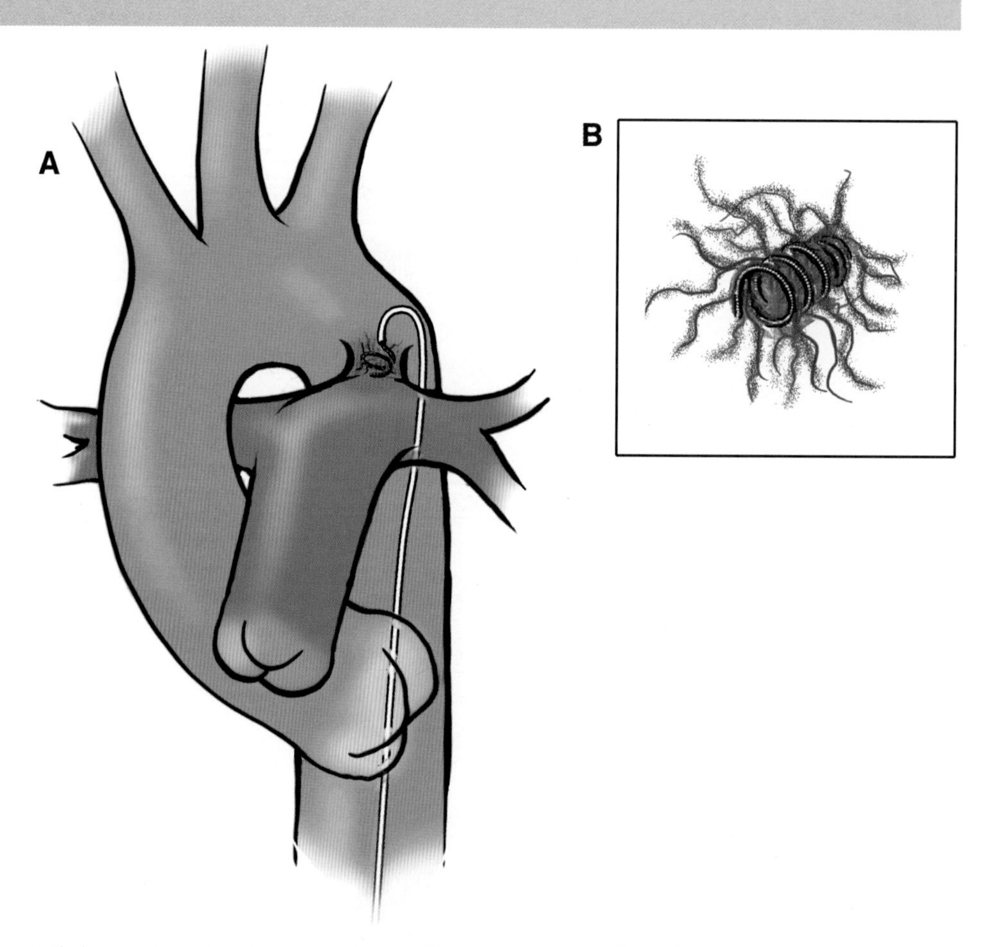

Coil closure of a patent ductus arteriosus is illustrated. *A*. A metallic coil with thrombogenic properties is placed within the ductus arteriosus, eliminating a left to right shunt. *B*. Closeup view of coil with thrombogenic Dacron threads.

FIGURE 4-3*A*

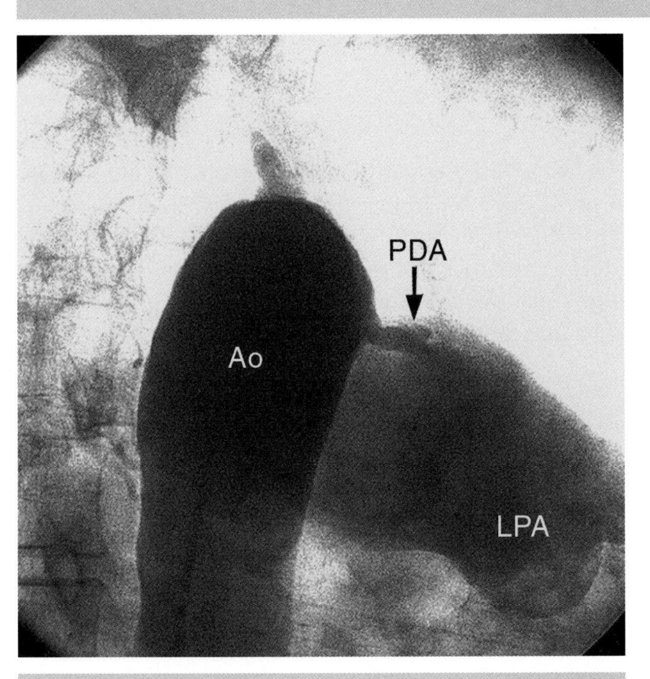

An angiogram performed in an adult with a patent ductus arteriosus (PDA). A proximal descending aortogram in the AP projection shows a long PDA with left-to-right shunting into a large pulmonary artery. Ao, aorta; PDA, patent ductus arteriosus; LPA, left pulmonary artery.

FIGURE 4-3*B*

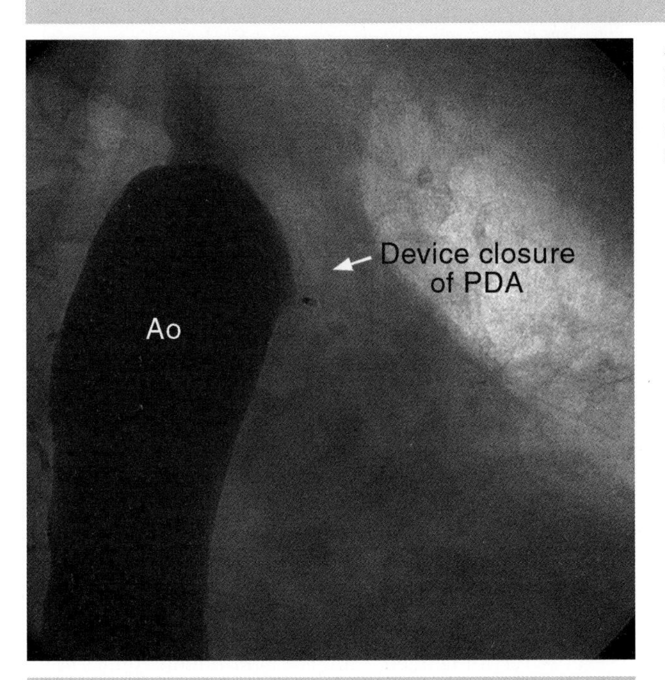

An aortogram following percutaneous closure of the patent ductus arteriosus (PDA) from the same patient as in Fig. 4-3*A*. The PDA has been closed by a PDA closure device. The white arrow points to the position of the device within the ductus. Ao, aorta.

prevention of BE. In older patients with very small defects, medical observation may be considered.

SURGICAL REPAIR

The anatomy of the ductus arteriosus may vary in terms of its length and width. A short, wide ductus may be ligated and not divided for technical reasons, especially when surgery is carried out during infancy. Older adults with moderate pulmonary hypertension can develop calcification in the ductus arteriosus that makes simple ligation infeasible. In these patients, closure of the ductus may require a median sternotomy with cardiopulmonary bypass to permit safe and adequate repair.

CATHETER CLOSURE

Cardiac-catheterization-based techniques for PDA closure are being used increasingly. Coil embolizations are utilized for small defects that meet specific anatomic criteria. Larger defects can be closed by using various other percutaneous devices. Some patients have been described with intrusion of coils into the pulmonary artery or aorta after percutaneous closure. These individuals should be followed, but important obstruction is not expected to be a clinical issue. Antibiotic prophylaxis against BE is discontinued after six months if the defect is closed completely.

SILENT DUCTUS

With the advent of sensitive Doppler methods, a tiny left-to-right shunt through a PDA may be seen in patients who have had an echocardiogram performed for other reasons. In most patients it is not necessary to intervene for these trivial shunts. Bacterial endocarditis in an undiagnosed silent ductus is extremely rare, and on a risk-benefit basis, it seems best simply to observe these patients with appropriate BE prophylaxis, as recommended by the American Heart Association.

LONG-TERM FOLLOW-UP

Once a PDA has been eliminated, the patient does not require cardiologic follow-up, and bacterial endocarditis prophylaxis is not needed. Rarely, a patient who had a ductus arteriosus ligated during childhood will present with a continuous murmur, indicating that the ductus has recanalized. When the ductus has been divided, of course, recanalization is not possible. Residual ductal shunts may be encountered in patients who have had coil embolization procedures. This has been reported to occur in the range of 5 to 10% of these patients but is expected to lessen in frequency as technology evolves. Small residual leaks noted immediately after the procedure usually close during early follow-up. If a small residual shunt remains, BE prophylaxis is recommended. Patients with ductal right-to-left shunts and pulmonary vascular disease are managed within the context of pulmonary vascular obstructive disease (Chap. 16).

SUMMARY

Adults with PDA and left-to-right shunts occasionally are encountered. A small PDA will have physical findings that include a machinery murmur at the left middle and upper sternal border, although occasionally the diastolic component is difficult to define. With shunts that are moderate in size, the pulse pressure may be wide and the precordium may be hyperdynamic. Some patients who have a history of previous intervention for PDA may have small residual shunts.

Catheter or surgical closure of a small but significant PDA is recommended to prevent BE. Larger defects require closure to prevent late heart failure. A patient with a PDA in the presence of pulmonary vascular obstructive disease may have a balanced or right-to-left shunt. The severity of pulmonary vascular obstruction defines the management. Very small shunts without clinical findings (silent ductus) may be observed medically with appropriate antibiotic prophylaxis to prevent endocarditis.

Algorithm 4–1
PDA

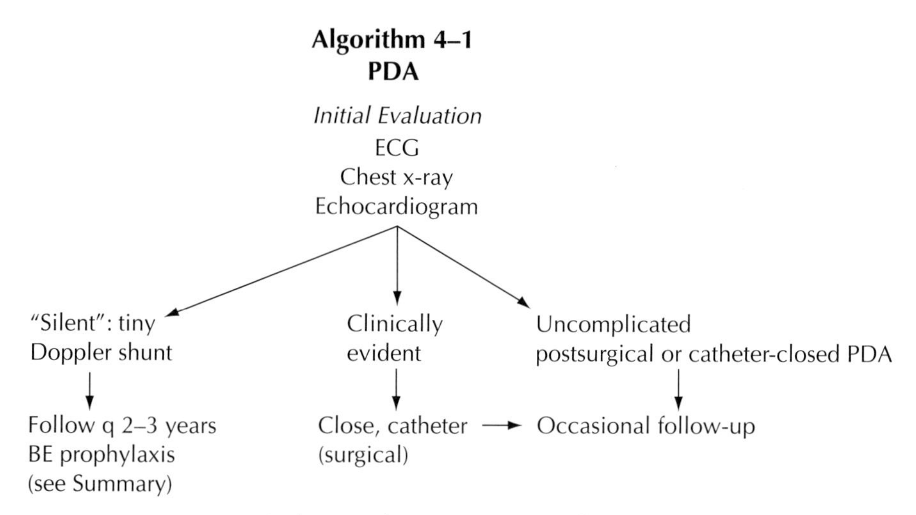

KEY: ECG, electrocardiogram; PDA, patent ductus arteriosus.

BIBLIOGRAPHY

Andrade A, Vargas-Barron J, Rijlaarsdan M, et al: Utility of transesophageal echocardiography in the examination of adult patients with patent ductus arteriosus. *Am Heart J* 130:543, 1995.

Bell-Thomson J, Jewell E, Ellis FH Jr, Schwaber JR: Surgical technique in the management of patent ductus arteriosus in the elderly patient. *Ann Thorac Surg* 30:80, 1980.

Blazer DT, Spray TL, McMullin O, et al: Endarteritis associated with a clinically silent patent ductus arteriosus. *Am Heart J* 125:1192, 1993.

Campbell M: Patent ductus arteriosus: Some notes on prognosis and on pulmonary hypertension. *Br Heart J* 17:511, 1955.

Coggin CJ, Parker KR, Keith JD: Natural history of isolated patent ductus arteriosus and the effect of surgical correction: Twenty years' experience at the Hospital for Sick Children, Toronto. *Can Med Assoc J* 102:718, 1970.

Dessy H, Hermus JP, van den Henvel F, et al: Echocardiographic and radionuclide pulmonary blood flow patterns after transcatheter closure of patent ductus arteriosus. *Circulation* 94:126, 1996.

Espino-Vela J, Cardenas N, Cruz R: Patent ductus arteriosus: With special reference to patients with pulmonary hypertension. *Circulation* 38(Suppl):45, 1968.

Fisher RG, Moodie DS, Sterba R, Gill CC: Patent ductus arteriosus in adults—long-term follow-up: Nonsurgical versus surgical treatment. *J Am Coll Cardiol* 8:280, 1986.

Gersony WM, Peckham GJ, Ellison RC, et al: Effects of indomethacin in premature infants with patent ductus arteriosus: Results of a collaborative study. *J Pediatr* 102:895, 1983.

Harrison DA, Benson LN, Lazzam C, et al: Percutaneous catheter closure of the persistently patent ductus arteriosus in the adult. *Am J Cardiol* 77:1094, 1996.

Hijazi AM, Geggel RL: Natural history of persistent ductus arteriosus. *Br Heart J* 30:4, 1968.

Hijazi AM, Geggel RL: Results of anterograde transcatheter closure of patent ductus arteriosus using single or multiple Gianturco coils. *Am J Cardiol* 74:925, 1994.

John S. Muralidharan S, Jairaj PS, et al: The adult ductus: Review of surgical experience with 131 patients. *J Thorac Cardiovasc Surg* 82:314, 1981.

Kelly DT: Patent ductus arteriosus in adults. *Cardiovasc Clin* 10:321, 1979.

Khan A, Yousef SA, Mullins CE, Sawyer W: Experience with 205 procedures of transcatheter closure of ductus arteriosus in 182 patients with special reference to residual shunts and long term follow-up. *J Thorac Cardiovasc Surg* 104:1721, 1992.

Lund JT, Jensen MB, Hjelms E: Aneurysm of the ductus arteriosus: A review of the literature and the surgical implications. *Eur J Cardiothorac Surg* 5:566, 1991.

Ottenkamp J, Hess J, Talsma MD, Buis-Liem TN: Protrusion of the device: A complication of the catheter closure of the patent ductus arteriosus. *Br Heart J* 68:301, 1992.

Porstmann W, Wierny L, Warnke H, et al: Catheter closure of patent ductus arteriosus: 62 cases treated without thoracotomy. *Radiol Clin North Am* 9:203, 1971.

Rashkind WJ, Mullins CE, Hellenbrand WE, Tait MA: Nonsurgical closure of patent ductus arteriosus: Clinical application of the Rashkind PDA Occluder System. *Circulation* 75:583, 1987.

Rothenberg SS, Chang JH, Toews WH, Washington RL: Thorascopic closure of patent ductus arteriosus: A less traumatic and more cost effective technique. *J Pediatr Surg* 30:1057, 1995.

Rudolph AM, Scarpelli EM, Golinko RJ, Gootman N: Hemodynamic basis for clinical manifestations of patent ductus arteriosus. *Am Heart J* 68:447, 1964.

Schrader R, Kadel C: Persistent ductus arteriosus—is closure indicated also in asymptomatic adults with small ductus and minor shunt. *Z Kardiol* 82:563, 1993.

Takenaka K, Sakamoto T, Shiota T, et al: Diagnosis of patent ductus arteriosus in adults by biplane transesophageal color Doppler flow mapping. *Am J Cardiol* 68:691, 1991.

CHAPTER 5

RIGHT VENTRICULAR OUTFLOW OBSTRUCTION

Right ventricular outflow tract obstruction may be present at the valvar, supravalvar, or subpulmonary levels. When an associated large ventricular septal defect (VSD) is present, the defect usually is classified as tetralogy of Fallot. Valvar pulmonary stenosis is the most common and accounts for 8 to 10% of all patients with congenital heart disease.

Subpulmonary (infundibular) stenosis is most often secondary to valvar obstruction. In the absence of valvar stenosis, infundibular stenosis almost always is associated with a VSD. Patients with branch stenoses of the pulmonary arteries, multiple peripheral arterial stenoses, or, rarely, a supravalvar component are considered to fall under the category of peripheral pulmonary artery stenoses. These lesions most often occur as a result of congenital rubella or as part of a syndrome of supravalvar aortic stenosis, mild mental retardation, "elfin" facies, and infantile hypercalcemia (Williams syndrome) (Chap. 6). Stenosis or narrowing of the main pulmonary artery or major branches also may be seen as a component of tetralogy of Fallot (Chap. 10).

VALVAR PULMONARY STENOSIS

In valvar pulmonary stenosis, the valve is usually conical or dome-shaped with fusion of the leaflet commissures. A bicuspid valve is present in 20% of cases. In 15% of patients with valvar pulmonary stenosis, a dysplastic pulmonary valve is present that causes obstruction from deformed, thickened, and rigid cusps (Fig. 5-1). A dysplastic pulmonary valve is most often seen in patients with Noonan's syndrome (Fig. 5-2).

Valvar pulmonary stenosis frequently is associated with a patent foramen ovale and occasionally an atrial septal defect. Poststenotic dilatation of the main pulmonary artery and left pulmonary artery are common and may be related to the direction of the

FIGURE 5-1

Right ventricular angiogram demonstrates valvar pulmonary stenosis. The pulmonary valve is extremely thickened, and there is poststenotic dilatation of the main pulmonary artery. The right ventricle is hypertrophied and heavily trabeculated. RV, right ventricle; PV, pulmonary valve; MPA, main pulmonary artery.

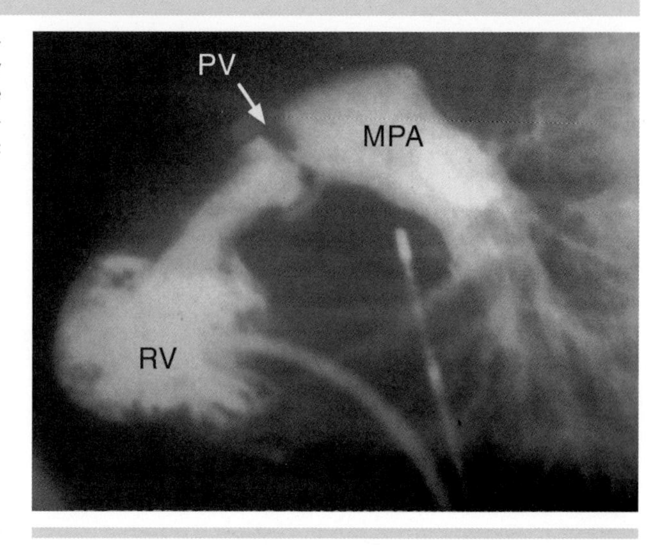

FIGURE 5-2

Right ventricular angiogram shows a dysplastic pulmonary valve (small black arrows) and poststenotic dilatation of the main pulmonary artery. The right ventricle is hypertrophied and heavily trabeculated. The white arrow indicates stenosis of a branch of the right pulmonary artery. RV, right ventricle; TV, tricuspid valve; MPA, main pulmonary artery; LPA, left pulmonary artery.

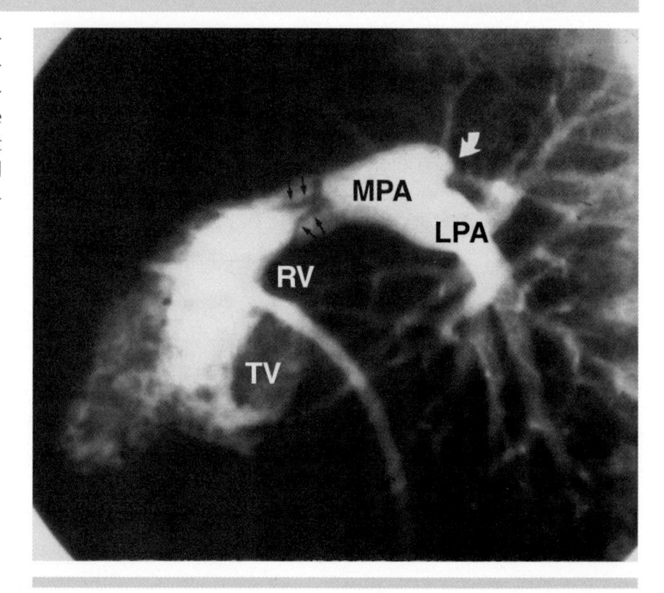

high-velocity jet through the stenotic valve. Varying degrees of right ventricular outflow muscular hypertrophy usually are present in cases of severe pulmonary stenosis.

CLINICAL FEATURES

The diagnosis of valvar pulmonary stenosis most often is made after the discovery of a systolic murmur at the left upper sternal border in an asymptomatic child. The natural history of this lesion depends on both the severity of the obstruction and its progression over time.

Critical Pulmonary Stenosis in Neonates

A small group of neonates with pulmonary stenosis have such severe valvar obstruction that pulmonary, as well as systemic, blood flow is dependent on right-to-left shunting across the foramen ovale and left-to-right shunting through a patent ductus arteriosus. In some patients, there is virtual pulmonary atresia. The right ventricle may be small, and the presentation and clinical course may mimic pulmonary atresia with an intact ventricular septum, although associated coronary artery abnormalities are not present. Infants with critical pulmonary stenosis are cyanotic and critically ill. They require pulmonary valvotomy, usually by balloon angioplasty, sometimes after temporary treatment with prostaglandin to maintain patency of the ductus arteriosus.

Children and Adults

When pulmonary stenosis presents beyond the neonatal period, clinical manifestations are usually absent. In these patients, the severity of pulmonary stenosis may be judged by the pulmonary valve gradient and/or right ventricular systolic pressure. When the cardiac output is normal, the severity is often referred to as follows: peak <25 mm Hg, trivial; 25–50 mm Hg, mild; 50–70 mm Hg, moderate; >70 mm Hg, severe.

The valve gradient during childhood may remain the same or may increase, depending on the growth of the pulmonary valve orifice relative to body growth over time. Patients with minimal pulmonary stenosis rarely progress to significant obstruction, although a stenotic pulmonary valve may calcify in older adults and can result in additional obstruction.

Right ventricular hypertrophy typically is present when pulmonary stenosis is moderate or greater. It is usually most pronounced in the infundibular region, where an obstructive component sometimes contributes to the gradient. Systolic function of the right ventricle usually is preserved. Congestive heart failure is unusual beyond the neonatal period except in patients with long-standing severe right ventricular outflow tract obstruction who have not had supervised medical care. When right ventricular pressure is suprasystemic, mild cyanosis may be present secondary to right-to-left shunting at the atrial level from elevated right atrial pressure. This manifestation, which is classically present in infants with critical pulmonary stenosis, is rare in older patients.

Most patients with isolated pulmonary stenosis are asymptomatic. An occasional patient with at least moderately severe pulmonary stenosis may experience exertional dyspnea and fatigue. Exertional chest pain has been reported in patients with severe pulmonary stenosis.

Natural History

A significant amount of information regarding pulmonary stenosis is available from the Natural History Study of Congenital Heart Defects (NHS-2). Patients with this lesion were followed since enrollment between 1958 and 1973 and were reassessed between 1983 and 1986.

In this study, patients with a PSG <50 mm Hg were managed medically, those with a PSG between 50 and 79 mm Hg received either medical or surgical treatment, and those with a PSG >80 mm Hg were treated surgically. Among patients treated medically, 19% and 58% with an initial PSG between 25 and 49 and 50 and 79 mm Hg, respectively, underwent surgery within 10 years. Survival of patients in the NHS was excellent; there were 22 deaths among 586 enrolled patients, and the majority were related to surgery in critically ill infants and occurred in an earlier era.

In the NHS-2 cohort of 116 medically treated and 215 surgically treated patients, 97% were in New York Heart Association (NYHA) class I and 89% had a normal electrocardiogram. Pulmonary insufficiency was present in a large proportion of the surgically treated patients but was not indicative of an adverse outcome. The average gradient in the medically treated group was 17 mm Hg; in the postoperative group, it was 10 mm Hg. The major conclusion that is relevant to adults with this lesion is that patients with both mild and moderate pulmonary stenosis as well as postoperative patients do very well and can anticipate excellent long-term survival. Most patients with a gradient between 50 and 79 mm Hg ultimately require intervention. Those with severe pulmonary stenosis do best if operated on early in life.

Physical Examination

The diagnosis and severity of valvar pulmonary stenosis can be assessed by physical examination. When the obstruction is severe in adults, a giant A wave can be detected in the jugular venous pulse secondary to decreased right ventricular compliance. A right ventricular impulse and a left upper sternal border thrill may be palpated. The first heart sound is normal and is followed closely by a pulmonary ejection click when the pulmonary valve is mobile and the stenosis is mild to moderate. The click is heard at the left middle to upper sternal border and differs from the click of aortic stenosis, which is best heard at the apex. Another distinguishing feature is the decrease in intensity of the pulmonary click during inspiration. As pulmonary stenosis increases, the pulmonary valve opens earlier and the click moves closer to the first heart sound. When obstruction is severe, a click is not heard.

The second heart sound is abnormally split in patients with pulmonary stenosis. As the gradient increases, right ventricular ejection time increases, producing additional delay in pulmonary closure and increased splitting of S_2. However, since pulmonary artery pressure becomes extremely low (8 to 12 mm) with moderate and severe obstruction, P_2 is no longer audible and the second heart sound becomes single.

The systolic ejection murmur of pulmonary stenosis is loudest at the second left interspace and is transmitted to the suprasternal and infraclavicular area and the left side of the neck. The murmur may be as loud as grade 3 or 4. The shape and duration of the murmur are related to the severity of pulmonary stenosis. In mild pulmonary stenosis, the murmur is crescendo-decrescendo and ends before the aortic closure sound. In moderate to severe pulmonary stenosis, the murmur peaks later in systole and obscures the aortic closure sound. When the stenosis is extremely severe, the murmur peaks even later and goes beyond A_2 and no second sound is heard. A right ventricular S_4 is associated with at least moderate pulmonary stenosis.

In patients with infundibular pulmonary stenosis, the murmur is maximal at the fourth left interspace and may be similar in location to a VSD.

Noninvasive Evaluation

The *electrocardiogram* is useful in assessing the severity of pulmonary stenosis. A normal electrocardiogram is present in most patients with mild pulmonary stenosis. Greater degrees of pulmonary stenosis are reflected by a rightward mean frontal QRS axis and increased right ventricular forces or an RSR^1 pattern in the right precordial leads.

In severe pulmonary stenosis, a pure R wave, QR, or RS is usually present in the right precordial leads with increased R-wave amplitude. The T wave may be upright, but with severe obstruction, an RV strain pattern may be seen.

The *chest x-ray* in valvar pulmonary stenosis usually shows dilatation of the left pulmonary artery and main pulmonary artery. This is not related to the severity of obstruction. The right atrium and right ventricle are usually normal in size except in the unusual patient with severe pulmonary stenosis who has developed right ventricular failure. In these cases, significant tricuspid insufficiency may also be present.

Echocardiography in patients with pulmonary stenosis provides essential information, including: (1) pulmonary valve morphology, (2) assessment of chamber size, degree of right ventricular hypertrophy, and secondary infundibular obstruction, (3) calculation of a predicted gradient across the right ventricular outflow tract, and (4) exclusion of additional lesions. Doppler studies predict the gradient across the right ventricular outflow tract and may be confirmed by the gradient between the right ventricle and the right atrium if there is enough tricuspid insufficiency to obtain this measurement. The configuration of the ventricular septum in systole also provides information regarding the relative pressures between the right and left ventricles. Systolic flattening of the septum generally implies that right ventricular pressure is nearly systemic or greater.

MANAGEMENT

The management of pulmonary stenosis is determined by assessment of the severity of obstruction, since symptomatic patients are encountered infrequently. In the presence of a normal cardiac output, the right ventricular–pulmonary artery (RV-PA) gradient is the main determinant of whether intervention is required.

Patients with minimal pulmonary stenosis (RV-PA gradient <25 mm) should be followed medically and should not be restricted. Progression to hemodynamically significant pulmonary stenosis is not expected. While dental prophylaxis is recommended, bacterial endocarditis (BE) is a rare complication of this lesion. A significant number of patients with gradients between 25 and 50 mm Hg as measured in childhood eventually require intervention. Children and young adults with moderately severe (50 to 79 mm Hg) and severe (>80 mm Hg) pulmonary stenosis currently are managed with balloon valvuloplasty. The procedure generally is performed shortly after diagnosis. The rare patient in whom balloon valvuloplasty is unsuccessful can be treated by surgical valvotomy. Valve replacement may be indicated for the rare older patient with a heavily calcified valve.

Management decisions for an asymptomatic patient with a moderate predicted gradient by Doppler assessment may be difficult. Before the development of balloon valvuloplasty, these patients would have been managed medically. With the success and safety of balloon valvuloplasty for this lesion, a patient with a measured gradient in the range of 50 mm Hg may be considered a candidate for intervention. However, since the predicted gradient with an echocardiogram may overestimate the true gradient, it is important to corroborate these findings with the assessment of the right ventricle, physical examination, and electrocardiography (ECG) to avoid an unnecessary cardiac catheterization.

Balloon Valvuloplasty

Before the use of balloon valvuloplasty in 1982, patients with significant valvar pulmonary stenosis required surgical valvotomy. With the effectiveness and safety of balloon valvuloplasty established, this treatment is now being used in patients with borderline gradients who might have been managed medically in the preballoon era. Balloon valvuloplasty also may be attempted when the pulmonary valve is dysplastic, but in this situation the procedure is less effective than surgical valvotomy. Surgery also may be required in the presence of severe infundibular stenosis associated with severe pulmonary valve stenosis.

The pulmonary valve gradient usually can be reduced by at least 50% with balloon valvuloplasty in the majority of patients. Further reductions in the gradient may occur with time-related resolution of the mild-to-moderate infundibular stenosis. A second valvuloplasty is not required if there was adequate relief of obstruction during the first valvuloplasty. Studies have demonstrated persistent relief of obstruction during a 5-year follow-up period.

Evidence for a successful balloon valvuloplasty or surgical valvotomy should be apparent on examination by the disappearance of a precordial thrill on palpation and a decrease in the duration and intensity of the systolic ejection murmur. A murmur of pulmonary insufficiency is present in most patients, but its presence rarely causes hemodynamic problems. The clinical outcome in these patients is excellent, and the need for a late operation is rare. Several studies have documented long-term relief of obstruction after successful relief of pulmonary stenosis.

The results may be less favorable in patients with right ventricular hypoplasia, which may be complicated by right-to-left shunting at the atrial level, right-sided heart failure, and residual pulmonary stenosis. Similarly, adults with untreated, long-standing severe pulmonary stenosis may experience persistent right ventricular dysfunction postoperatively because of a noncompliant and hypertrophied right ventricle, with tricuspid insufficiency, elevated systemic venous pressure, and diminished cardiac output.

Surgical Repair

If balloon valvuloplasty is ineffective in reducing the gradient, surgical valvotomy may be performed with effective relief of obstruction. While closed valvotomy avoids the need for cardiopulmonary bypass, more precise correction of valvar stenosis is afforded by an open procedure that permits infundibular resection or transannular patching, if necessary.

A rare adult may require pulmonary valve replacement as a result of (1) significant obstruction with late calcification of the pulmonary valve or (2) right ventricular dilatation and diminished function that may be related to chronic pulmonary insufficiency after surgical valvotomy.

Infundibular stenosis can complicate valvar pulmonary stenosis, and it may be difficult in some cases to determine whether this is secondary to valvar obstruction and will regress after valvotomy or whether subvalvar obstruction is contributing to the gradient and should be resected. Moderate infundibular stenosis secondary to valvar pulmonary stenosis generally is not a contraindication for balloon valvuloplasty, but in some cases surgery is a safe and effective alternative. Infundibular resection and patch enlargement of the outflow tract may be mandatory in severe cases when right ventricular pressure is suprasystemic or when right ventricular hypoplasia is present.

LONG-TERM FOLLOW-UP

A postoperative or postballoon valvuloplasty patient is almost invariably asymptomatic. A short systolic ejection murmur and a soft diastolic murmur are usually audible. The ECG will show a right ventricular conduction delay. The echocardiogram will reveal some deformity of the pulmonary valve with varying degrees of pulmonary valve insufficiency. Antibiotic prophylaxis should be continued. The prognosis for an uncomplicated post-repair life is excellent.

Physical examination is helpful in determining the patient's status. A short systolic ejection murmur is audible along the left middle and upper sternal border, associated with a short medium-pitched diastolic murmur. It may not be possible to recognize physiologic splitting of the second sound. There may be a residual variable systolic ejection click at the left upper sternal border. In patients with a long systolic murmur along the left sternal border, the possibility of residual stenosis must be considered. These patients have little or no diastolic murmur. When significant pulmonary valve insufficiency is present, there is usually no significant residual stenosis.

The ECG will show an RSR′ pattern in VI or complete right bundle branch block. The echocardiogram may show right ventricular chamber dilatation with color Doppler evidence of pulmonary valve insufficiency. A gradient as high as 30 to 50 mm Hg may be present in patients with pulmonary valve insufficiency because of the increased stroke volume. Right ventricular function and the status of the tricuspid valve should also be determined. The vast majority of patients tolerate postoperative pulmonary valve regurgitation without difficulty and require no further treatment.

Patients with greater degrees of right ventricular enlargement require more frequent follow-up, and rare patients with right ventricular dysfunction and/or tricuspid insufficiency and significant pulmonary regurgitation are candidates for pulmonary valve replacement. Periodic exercise testing and 24-h Holter recordings may be useful in identifying the occasional patient with postoperative rhythm disturbances. Antibiotic prophylaxis for dental care is recommended.

PULMONARY ATRESIA WITH INTACT VENTRICULAR SEPTUM

Pulmonary atresia with intact ventricular septum is a defect in which there is no connection between the right ventricular outflow tract and the pulmonary artery. The great majority of these patients have hypoplasia of the right ventricular chamber associated with severe right ventricular hypertrophy; myocardial sinusoids are often present, connecting the right ventricle with the coronary arteries. Pulmonary blood flow is maintained in a neonate with this defect through a patent ductus arteriosus. Blood reaches the left side of the heart by means of a patent foramen ovale. When the ductus closes spontaneously over the first several days of life, the patient becomes severely cyanotic, and survival beyond 1 week of age is extremely rare. Thus, patients with this entity encountered during adult life are those in whom surgical intervention was carried out initially in the early neonatal period; most often, multiple procedures were required.

Initial management in neonatal life consists of a prostaglandin infusion to keep the ductus open and is usually followed by a shunt and, if feasible, RV decompression. There is an assessment concerning the adequacy of the right ventricular chamber and tricuspid valve for a biventricular repair (Figs. 5-3*A* and *B*). In addition, it must be determined whether a portion of the coronary circulation is dependent on RV flow through myocardial sinusoids.

Some infants with pulmonary atresia and an intact ventricular system have severe coronary obstruction with coronary perfusion via myocardial sinusoids from the high-pressure right ventricle. Decompression of the right ventricle during surgery in such cases can have catastrophic consequences. In these patients, a Fontan procedure is required that allows the right ventricle to provide myocardial blood flow via sinusoids connecting to the distal coronary arteries (Fig. 5-4). In these cases there is proximal obstruction of the coronary arteries.

Survivors of pulmonary atresia beyond childhood include patients with both single and two-ventricle repairs. In some patients, the right ventricular outflow tract has been reconstructed, although many patients continue to have some right-to-left shunting across the foramen ovale and are cyanotic. Others may have had a Glenn anastomosis (superior vena cava to right pulmonary artery), which channels upper extremity systemic venous return directly to the right lung, preserving the small right ventricle to deliver pulmonary blood flow to the left lung. Occasionally, the superior vena cava anastomosis is connected to provide bidirectional pulmonary blood flow in preparation for a Fontan operation in which all the systemic venous blood returns to the lungs directly, completely bypassing a diminutive right ventricle (Chap. 12). Whereas very few of these patients have survived

FIGURE 5-3

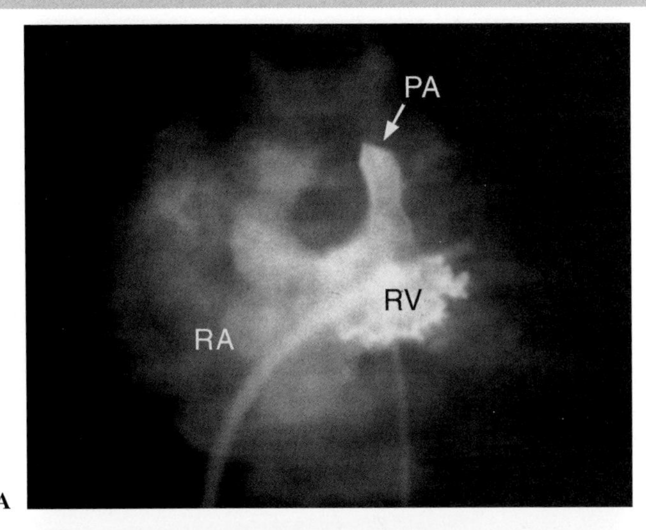

A

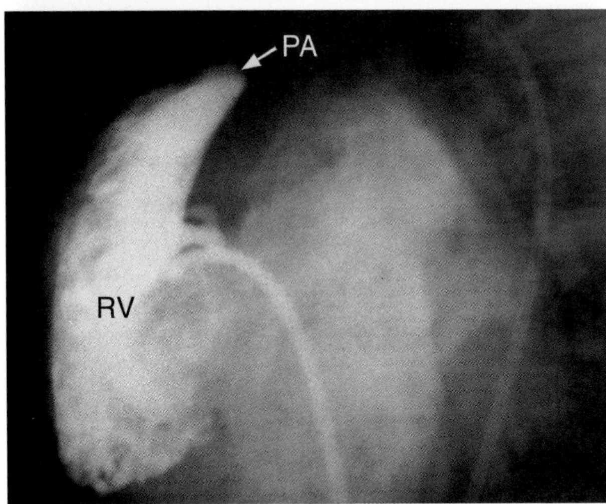

B

A. A right ventricular angiogram in a patient with pulmonary atresia and intact ventricular septum which displays a small trabeculated right ventricular chamber with tricuspid insufficiency and a blind right ventricular outflow. The pulmonary artery is not seen but is filled later from a ductus arteriosus. RV, right ventricle; RA, right atrium; PA, pulmonary atresia. *B*. Patient with pulmonary atresia and intact ventricular septum with a large right ventricular chamber. There is a blind right ventricular outflow. RV, right ventricle; PA, pulmonary atresia.

to late childhood or adolescence in the past, better management strategies today have resulted in improved survival. Careful observation for coronary ischemia is important for all survivors of pulmonary atresia, whether a two-ventricle or single-ventricle repair has been performed (Chap. 9).

PERIPHERAL PULMONARY STENOSIS

Peripheral pulmonary stenosis occurs as part of entities such as Williams syndrome (Chap. 6), rubella cardiovascular disease, and some forms of severe tetralogy of Fallot

FIGURE 5-4

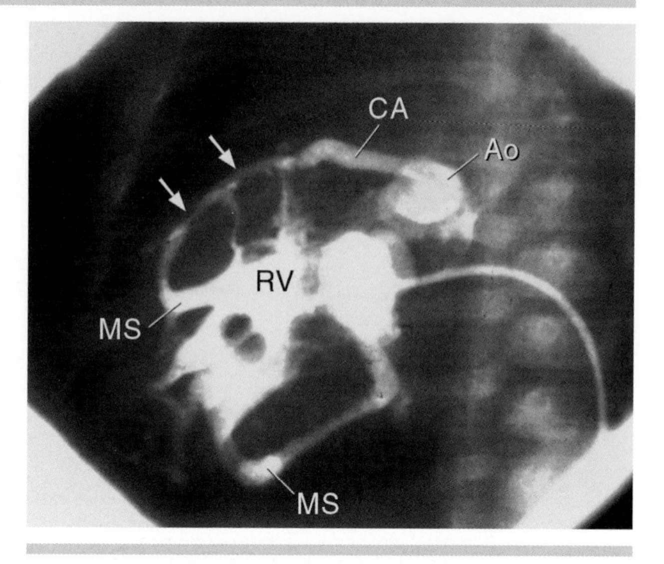

A right ventricular angiogram in a patient with pulmonary atresia and intact ventricular septum, which illustrates myocardial sinusoids connecting with the coronary arteries and retrograde filling of the aorta. Arrows indicate narrow segments of coronary vessels. RV, right ventricle; CA, coronary artery; Ao, aorta; MS, myocardial sinusoids.

(Chap. 11). Peripheral pulmonary stenosis also occurs as an isolated lesion (Fig. 5-5). Some cases are diagnosed in early infancy, and most are mild to moderate in terms of the degree of obstruction of right ventricular blood flow and associated right ventricular hypertension. Even patients with significant obstruction often improve with time. Although some degree of right ventricular hypertension will be present because of peripheral pulmonary stenoses, no treatment is required and the prognosis appears to be excellent. Rarely, a child or young adult is encountered with severe isolated peripheral pulmonary stenosis who may develop right ventricular dysfunction that leads to right-sided heart failure. Management of these patients is often difficult. Surgical intervention for proximal lesions may be possible, but often the gradients across obstructed branches are merely shifted distally. The same may be true for interventional balloon angioplasty or stenting. However, a number of cases have been reported where, often after multiple interventions, dilatation of obstructive pulmonary artery branches has been sufficient to significantly lower the degree of obstruction and right ventricular hypertension.

DOUBLE-CHAMBER RIGHT VENTRICLE

Double-chamber right ventricle refers to an obstruction in the midportion of the right ventricle that essentially divides the chamber into two components: a high-pressure lower chamber and a normal-pressure upper chamber. The inflow area is obstructed by fibromuscular tissue and right ventricular hypertrophy. In virtually all cases, there is an associated VSD that is usually small. If left untreated, the VSD may close completely as fibromuscular tissue proliferates, leaving isolated right ventricular outflow obstruction. When this lesion was first recognized 20 to 30 years ago, many of the patients were older

FIGURE 5-5

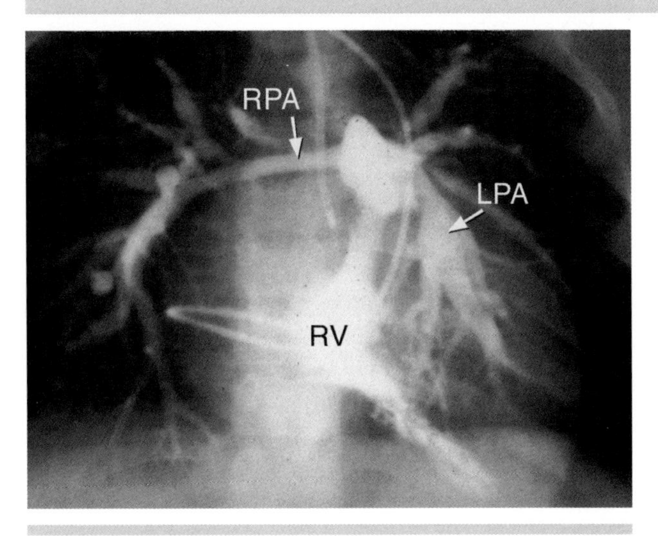

Right ventricular angiogram in a patient with peripheral pulmonary stenosis. Note the narrow right pulmonary artery with multiple peripheral pulmonary artery stenoses. The right ventricle is markedly hypertrophied. RPA, right pulmonary artery; RV, right ventricle; LPA, left pulmonary artery.

and had no VSD. In the era of echocardiography, most patients are diagnosed early, and it is unusual to see a patient without an associated VSD.

Treatment of this entity is surgical. Relief of obstruction in the mid portion of the right ventricle is easily achieved, and unlike other types of subvalvular obstruction of either the left or the right ventricular outflow tract, recurrences are rare. It is of interest that during surgery, when the obstructive tissue is excised, a VSD is almost invariably noted, even in patients in whom the septum had been noted to be intact by echocardiography. After relief of the obstruction and closure of the VSD, patients with double-chamber right ventricles have an excellent prognosis in terms of longevity and unrestricted activities.

SUMMARY

Patients with pulmonary stenosis present in adult life having had no previous operative or interventional procedures or after earlier interventions. In either case, the important issue is the severity of stenosis. Pulmonary insufficiency is rarely a late issue. These patients are usually symptomatic. Principles of management can be summarized on the basis of the RV-PA gradient.

Mild Pulmonary Stenosis (RV-PA Gradient <50 mm Hg)

Patients with trivial or mild pulmonary stenosis do not require valvuloplasty or surgery. The clinical features, ECG, and echocardiogram should delineate the mild abnormality of the pulmonary valve and document the absence of other lesions. The physical examination reveals only a short systolic ejection murmur at the left upper sternal body (LUSB), a normally split-second sound, and occasionally a variable systolic ejection click. The ECG is normal; right ventricular hypertrophy is absent. Echocardiographic examination reveals normal right ventricular function, no tricuspid insufficiency, no right ventricular hypertrophy, normal configuration of the ventricular septum, and only a small predicted gradient by Doppler examination. Cardiac catheterization is not required. Patients with mild pulmonary stenosis need not be restricted in their routine activities, which can include participation in sports and childbearing. Although bacterial endocarditis is extremely rare, antibiotic prophylaxis is recommended. Cardiac arrhythmias generally are not expected.

Patients with gradients less than 25 mm Hg have not been documented to progress in severity either during childhood or in adult life. However, gradients in the range of 25 to 50 mm Hg represent significantly more anatomic narrowing and, with time and possible right ventricular outflow muscular hypertrophy, could reach gradients at the higher levels of severity. Patients with trivial stenosis require only minimal follow-up and can be reassured that intervention will not be necessary. Those with gradients close to the moderate range must be followed for the possibility of increasing obstruction over time.

Severe Pulmonary Stenosis (RV-PA Gradient >70 mm Hg)

In the presence of pure pulmonary valve stenosis without severe associated infundibular hypertrophy or valve dysplasia or calcification, balloon valvuloplasty is the treatment of choice.

Cardiac examination reveals an RV impulse and a late peaking systolic ejection murmur at the left middle and upper sternal border that obscures A_2. A click is absent. An ECG shows right ventricular hypertrophy, and an echocardiogram delineates the anatomy of the right ventricular outflow tract and the predicted gradient across the right ventricular outflow tract. On the basis of these findings and confirmatory hemodynamic and angiographic data, balloon valvuloplasty is performed. If balloon valvuloplasty cannot be done successfully because of severe infundibular hypertrophy or pulmonary valve dysplasia, surgical valvotomy is carried out. When severe associated infundibular stenosis is present, surgical resection of infundibular muscle is performed at the time of operation. In rare patients with long-standing severe pulmonary stenosis, right ventricular dysfunction and tricuspid insufficiency may be present, and pulmonary valve and/or tricuspid valve replacement may be required.

Moderate Stenosis (RV-PA Gradient 50 to 70 mm Hg)

Asymptomatic patients with RV-PA gradients between 50 and 69 mm Hg and no contraindications are appropriate candidates for balloon valvuloplasty. In patients with a gradient at the lower end of this range, associated findings, such as symptoms, degree of right ventricular hypertrophy, and the possibility of future pregnancy, will contribute to the decision making about the timing of intervention. Overestimation of gradient by Doppler prediction may be a factor.

Algorithm 5–1
PS—Unoperated

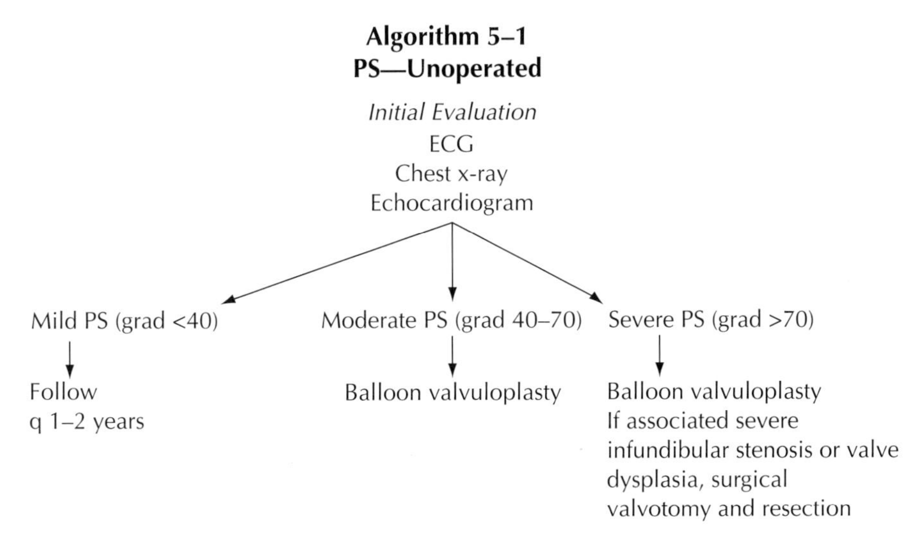

KEY: ECG, electrocardiogram; grad, gradient; PS, pulmonary stenosis.

Algorithm 5–2
PS—Operated

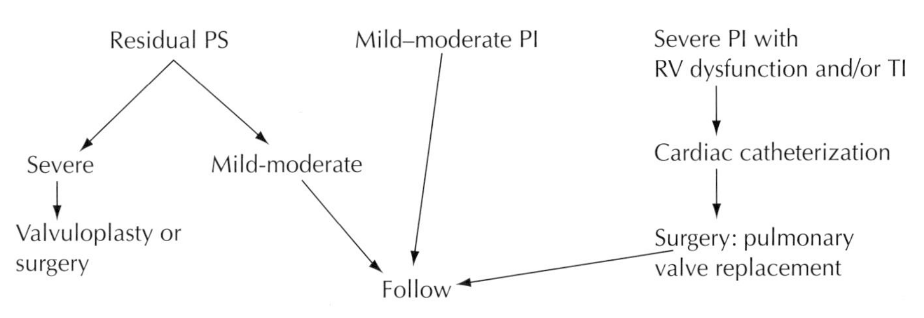

KEY: PI, pulmonary insufficiency; PS, pulmonary stenosis; RV, right ventricle; TI, tricuspid insufficiency.

BIBLIOGRAPHY

Ben-Shacher G, Cohen MH, Sivakof MC: Development of infundibular obstruction after percutaneous pulmonary balloon valvuloplasty. *J Am Coll Cardiol* 11:161, 1985.

Benson LN, Smallhorn JS, Freedom RM, et al: Pulmonary valve morphology after balloon dilation of pulmonary valve stenosis. *Cathet Cardiovasc Diagn* 11:161, 1985.

Bove EL, Kavey RE, Byrum CJ, et al: Improved right ventricular function following late pulmonary valve replacement for residual pulmonary insufficiency or stenosis. *J Thorac Cardiovasc Surg* 90:50, 1985.

Chen C-R, Cheng TO, Huang T, et al: Percutaneous balloon valvuloplasty for pulmonic stenosis in adolescents and adults. *N Engl J Med* 335:21, 1996.

Fawzy ME, Galal O, Dunn B, et al: Regression of infundibular pulmonary stenosis after successful balloon pulmonary valvuloplasty in adults. *Cathet Cardiovasc Diagn* 21:77, 1990.

Fogelman R, Nykanen D, Smallhorn JF, et al: Endovascular stents in the pulmonary circulation: Clinical impact on management of medium-term follow-up. *Circulation* 92:881, 1995.

Gersony WM, Bernhard WF, Nadas AS, Gross RE: Diagnosis and surgical treatment of pulmonic stenosis. *Circulation* 13:765, 1967.

Hayes CJ, Gersony WM, Driscoll DJ, et al: Second Natural History Study of Congenital Heart Defects: Results of treatment of patients with pulmonary valvar stenosis. *Circulation* 87(Suppl I):I-28I, 1993.

Hermann HC, Hill JA, Krol J, et al: Effectiveness of percutaneous balloon valvuloplasty in adults with pulmonic valve stenosis. *Am J Cardiol* 68:1111, 1991.

Hosking MC, Thomaidis A, Hamilton B, et al: Clinical impact of balloon angioplasty for branch pulmonary artery stenosis. *Am J Cardiol* 69:1467, 1992.

Kan JS, White RI, Mitchell SE, Gardner TJ: Percutaneous balloon valvuloplasty: A new method of treatment of congenital pulmonary valve stenosis. *N Engl J Med* 307:540, 1982.

Kaul UA, Singh B, Tyagi S, et al: Long-term results after balloon pulmonary valvuloplasty in adults. *Am Heart J* 126:1152, 1993.

Koretzky ED, Moller JH, Korns ME, et al: Congenital pulmonary stenosis resulting from dysplasia of the valve. *Circulation* 40, 1969.

McCrindle BW: Independent predictors of long-term results after balloon pulmonary valvuloplasty: Valvuloplasty and Angioplasty of Congenital Anomalies (VACA) Registry investigators. *Circulation* 89:1751, 1994.

McCrindle BW, Kan JS: Long-term results after balloon pulmonary valvuloplasty. *Circulation* 83:1915, 1991.

Mendelson AM, Bove EL, Lupinetti FM, et al: Intraoperative and percutaneous stenting of congenital pulmonary artery and vein stenosis. *Circulation* 88(2):210, 1993.

Musewe NN, Robertson MA, Benson LN, et al: The dysplastic pulmonary valve: Echographic features and results of balloon dilatation. *Br Heart J* 57:364, 1987.

Nadas AD: Pulmonic stenosis: Indications for surgery in children and adults. *N Engl J Med* 287:1196, 1972.

Nugent EW, Freedom RM, Nora JJ, et al: Clinical course in pulmonary stenosis. *Circulation* 56(Suppl I):38, 1977.

O'Connor BK, Beekman RH, Lindauer AM, Rocchini A: Intermediate-term outcome after pulmonary balloon valvuloplasty: Comparison with a matched surgical control group. *J Am Coll Cardiol* 20:169, 1992.

O'Laughlin MP, Perry SB, Lock JE, Mullins CE: Use of endovascular stents in congenital heart disease. *Circulation* 83:1923, 1991.

Pepine CJ, Gessner IH, Feldman RL: Percutaneous balloon valvuloplasty for pulmonary valve stenosis in the adult. *Am J Cardiol* 50:1442, 1982.

Rothman A, Perry JB, Keane JF, Lock JE: Early results and follow-up of balloon angioplasty for branch pulmonary artery stenosis. *J Am Coll Cardiol* 15:1109, 1990.

Rowland TW, Rosenthal A, Castandea AR: Double-chamber right ventricle: Experience with 17 cases. *Am Heart J* 89:445, 1975.

Sadr-Ameli MA, Sheikholeslami F, Firoozi I, Azarnik H: Late results of balloon pulmonary valvuloplasty in adults. *Am J Cardiol* 82:398, 1998.

Sherman W, Hershman R, Alexopoulos D, et al: Pulmonic balloon valvuloplasty in adults. *Am Heart J* 119:187, 1990.

Stanger P, Cassidy SC, Girod DA, et al: Balloon pulmonary valvuloplasty: Results of the Valvuloplasty and Angioplasty of Congenital Anomalies Registry. *Am J Cardiol* 65:775, 1990.

Teupe CH, Burger W, Schrader R, Zeiher AM: Late (five to nine years) follow-up after balloon dilation of valvular pulmonary stenosis in adults. *Am J Cardiol* 80:240, 1997.

CHAPTER 6

LEFT VENTRICULAR OUTFLOW TRACT OBSTRUCTION

I. VALVAR AORTIC STENOSIS

Congenital aortic stenosis accounts for 3 to 6% of all cases of congenital heart disease. The basic abnormality in valvar aortic stenosis is a fusion of the valve commissures that results in rigidity of the valve leaflets and a reduced aortic orifice. The valve is usually bicuspid, occasionally tricuspid, and in rare instances dome-shaped or unicuspid. The aortic valve annulus is sometimes small, and this poses a particular problem in patients with severe obstruction. Associated anomalies are present in approximately 20% of patients with this lesion. The most common anomaly is coarctation of the aorta.

Unobstructed bicuspid aortic valve (Fig. 6-1) is the most common congenital cardiac anomaly and has no clinical relevance unless it is associated with progressive late stenosis or regurgitation. A small subset of patients may have associated dilatation of the ascending aorta. The diagnosis usually is made by echocardiography, often after an aortic click has been noted.

CLINICAL FEATURES

The diagnosis of aortic stenosis usually is made after birth with the discovery of a systolic murmur at the right and left upper sternal border. The severity of aortic stenosis can vary from mild to severe obstruction. The most severe form occurs in neonates with critical stenosis. In this situation, blood flow through the aortic valve is inadequate and results in low cardiac output, elevated left atrial pressure, and persistent pulmonary hypertension. Right-to-left shunting via the ductus arteriosus into the descending aorta may be necessary to support systemic cardiac output. Prostaglandin is used to keep the ductus arteriosus open after birth. Relief of obstruction is essential to survival.

FIGURE 6-1

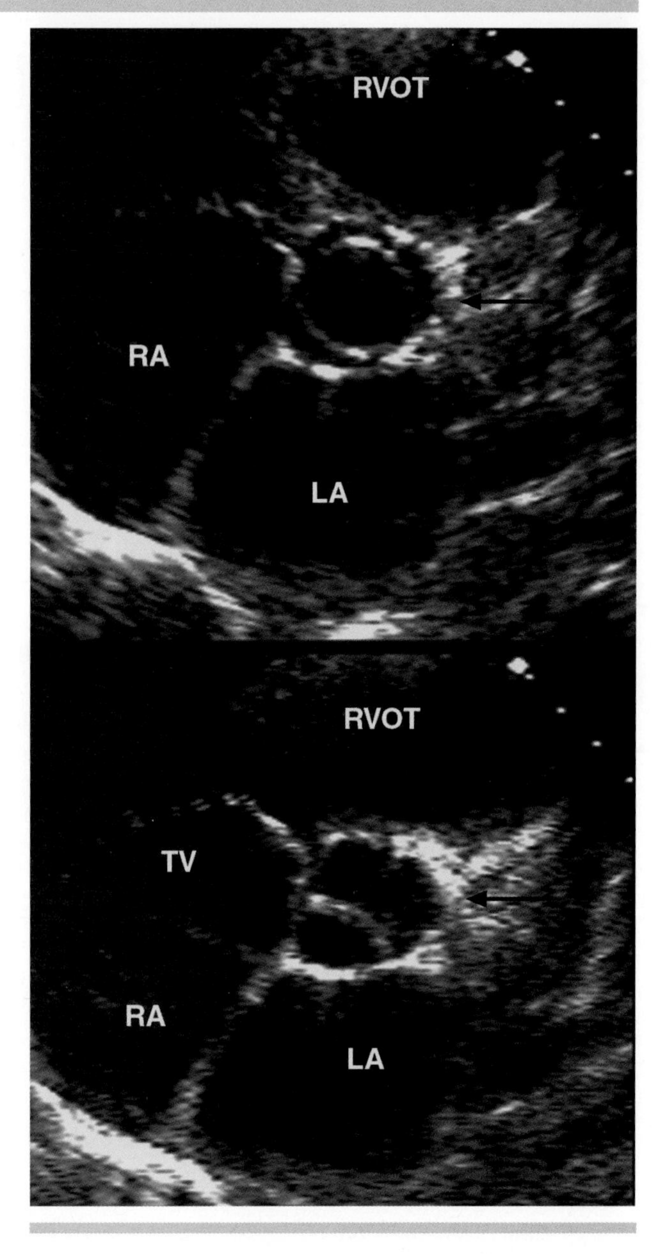

Parasternal short-axis view in systole (top) and diastole (bottom) from a patient with a bicuspid aortic valve. In systole, the cusps have a fish-mouthed shape. In diastole, there is an eccentric closure line. Arrows in both pictures point to the aortic valve. RVOT, right ventricular outflow tract; RA, right atrium; LA, left atrium; TV, tricuspid valve.

In the vast majority of patients with aortic stenosis, the obstruction is not severe enough to cause symptoms during infancy. Symptoms in children or adults are the result of progression to severe stenosis. Valve calcification may be an important factor. The symptoms consist of exertional dyspnea, angina, and syncope. Dyspnea is caused by elevated left atrial pressure that is due to reduced left ventricular compliance secondary to left ventricular pressure overload and hypertrophy. In the most severe cases, anginal-type pain may occur and is presumed to result from inadequate subendocardial blood flow. Exercise-induced light-headedness, or syncope, may be due to inadequate cardiac output with exertion or a ventricular tachyarrhythmia. Sudden death in children and young adults is usually confined to patients with severe obstruction; the mechanism is presumed to be ventricular fibrillation. Symptoms most often are related to the severity of obstruction. However, some patients with moderately severe or severe obstruction may appear to be asymptomatic because they have limited their physical activities.

Progression of aortic stenosis may occur at any age but is most commonly seen during childhood and adolescence, when the disparity between the aortic valve orifice and the growth of the patient is greatest. Progressive obstruction in older adults almost invariably is the result of aortic valve calcification.

The severity of aortic stenosis is classified according to the aortic valve gradient and the calculated valve area. The valve area is directly related to the cardiac output and inversely related to the square root of the mean aortic valve gradient. This is expressed by the Gorlin formula: aortic valve area (cm^2) = $F/44.3\sqrt{\text{aortic valve gradient}}$, where F (flow) (mL/s) = cardiac output (mL/min)/SEP (s/min). SEP (systolic ejection period) is derived by measuring aortic valve opening to closing per beat and multiplying by the heart rate. It is important to recognize that there are pitfalls in the determination of valve area that are most pronounced when cardiac output is low. In addition, the calculation will be underestimated in the presence of aortic regurgitation, since the actual flow per beat is greater than the flow calculated from the systemic cardiac output.

In children and adolescents with aortic stenosis and normal cardiac output, the peak-to-peak aortic gradient generally is used to assess the severity of aortic stenosis. Gradients $<$25 mm Hg are referred to as mild, those 25 to 50 mm Hg as moderate, those 50 to 75 mm Hg as moderately severe, and those $>$75 mm Hg as severe. In echocardiography, the mean predicted gradient may be more useful than the peak predicted gradient in that it may better correlate with the peak gradient measured at cardiac catheterization.

Physical Examination

The diagnosis of aortic stenosis can be made by physical examination, with particular emphasis on palpation of the chest, carotid pulse contour, and the location and quality of the murmur. When aortic stenosis is at least moderately severe, palpation usually reveals a left ventricular (LV) lift, laterally displaced apical impulse, and a systolic thrill at the base, predominantly along the right upper sternal border. A suprasternal thrill and a carotid thrill are commonly present in patients with congenital aortic stenosis, but this finding does not by itself imply severe obstruction.

Abnormalities of the carotid pulse include diminished volume, delayed upstroke, and a carotid shudder. Although these findings are common in older patients with significant aortic stenosis, similar degrees of obstruction in adolescents and young adults may be associated with a normal carotid contour. Auscultation reveals a normal first heart sound. The second heart sound may be unremarkable in patients with mild or moderate aortic stenosis but is usually abnormal in those with severe obstruction. Delayed closure of the aortic valve results in abnormal splitting of S_2 with little to no inspiratory widening between the aortic and pulmonary components. Paradoxical splitting may be noted with very severe disease. In young patients with aortic stenosis, the second heart sound may be unremarkable even with significant obstruction.

A systolic ejection click is frequently audible in patients with congenital aortic stenosis. The click is best heard at the cardiac apex and implies a mobile aortic valve and mild or moderate aortic stenosis. An S_4 is associated with LV hypertrophy (LVH) and a noncompliant left ventricle.

The systolic murmur of aortic stenosis is rough and ejection-type and is best heard at the right and left upper sternal border. The murmur radiates to the jugular notch and carotid arteries as well as to the left sternal border and apex. The murmur is usually grade III even with mild aortic stenosis but becomes louder and more late-peaking as the severity of aortic stenosis increases. However, this finding is not as consistent as it is with pulmonary stenosis.

A diastolic murmur of aortic insufficiency may be audible but is rarely hemodynamically significant unless the patient has had bacterial endocarditis. An occasional patient with a nonobstructed bicuspid aortic valve can present with isolated aortic insufficiency even without a history of bacterial endocarditis.

If severe aortic stenosis is not relieved, it eventually will result in LV failure and low cardiac output. At this stage, the systolic murmur becomes softer and more difficult to recognize as aortic stenosis. The diagnosis of severe aortic stenosis may be suspected clinically in the presence of diminished carotid pulses, LV failure, and LVH. The difficulties in establishing the diagnosis at a later stage have been largely overcome since the advent of echocardiography.

The murmur of aortic stenosis usually can be distinguished from other lesions on examination. The murmur of pulmonary stenosis is maximal at the left upper sternal border and is associated with a delayed or absent pulmonary closure sound. The murmur of subaortic stenosis is maximal at the left midsternal border and is not associated with a click. The systolic murmur of idiopathic hypertrophic subaortic stenosis (IHSS) also may be loudest along the left midsternal border, but characteristic carotid pulses and a prominent pansystolic murmur at the apex distinguish this condition from valvar aortic stenosis. Supravalvar aortic stenosis may be difficult to distinguish from valvar aortic stenosis. The diagnosis may be suspected from the absence of a click and the presence of differential blood pressures in the upper extremities. About one-half of these patients have Williams syndrome, which is characterized by the presence of "elfin facies," mental retardation, peripheral pulmonary stenoses, and other arterial stenoses such as coronary or renal.

Noninvasive Evaluation

The *chest x-ray* in aortic stenosis typically shows a normal-size heart with poststenotic dilation of the ascending aorta. *Electrocardiographic* (ECG) abnormalities are related to the severity of aortic stenosis. Moderate obstruction usually is associated with increased LV voltage and left atrial enlargement. Severe obstruction typically results in the development of an ST "strain" pattern. It should be recognized, however, that severe obstruction occasionally may be present despite a normal ECG.

Exercise testing may be useful in children and adolescents to assess the ECG response to exercise as well as the symptoms. Exercise-induced abnormalities indicative of significant aortic stenosis include an abnormal blood pressure response, >2-mm ST depression, and the development of ventricular arrhythmias. Exercise testing is contraindicated in patients with severe aortic stenosis and always must be used cautiously in any patient with left ventricular outflow obstruction.

Echocardiography has greatly simplified the diagnosis and management of patients with aortic stenosis by providing information regarding valve gradient and mobility, annulus size, anatomy of the left ventricular outflow tract (LVOT), and LVH. In adults, predicted mean valve gradient correlates best with the gradient measured at catheterization. Ventricular function must be assessed. Children and adolescents with aortic stenosis often display hyperdynamic LV function. Associated lesions such as subaortic stenosis, ventricular septal defect, and mitral valve abnormalities must be documented. Serial studies are useful in following changes in aortic peak and mean valve gradients over time and the degree of LVH.

Cardiac Catheterization

Before the development of echocardiography, cardiac catheterization frequently was performed in young patients in whom at least moderate aortic stenosis was suspected. In recent years, echocardiography has markedly reduced the need for diagnostic cardiac catheterization. Invasive studies are now performed most frequently in conjunction with balloon valvuloplasty in adolescents and young adults with moderate or severe obstruction.

Diagnostic cardiac catheterization still may be required when there is discordance between the clinical findings and the echocardiogram or when additional hemodynamic information is needed, especially when additional lesions are present. The procedure will answer specific questions regarding aortic–LV gradients and cardiac output, associated lesions such as an intracardiac shunt, mitral regurgitation, coarctation, and aortic annulus size. A jet of nonopacified blood across the stenotic valve is nicely demonstrated by aortic angiography (Fig. 6-2).

Coronary artery anomalies most often are not associated with congenital valvar aortic stenosis. However, patients with a bicuspid aortic valve frequently have a short left main coronary artery and a dominant circumflex artery. Coronary arteriography generally is reserved for patients >40 years of age unless premature coronary artery disease is suspected.

MANAGEMENT

The management of aortic stenosis depends on both the symptoms and the severity of aortic valve obstruction. Patients with mild aortic stenosis are asymptomatic and have gradients <25 mm Hg with normal cardiac output. The ECG is normal, and there is no echocardiographic evidence of LVH. These patients should be followed periodically, since increased valve rigidity may lead to increased obstruction over time. Progressive stenosis is even more likely in patients with gradients between 25 and 50 mm Hg. Prophylaxis against endocarditis is essential.

An aortic gradient >50 mm Hg is at least moderate in severity. At this level, only a minority of patients report symptoms of exertional dyspnea or chest pain. However, once

FIGURE 6-2

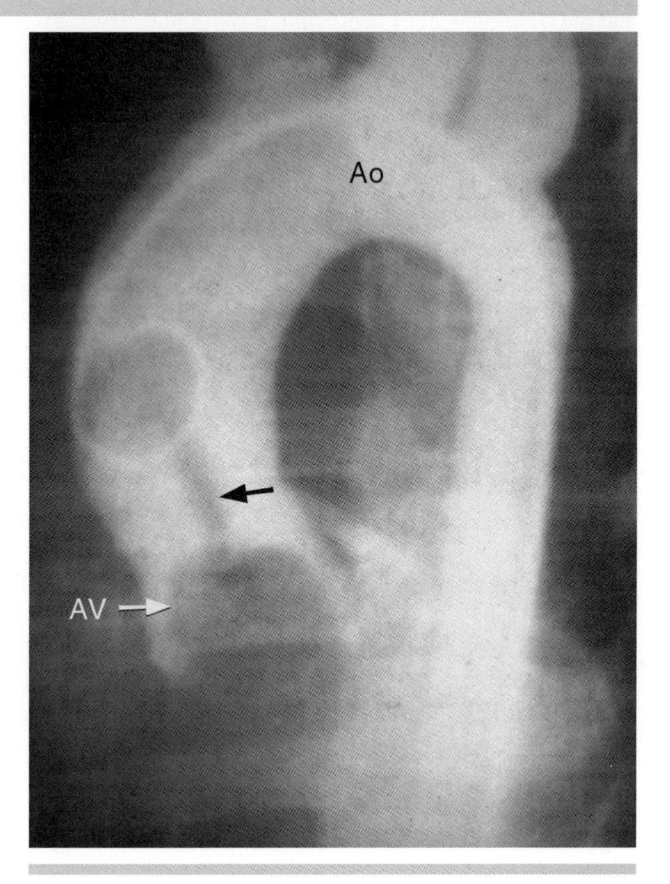

Aortogram in a patient with valvar aortic stenosis. Note the domed aortic valve. A jet of unopacified blood enters the ascending aorta (black arrow). Ao, aorta; AV, aortic valve.

this degree of obstruction is reached, a small decrease in the aortic valve orifice will result in a large and sometimes rapid increase in the aortic valve gradient and LV systolic pressure. This occurs because the valve area is directly related to the cardiac output and inversely proportional to the square root of the pressure gradient. The possibility of rapid progression underscores the need for close follow-up of patients with moderate aortic stenosis. These patients should be advised against participating in competitive sports.

Balloon Valvuloplasty

Once symptoms develop, relief of aortic valve obstruction is imperative. In children and adolescents, balloon valvuloplasty is considered the procedure of choice and has replaced surgical valvotomy over the last 10 to 15 years. Balloon valvuloplasty for congenital aortic stenosis was first reported in 1984. Since that time, the number of young patients referred for surgical valvotomy has declined steadily. Although a direct comparison between the two procedures is not feasible, there is general agreement that both forms of valvuloplasty provide similar results in terms of relief of valve obstruction and postprocedural aortic insufficiency. Balloon valvuloplasty has been a safe procedure when performed at experienced centers.

The precise gradient for which balloon valvuloplasty should be performed has not been firmly established. Before balloon valvuloplasty was available, surgical valvotomy was performed in patients with gradients >75 mm Hg. In symptomatic patients and those with evidence of severe LVH, surgical valvotomy was undertaken for gradients as low as 40 to 50 mm Hg. Today, balloon valvuloplasty generally is performed somewhat earlier than surgical valvotomy in asymptomatic patients with a peak-to-peak gradient of at least 50 mm Hg but is not carried out if significant aortic insufficiency is already present. Balloon aortic valvuloplasty usually is not feasible in adults with heavily calcified valves.

Successful balloon valvuloplasty typically results in a 60 to 70% reduction in peak-to-peak systolic gradient across the aortic valve with a 25 to 30% incidence of significant aortic regurgitation. The aortic regurgitation is generally mild, but it may be more severe in some patients, producing an additional volume load on a ventricle with preexisting LVH. In addition, eventual recurrence of stenosis after balloon valvuloplasty is common, and post-procedural patients must continue to be followed closely. Cardiac catheterization studies at one year have shown average residual peak gradients between 35 and 45 mm Hg.

Surgical Repair

Valvotomy

If a balloon valvuloplasty is not feasible or is unsuccessful, aortic valve surgery usually is advised. A surgical valvotomy is carried out, during which the surgeon can incise the valve commissures under direct vision. Aortic valve replacement is usually unnecessary at the first operation for congenital aortic stenosis unless the valve is calcified or hemodynamically significant aortic regurgitation is already present or was created during previous surgery or balloon valvuloplasty.

The surgical benefit of aortic valvotomy is well established. In the Natural History Study, 66% of 130 patients who underwent cardiac catheterization 6.5 years after surgical valvotomy had a residual gradient <50 mm Hg and only 6% had severe regurgitation. In another study, 44% of the patients required reoperation within 22 years of aortic valvotomy. Valve replacement was required in virtually all these patients, nearly half for aortic regurgitation. Thus, it should be emphasized that valvotomy is a palliative procedure; residual obstruction or regurgitation and/or progressive valve calcification eventually will lead to aortic valve replacement.

Follow-Up After Valvuloplasty or Surgical Valvotomy

Many young adults with congenital aortic stenosis have had aortic valvuloplasty during childhood. It is often difficult to assess the degree of residual aortic valve disease after valvuloplasty by examination alone. Since most patients continue to have an aortic valve gradient of 25 to 45 mm Hg, a prominent systolic murmur is frequently present as well as varying degrees of aortic insufficiency. A right upper sternal border thrill may no longer be present after successful valvuloplasty; however, a suprasternal thrill and a carotid shudder typically remain. The systolic murmur is usually shorter and less harsh, but if aortic insufficiency is superimposed, the additional volume across the LV outflow tract will accentuate the murmur of stenosis. The murmur of aortic insufficiency is usually grade I to II and short to moderate in duration. A more pronounced murmur with a wide pulse pressure is indicative of hemodynamically significant aortic insufficiency.

Although Doppler echocardiography is helpful in assessing the results of an aortic valvuloplasty, the peak gradients may overestimate the gradient that would be measured during cardiac catheterization. Persistence of LVH may be indicative of significant residual obstruction and/or insufficiency. If significant residual obstruction is suspected, cardiac catheterization may be necessary.

A successful aortic valvuloplasty should prevent symptoms related to aortic stenosis. The development of symptoms should initiate prompt reevaluation for residual or recurrent obstruction and consideration of aortic valve replacement.

Aortic Valve Replacement

The timing of aortic valve replacement in young patients can be challenging. In contrast to calcific aortic stenosis in adults, in whom valve replacement typically is deferred until the onset of symptoms, the recommendations for children and adolescents with congenital aortic stenosis in whom balloon or surgical valvuloplasty is no longer feasible historically have been based on the severity of obstruction even in the absence of symptoms. Several reasons have been advanced to justify the difference in management. First, there is the possibility that children with severe aortic stenosis may experience sudden death as the first clinical manifestation of this lesion, although this is extremely rare in asymptomatic patients. Second, there is concern that chronic LVH will have a deleterious effect on long-term survival because of eventual heart failure and/or ventricular arrhythmias. Finally, in practical terms, the difficulty in restricting physical activities in young patients makes early relief of obstruction more important.

In the past, surgery often was deferred because the options for valve replacement in children and adolescents were limited to a mechanical valve requiring chronic anticoagulation or a homograft or tissue valve that had limited longevity before requiring a reoperation. Since the porcine aortic valve has been associated with rapid calcification in young patients and at best may produce 10 years of benefit, it is rarely used for adolescents or young adults. The newer Carpentier-Edwards bovine pericardial valve may last several years longer than the porcine valve in adults, but the longevity of this valve in children and adolescents has not been determined. Aortic valve replacement in a woman who wishes to become pregnant creates unique difficulties. Since warfarin may produce fetal abnormalities when used during the first trimester, there is little enthusiasm for recommending a mechanical valve in these patients.

In view of the difficulties associated with both the mechanical valve and the biological valves, the Ross operation (pulmonary autograft) has been advocated for young patients who require aortic valve replacement (Fig. 6-3). In the Ross procedure, the patient's native pulmonary root is removed and reimplanted into the aortic position, the coronary arteries are anastomosed into the neoaortic root, and a pulmonary homograft is used to

FIGURE 6-3

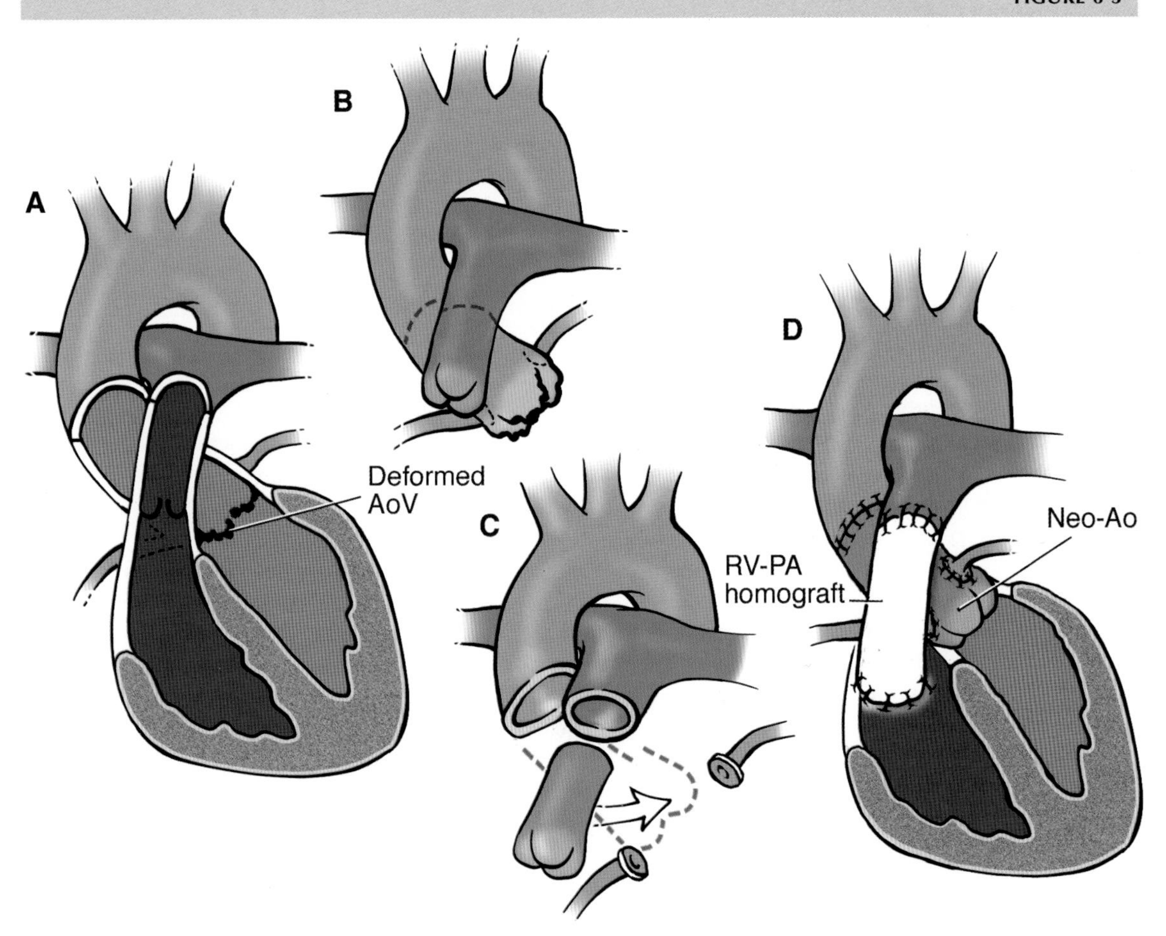

The Ross operation. In order to avoid prosthetic valve replacement of a deformed aortic valve, a pulmonary autograft is used to replace the aortic valve by: *A.* removing the proximal pulmonary artery and pulmonary valve and using this segment as a neoaortic valve and root. *B.* The pulmonary and aortic roots are incised (red dashed lines). *C.* The coronary arteries are detached from the aortic root and the aortic valve is removed. *D.* The pulmonary root is placed in the aortic position and the coronary arteries are attached. AoV, aortic valve; Neo-Ao, neoaortic valve; PA, pulmonary artery; RV, right ventricle.

replace the pulmonary valve. The operation avoids the need for anticoagulation, and there appears to be a very low incidence of native pulmonary valve deterioration in the aortic position. Late reoperation for degeneration of the homograft in the pulmonary position may be required, but these conduits may last longer in the presence of a normal right ventricle. Whereas the pulmonary autograft operation does offer a young patient the potential for excellent long-term survival without the risks of anticoagulation and possibly another aortic valve replacement, this operation is technically demanding, and surgical expertise is critically important to the success of the procedure. The surgical issues include potential damage to the septal artery during the harvesting of the pulmonary autograft and proper placement of the pulmonary autograft to avoid aortic regurgitation. The Ross procedure has become the preferred operation in many centers when aortic valve replacement is required in children and young adults. Since anticoagulation is not necessary after surgery, this procedure is especially desirable for women who plan to become pregnant. However, the complexity of the operation is apt to limit its general use in older patients.

LONG-TERM FOLLOW-UP OF ADULTS AFTER AORTIC VALVE REPLACEMENT

Aortic valve replacement for aortic stenosis results in regression of LVH and improvement in LV systolic function in patients with preoperative LV dysfunction. Symptoms of dyspnea, chest pain, and syncope are eliminated. Persistent symptoms should prompt a search for other causes, such as arrhythmia and associated intracardiac lesions.

A grade II systolic ejection murmur is typically present along the left sternal border after aortic valve replacement. A louder murmur should prompt an echocardiogram to determine the status of the LVOT. The systolic ejection murmur along the left sternal border also may represent turbulence across the right ventricular outflow tract in Ross patients. In older patients, the improvement in carotid pulse is readily appreciated. A murmur of significant aortic insufficiency is unusual after mechanical, tissue valve, or pulmonary autograft insertion and generally indicates the presence of a paravalvar leak.

Late development of aortic regurgitation in a patient with a porcine, pericardial, or homograft valve generally heralds the onset of valve failure. Calcification of a donor valve and/or aortic root is commonly seen.

SUMMARY

Valvar aortic stenosis is a common congenital heart defect with varying severity. The disease may present in the neonatal period as severe left ventricular outflow tract obstruction, which, if untreated, leads to mortality within days or weeks. At the other extreme, a patient with a bicuspid aortic valve with mild turbulence and a trivial aortic–left ventricular gradient may live a normal life, with some needing relief of late calcific aortic stenosis. Moderate aortic stenosis recognized in childhood must be followed closely, especially during puberty, when body growth is rapid, and as more cardiac output is required, moderate obstruction becomes severe.

Cardiologists should follow young adults carefully, as the degree of severity of obstruction may increase with time. An asymptomatic patient with a normal ECG and no LVH and with only a mild predicted gradient on echocardiography should be followed yearly. Patients with moderate gradients and mild LVH need even closer follow-up, and if the gradient reaches the range of 50 mm or more, balloon valvuloplasty should be considered in patients with noncalcified valves. Otherwise, surgery is necessary to relieve severe calcific aortic stenosis.

Physical examination in the usual patient with aortic stenosis reveals a suprasternal notch thrill; a right upper sternal border systolic thrill suggests severe disease, whereas the presence of a suprasternal notch thrill does not necessarily imply severe obstruction. A loud, rough systolic ejection murmur is heard best at the right base and radiates well to the carotid arteries and left sternal border. Often, an apical systolic ejection click is noted. Some patients have a high-pitched protodiastolic murmur of aortic insufficiency that is heard best along the left midsternal border. It is important to determine in patients with both stenosis and insufficiency which is the more dominant defect. This has important implications for the type and timing of intervention. Patients with significant associated aortic insufficiency are not candidates for balloon valvuloplasty and often must be evaluated on the basis of the severity of the aortic insufficiency, becoming eventual candidates for a Ross operation or prosthetic valve replacement. The echocardiogram is extremely helpful in determining the status of the aortic valve in terms of the predicted gradient, evaluation of the degree of aortic insufficiency, the presence of LVH, and evaluation of ventricular function.

Valvar aortic stenosis is differentiated from subvalvar disease by the position of the murmur (basilar rather than left midsternal border), the absence of a systolic ejection click, and, more definitively, the evaluation of the LVOT by echocardiographic examination.

Post–aortic valvuloplasty or postsurgical patients also must be followed closely, since restenosis is not uncommon with calcification. In general, a postoperative patient should

Algorithm 6–1
Valvar Aortic Stenosis—Unoperated

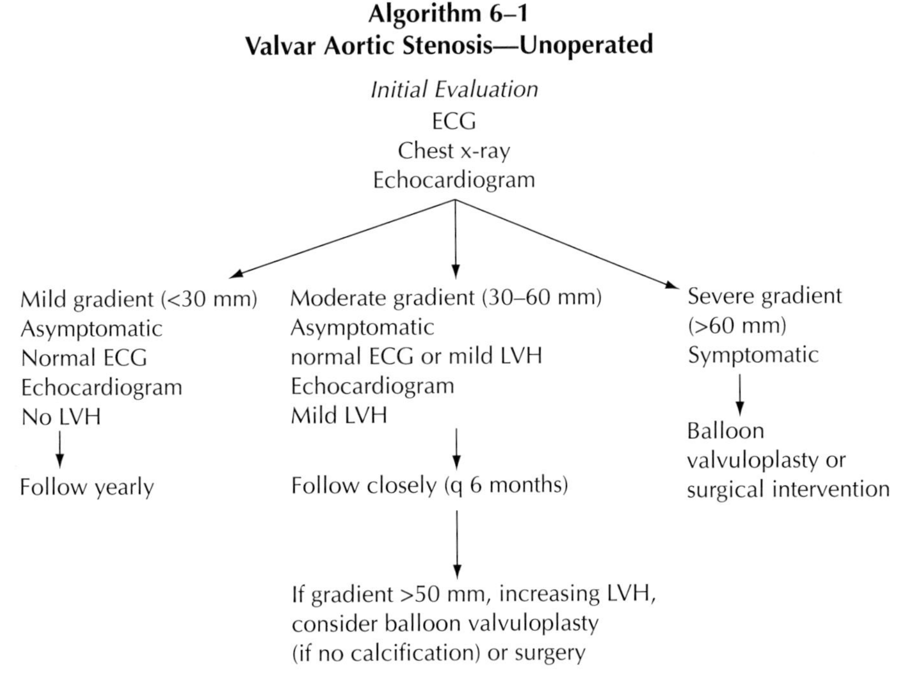

KEY: ECG, electrocardiogram; LVH, left ventricular hypertrophy.

Algorithm 6–2
Valvar Aortic Stenosis
"Operated" (Catheter or Surgical Valvuloplasty)

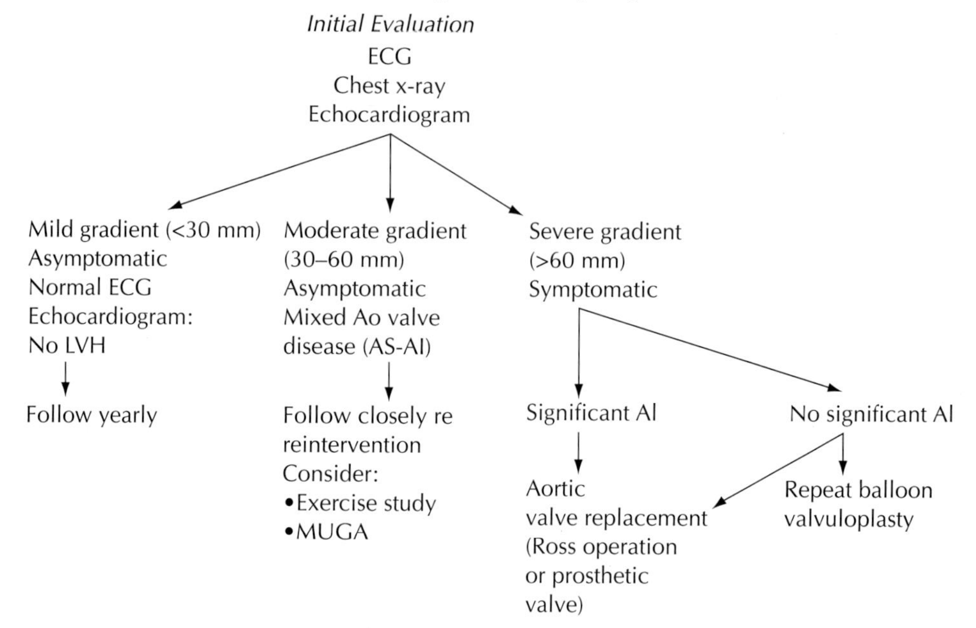

KEY: AI, aortic insufficiency; Ao, aortal; AS, aortic stenosis; ECG, electrocardiogram; LVH, left ventricular hypertrophy; MUGA, multiple-gated acquisition.

be followed in a manner similar to that for patients who have not had an intervention. Most often, after a previous intervention, the Ross operation or a prosthetic valve will be required.

II. NONVALVAR LEFT VENTRICULAR OUTFLOW TRACT OBSTRUCTION

Nonvalvar LV outflow includes several forms of subvalvar and supravalvar obstruction. Discrete membranous subvalvar aortic stenosis (DSVAS) occurs as a result of an obstructive fibromuscular ridge that impinges on the LV outflow tract (LVOT), causing varying degrees of obstruction. In addition, secondary LVH may add a muscular component to the stenosis. Hypertrophic cardiomyopathy (HCM) may result in LVOT obstruction (LVOTO) because of asymmetric hypertrophy of the ventricular septum, usually accompanied by systolic anterior motion of the mitral valve. The IHSS variant of HCM is a well known entity in adult cardiology in which there is often a genetic basis for this condition;

however, it is not considered to be among the classic forms of "congenital heart disease." Supravalvar stenosis may include a discrete region of obstruction just distal to the aortic valve and/or generalized hypoplasia of the ascending aorta. Supravalvar aortic stenosis may be associated with Williams syndrome, a diagnosis that includes a number of associated morphologic abnormalities. These patients often have associated multiple peripheral pulmonary stenoses. In adulthood, stenosis of other systemic arteries may be identified, including coronary, renal, and/or mesenteric vessels.

DISCRETE SUBVALVAR AORTIC STENOSIS

DSVAS is a condition that is noted in early childhood and that often progresses to severe LV outflow obstruction, not uncommonly within a few years of recognition. The disease is characterized by a fibrous ridge that develops just below the aortic valve. There appears to be a congenital basis for the condition, although it always appears to be an "acquired" lesion that is virtually never recognized in the neonatal period or in early infancy. A disparate angle between the muscular septum and the conal septum may be the predisposing factor.

DSVAS is recognized clinically by a harsh left midsternal border systolic murmur that is similar to the murmur heard with a ventricular septal defect. The bruit often is loudest at the left middle and lower sternal border, in contrast to valvar aortic stenosis, which is more prominent at the base. In addition, subvalvar aortic stenosis (SVAS) is not associated with a systolic ejection click. The diagnosis is confirmed by echocardiography, which usually reveals an intrusion into the LVOT, just below the aortic valve. Doppler examination shows turbulence originating below the aortic valve. This condition may be associated with some distortion of the aortic valve itself, and mild aortic regurgitation often is seen. DSVAS can also be associated with other defects, including ventricular septal defect, coarctation of the aorta, interrupted aortic arch, complex single-ventricle lesions, atrioventricular (AV) canal defect, and, rarely, tetralogy of Fallot. DSVAS occurs in unoperated patients but also may develop and progress after surgical correction of an associated lesion. The development of SVAS after repair of AV canal lesions is one of the most important considerations. This occurs in approximately 10% of patients. The anatomy of the LVOT may predispose these patients to subaortic obstruction months or years after successful repair of the original AV canal defect.

Clinical Features

The early clinical course of patients with DSVAS usually relates to an associated lesion, although the defect also may evolve as an isolated abnormality. In many patients with SVAS, echocardiography or cardiac catheterization early in life failed to reveal LVOTO. However, in later years, the typical obstructive ridge became prominent. Once significant stenosis occurs in a child, there may be rapid progression to severe obstruction within a year or two, requiring urgent surgical relief. However, many patients with mild-to-moderate stenosis remain stable for many years and reach adulthood without requiring surgery.

The diagnosis of isolated DSVAS rarely is made on the basis of symptomatology. Usually, a prominent murmur leads to echocardiographic investigation, and the diagnosis is made before the appearance of clinical signs or symptoms. This most often occurs in the first decade of life, but there are a number of patients, especially those with loud murmurs secondary to an associated lesion such as ventricular septal defect, in whom the diagnosis is not made until late childhood or even adulthood. A murmur is noted, and the ECG and echocardiogram reveal the obstruction along with various degrees of left ventricular hypertrophy, depending on the severity of the subaortic stenosis. Only rarely will a patient present with exertional dyspnea and signs of LV failure. Although mild aortic insufficiency is noted commonly, this is usually not a major clinical finding. The clinical picture of the associated lesions often is dominant in early life, and in these patients discrete subaortic stenosis may not become an issue until after surgical repair of the original congenital heart defect.

Physical Examination

There are both similarities and differences in the physical examination of a patient with discrete subvalvar obstruction and one with valvar aortic stenosis. In severe cases, cardiac examination of a patient with DSVAS includes an LV lift and an apical impulse that is displaced inferiorly and laterally. A systolic thrill may be present along the left middle and upper sternal border as opposed to the base in valvar aortic stenosis. In addition, turbulence in the suprasternal notch and over the carotid arteries is less prominent in patients with DSVAS than in those with valvar aortic stenosis. The carotid contour is most often normal. The second heart sound is similar to that noted in valvar aortic stenosis; it often is single in patients with severe obstruction but may be normal in milder cases. A striking difference in the cardiac examination of a patient with subvalvar stenosis compared with valvar stenosis is the absence of a systolic ejection click. The presence of an S_4 with severe obstruction is similar for the two entities.

The systolic murmur of subaortic stenosis is ejection-type and is heard best along the left midsternal border rather than along the base. The murmur is harsh, often without the extremely rough quality noted with valvar aortic stenosis. The murmur resembles the murmur of a ventricular septal defect more closely than that of valvar aortic stenosis, and in some cases both are present. A high-pitched protodiastolic murmur of aortic insufficiency may be audible but rarely represents severe incompetence.

The classic murmur of discrete subaortic stenosis is heard in a similar area to that of obstructive HCM, but in the latter case, there are characteristic carotid pulse abnormalities and usually a pansystolic murmur at the apex, indicating the presence of coexisting mitral insufficiency. In the modern era, noninvasive assessment can readily distinguish the level of LVOTO.

Noninvasive Evaluation

The *chest x-ray* usually shows a normal cardiac silhouette. Poststenotic dilatation of the ascending aorta is absent. As with valvar aortic stenosis, *ECG abnormalities* are related to the severity of obstruction, although on occasion, severe stenosis may be present without ECG changes. The rationale for exercise studies is similar to that for valvar aortic stenosis.

FIGURE 6-4

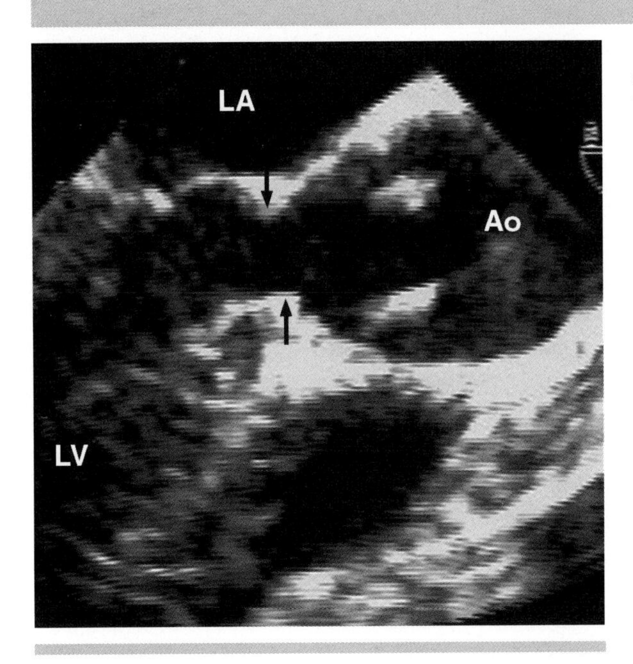

Parasternal long-axis view in a patient with subaortic stenosis. The arrows point to the narrowing in the subaortic region. Ao, aorta; LA, left atrium; LV, left ventricle.

Echocardiographic evaluation is the most important imaging modality for patients with DSVAS and is far more reliable than angiography. The echocardiogram displays a fibrous ridge of tissue intruding into the LVOT just below the aortic valve (Fig. 6-4). The study clearly differentiates this condition from other forms of LVOTO, including supravalvar aortic stenosis, valvular obstruction, and certain forms of accessory mitral valve tissue obstruction. The presence and degree of LVH also are determined. Some patients will have severe septal hypertrophy similar to a patient with IHSS, and in the pre-echo era, misdiagnosis was common. Obstructive HCM usually is associated with more extensive ventricular muscular hypertrophy as well as systolic anterior motion (SAM) of the mitral valve and mitral sufficiency. Doppler-predicted gradients are useful, although peak gradients often overestimate the actual resting gradient. Associated lesions also are evaluated by ultrasound study.

Cardiac Catheterization

As with valvar aortic stenosis, cardiac catheterization is often unnecessary for patients with discrete subvalvar stenosis. The most important aspects of a catheterization procedure are the hemodynamic assessment and the identification of associated defects. True gradients can be measured, and this is especially important when clinical and noninvasive assessment is indeterminate. Angiography may not be useful in delineating DSVAS, since a static view during the contrast injection may result in an angulation that obscures the thin ridge of tissue just below the aortic valve. The abnormality occasionally can be demonstrated (Fig. 6-5), but echocardiographic examination is far more reliable. Angiography also may show other associated abnormalities. Interventional catheterization procedures such as balloon valvuloplasty have not been effective for the management of DSVAS.

FIGURE 6-5

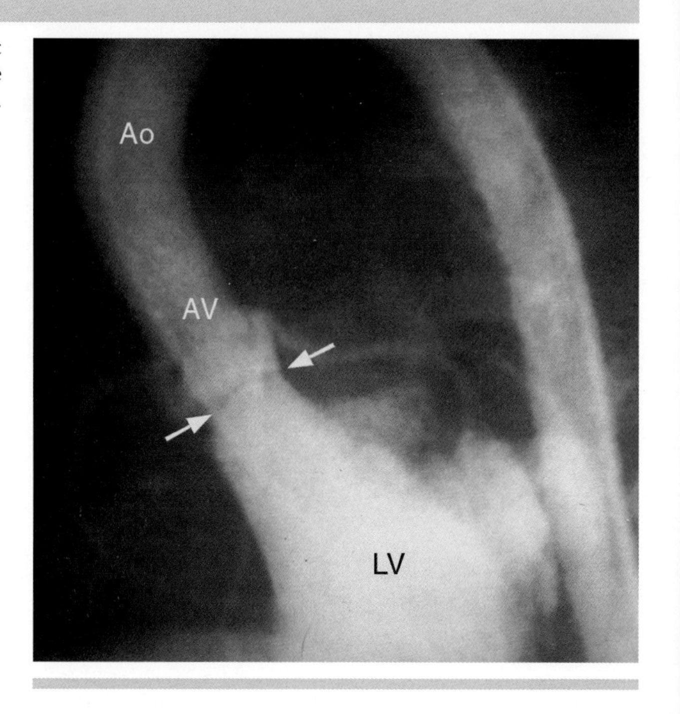

Left ventricular angiogram in a patient with subaortic stenosis. The arrows point to the lucency below the aortic valve, representing the subaortic membrane. AV = aortic valve, Ao = aorta, LV = left ventricle.

Management

The natural history of subaortic stenosis is variable. Rapid progression of subaortic stenosis documented during infancy leads to early surgical intervention. However, controversy exists about the precise indications for surgery in patients who have mild obstruction with low Doppler-predicted gradients across the LVOT. Although some centers advocate surgical intervention for pediatric patients when an anatomic defect is noted, regardless of the gradient, most agree that a gradient of 30 mm or more is required as an indication for surgery. Lesser gradients may or may not progress, and demonstration of the progression of obstruction is required by many centers before surgical intervention is planned. There are asymptomatic patients with trivial gradients and no evidence of significant LVH who remain stable for many decades. Thus, severity of obstruction is the main criterion for surgery. Another controversial issue is whether mild DSVAS will lead to aortic insufficiency (AI) by jet damage to the valve. Proponents of this theory consider milder degrees of obstruction an indication for early repair. However, in some cases greater degrees of AI have been seen after surgical relief of DSVAS than was present before the operation. Thus, "prevention" of AI is not considered by many centers to be a specific indication for surgery in the presence of insignificant obstruction with a minimal gradient.

Surgical Repair

The surgical approach to DSVAS has evolved over the years in an attempt to decrease the recurrence rate for this lesion, previously reported to be as high as 30 to 50%. In some cases, it is incomplete relief of obstruction at the time of the initial operation that results in progressive subaortic stenosis. In the presence of a ringlike obstruction below the aortic valve, removal of this tissue along the septal surface presents a risk for complete heart block. Furthermore, dissection in the region of the continuity between the aortic cusp and the mitral valve can cause mitral valve damage. Thus, to avoid these complications, early attempts at complete elimination of DSVAS often were incomplete. The result was either incomplete relief or regrowth of fibromuscular tissue. A wider resection accompanied by a myotomy or myomectomy of the secondarily hypertrophied ventricular septum has resulted in some improvement in outcome, but recurrences still happen. Another surgical technique that is used to treat DSVAS is a circumferential blunt dissection of the fibromuscular ring, in which the entire circle of fibromuscular tissue is removed. The removal of the fixed obstruction may be accompanied by myotomy or myomectomy in advanced patients who have marked secondary septal muscular hypertrophy. Although this has been an effective approach to SVAS with less likelihood of recurrence, regrowth of fibromuscular tissue nevertheless may occur, and second or even third interventions have been required.

Discrete subvalvar aortic stenosis may be associated with a narrow tunnel-like LV outflow (Fig. 6-6). In such cases, complete relief of obstruction is not possible, and a number of patients are encountered who have had multiple surgical procedures on the LVOT but still have significant gradients. Aortic valve replacement, most often by a Ross-Konno pulmonary autograft procedure, may well be necessary in such patients to totally elimi-

FIGURE 6-6

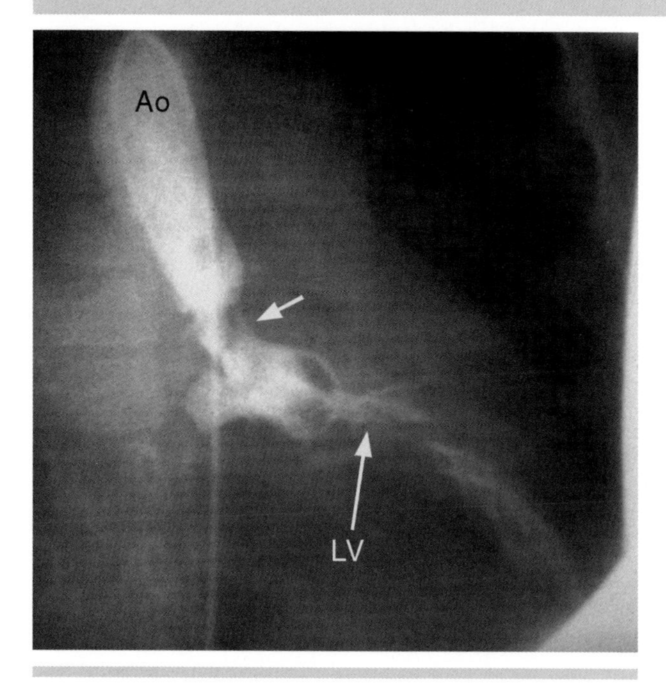

Left ventriculogram in a patient with tunnel outflow obstruction of the left ventricle. Note the severe narrowing of the subaortic region (arrow) and the markedly hypertrophied left ventricle with a small ventricular chamber. LV = left ventricle, Ao = aorta.

nate LV outflow obstruction. This involves the Ross operation in conjunction with enlargement of the LV outlet at the upper portion of the ventricular septum. In the past, apical-descending aortic conduits were utilized in extreme cases, and some adult patients may still be encountered who have had this operation (Fig. 6-7*A* and *B*).

Long-Term Follow-Up

Patients with subaortic stenosis require careful follow-up as adults. Even if a corrective operation has been carried out, the possibility of recurrent obstruction exists and patients should be reevaluated periodically for this possibility. The presence of a new systolic murmur or a soft murmur that has become more intense is an indication for echocardiographic examination to assess the LVOT. The state of the aortic valve also must be monitored, and if aortic regurgitation is progressive, decisions regarding reoperation may have to be made on the basis of the aortic valve rather than the subaortic obstructive disease. However, this situation is not encountered frequently in the adult population; although mild AI is often present, it tends to remain stable for many years.

SUPRAVALVAR AORTIC STENOSIS

Supravalvar aortic stenosis is a localized hourglass deformity immediately above the aortic sinuses that is demonstrated by echocardiography and/or angiography (Figs. 6-8 and 6-9). Less commonly, there is a more diffuse narrowing of the ascending aorta. Supravalvar aortic stenosis is encountered only rarely in adults and, when seen, may be one of the components of Williams syndrome, which also includes a classical "elfin face," mild mental retardation with usually an outgoing "cocktail party" personality, dental abnormalities, peripheral pulmonary stenosis (Fig. 5-5), and late development of other arterial stenoses. A chromosomal marker is present. Williams syndrome is associated with idiopathic infantile hypercalcemia. Within the first months of life, the serum calcium, which is elevated at birth, becomes normal and the major issue becomes the cardiovascular status and the accompanying anomalies. Associated peripheral pulmonary stenosis also is found in non-Williams patients, but the other syndromic features are not present.

Patients with supravalvar aortic stenosis may be classified as (1) sporadic, nonfamilial with normal facies and intelligence, (2) autosomal dominant with normal facies and normal intelligence, and (3) classic Williams syndrome. It is of interest that the non-Williams form of supravalvular aortic stenosis is associated with a positive family history in over one-half of the cases, whereas Williams syndrome usually appears sporadically. However, recently, parent-to-child transmission has been reported.

Among patients with Williams syndrome, the classic noncardiac features are present. Cardiac examination reveals a LV impulse; the prominence depends on the severity of obstruction and the resultant LVH. A harsh basilar systolic ejection murmur is present that radiates to the neck, accompanied by a suprasternal thrill. A diastolic murmur is not expected. Pulses are easily palpable but may vary in intensity in the upper extremities, with left arm pulses being more prominent. Characteristically, there are significant differences in blood pressure between the left and right arms as a result of an asymmetric jet of blood past the innominate artery, creating uneven distribution of flow (Bernoulli effect). The chest x-ray is often normal. The echocardiogram is usually definitive in outlining the

FIGURE 6-7*A*

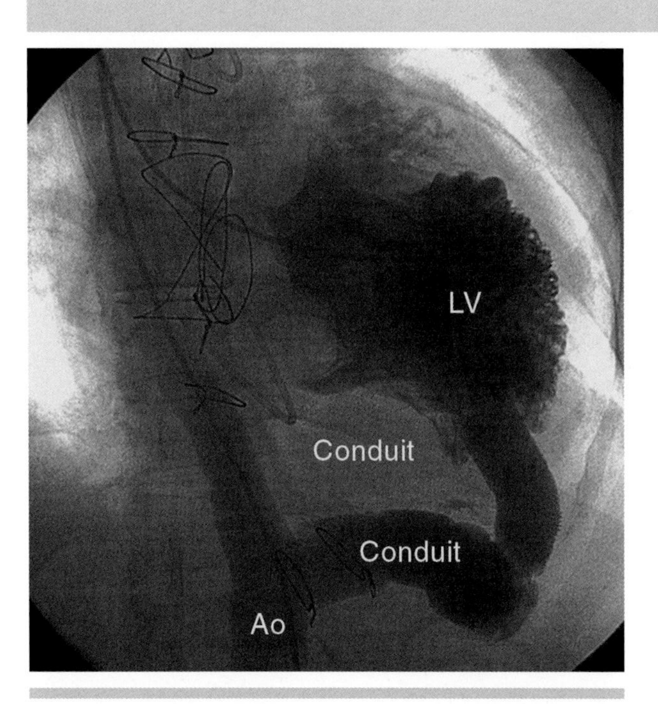

An RAO left ventriculogram in a patient with severe subaortic stenosis treated with an apical conduit. The catheter is positioned retrograde across the aortic valve into the left ventricle. A left ventriculogram shows filling of the left ventricle, apical conduit, and the descending aorta. There is no antegrade flow through the aortic valve because of severe subaortic obstruction. LV, left ventricle; Ao, aorta.

FIGURE 6-7*B*

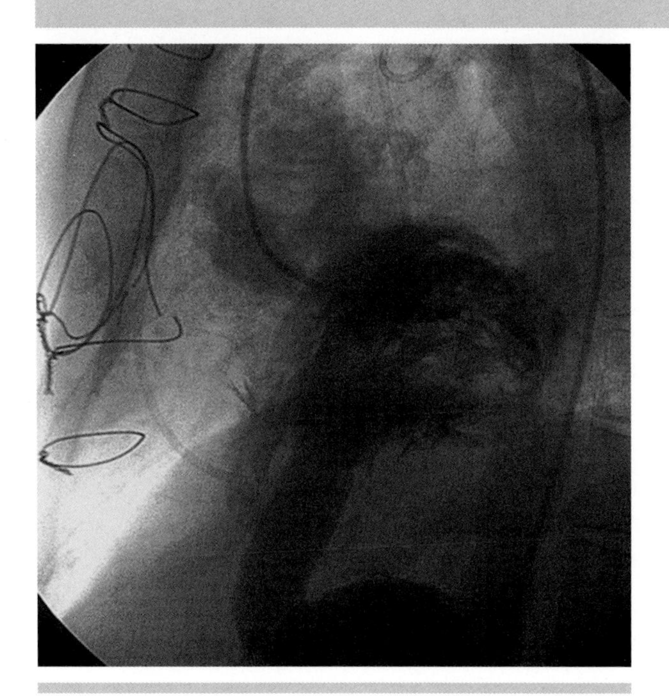

A lateral left ventriculogram from the patient in Figure 6-7*A*, which shows severe subaortic stenosis and filling of an apical conduit. The ascending aorta does not opacify.

FIGURE 6-8

Parasternal long-axis view showing an hour-glass-like narrowing just above the aortic sinuses typical of supravalvar aortic stenosis. LA, left atrium; LV, left ventricle; Ao, aorta.

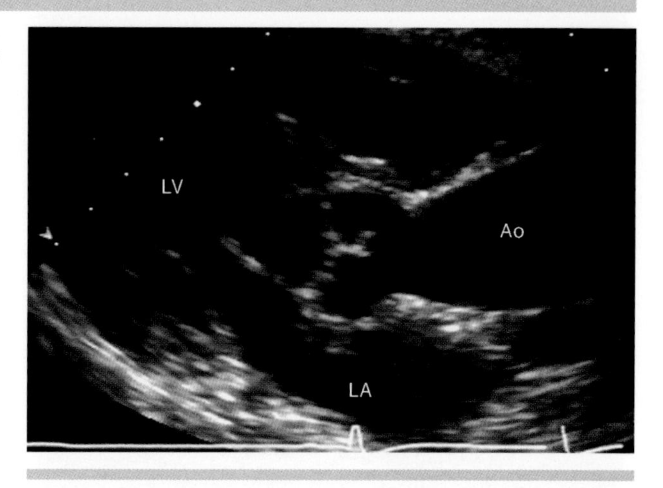

FIGURE 6-9

Left ventricular angiogram in a patient with supravalvar aortic stenosis. A shelflike obstruction (arrow) is noted above the dilated aortic sinuses. Mitral valve insufficiency is also demonstrated. Ao = aorta, AV = aortic valve, LV = left ventricle, LA = left atrium.

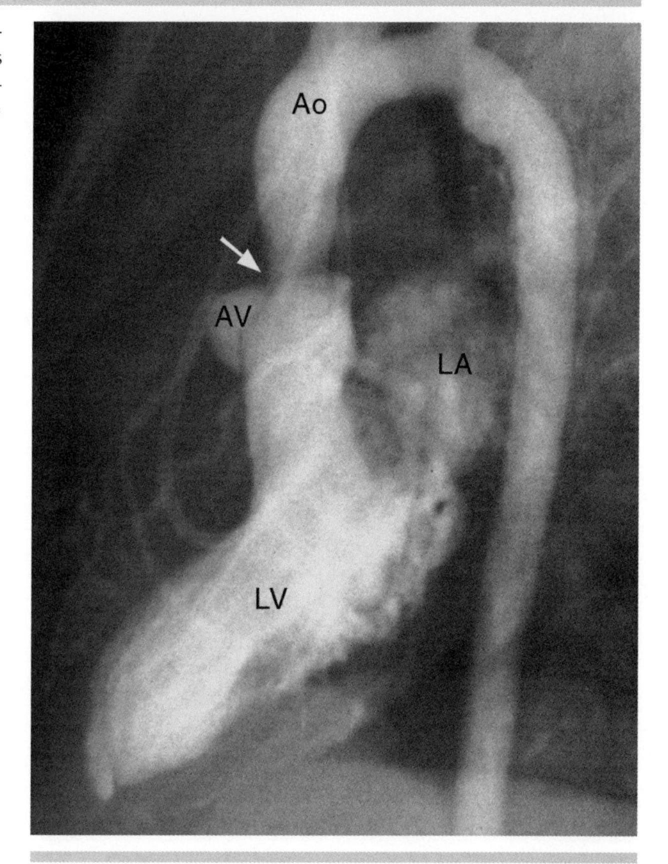

specific anatomy of the supravalvar stenosis and the severity of obstruction, although this region of the aorta may be difficult to image in larger adults.

Many patients with supravalvar stenosis have only mild obstruction that does not progress in severity with time. Those with severe stenosis (gradient >50) should undergo surgical repair. The procedure may be difficult since the operation may require reconstruction of the supravalvar area contiguous with the aortic sinuses, and injury to valve cusps must be avoided. Some patients have a long segment of narrowing of the ascending aorta. Relief of obstruction of the affected supravalvar region without injury to the valve is the surgical goal. In experienced hands, these patients can be repaired with a low incidence of recurrence. However, distortion of the aortic valve can result in AI in some patients.

Patients with supravalvar aortic stenosis should be followed for the possibility of progressive obstruction in the supravalvar area and with the knowledge that arterial stenoses in other arteries may appear. Renal artery stenosis has been described; unexplained hypertension should prompt an evaluation for this entity. In addition, coronary artery narrowing may become evident in adulthood among patients with supravalvar aortic stenosis.

SUMMARY

Nonvalvar LVOTO may occur below or above the aortic valve. These entities include discrete subvalvar aortic stenosis, hypertrophic cardiomyopathy with LVOTO, and supravalvar aortic stenosis.

Discrete subvalvar aortic stenosis is characterized by an obstructive fibrous ridge immediately below the aortic valve. This entity rarely is identified in early infancy but is often a progressive lesion later in childhood. When obstruction is severe, marked LV hypertension leads to LVH, and the ultimate complications are similar to those of valvar aortic stenosis. Mild AI often occurs in conjunction with this entity, probably as a result of distortion of the aortic valve from a jet lesion. DVAS often is associated with other defects, including ventricular septal defect, AV canal, coarctation of the aorta, and other, less common congenital heart defects. Obstruction often evolves years after repair of one of the predisposing defects. Many patients will have had one or more surgical interventions for DSVAS during childhood or adolescence. However, because of the variation in the progression of obstruction and a significant restenosis rate after surgery, this entity is encountered by adult cardiologists with some frequency.

Physical examination varies with the severity of the obstruction; a harsh left middle and lower sternal border systolic ejection murmur radiating to the base is audible in any patient with a significant gradient. The findings differ from those of valvar aortic stenosis because of the absence of a systolic ejection click and the prominence of the murmur along the left midsternal border rather than the base. The murmur of mild AI occasionally may be heard. The ECG can show LVH, and in cases of severe long-standing obstruction, a left ventricular strain pattern may be noted.

The echocardiogram is diagnostic. A ringlike intrusion of tissue is noted just below the aortic valve, sometimes with secondary hypertrophy of the ventricular septum. In some patients, this secondary feature is exaggerated so that if the obstructed ridge is not noted, a false diagnosis of hypertrophic cardiomyopathy with obstruction (IHSS) may be made. Cardiac catheterization is usually not necessary to make the diagnosis of DSVAS.

Surgery is indicated for significant LVOTO, and relief of obstruction may be required in the first years of life. Some children remain stable for many years but nevertheless require resection by late childhood. Occasionally, minimal ridges with minimal gradients, not associated with other congenital defects, with no evidence of LVH may be followed into adolescence and adulthood. Some cardiologists believe that early surgery with minimal LV–aortic gradients may be justified to prevent progressive AI. However, the evidence for this is lacking.

A number of surgical options for resection of DSVAS have been utilized; recurrence rates are significant. Many centers now carry out circumferential blunt dissection of the fibrous ring, with myotomy and/or myectomy in the most severe cases. The recurrence rate ranges from 10 to 30% in these patients, and periodic evaluation by physical examinations and echocardiograms is required to recognize possible reobstruction in a timely manner.

The relationship of DSVAS to AI is variable. Early resection of the fibrous ridge may improve the hemodynamics of the outflow tract. However, some patients have been recognized who develop aortic insufficiency after resection. Furthermore, hemodynamically significant aortic insufficiency has not been identified as a common complication of DSVAS in postoperative patients regardless of the timing of the initial resection.

Both operated and unoperated patients who present in adulthood should be followed in a similar manner. Asymptomatic patients with small gradients, no evidence of LVH, and minimal AI should be followed yearly. Patients with moderate to severe disease require surgical resection of the DSVAS. Patients who have undergone multiple recurrences may have a tunnel-like outflow obstruction with a small aortic annulus and may require a Ross-Konno operation to relieve LVOTO.

Supravalvar aortic stenosis occurs as a component of Williams syndrome with a number of associated abnormalities, including mental retardation, dental abnormalities, elfin facies, and small stature. These syndromic patients appear sporadically, but supravalvar aortic stenosis without Williams syndrome is more likely to be genetic. Both groups of patients can have associated peripheral pulmonary stenosis. In addition, stenoses of other arteries may occur later in life. Supravalvar aortic stenosis may be surgically repaired when large gradients are documented, and the results are generally good. Balloon angioplasty or stenting of other arterial obstructions may be required.

Algorithm 6–3
Non-Valvar Left Ventricular Outflow Tract Obstruction
DSVAS—unoperated or operated

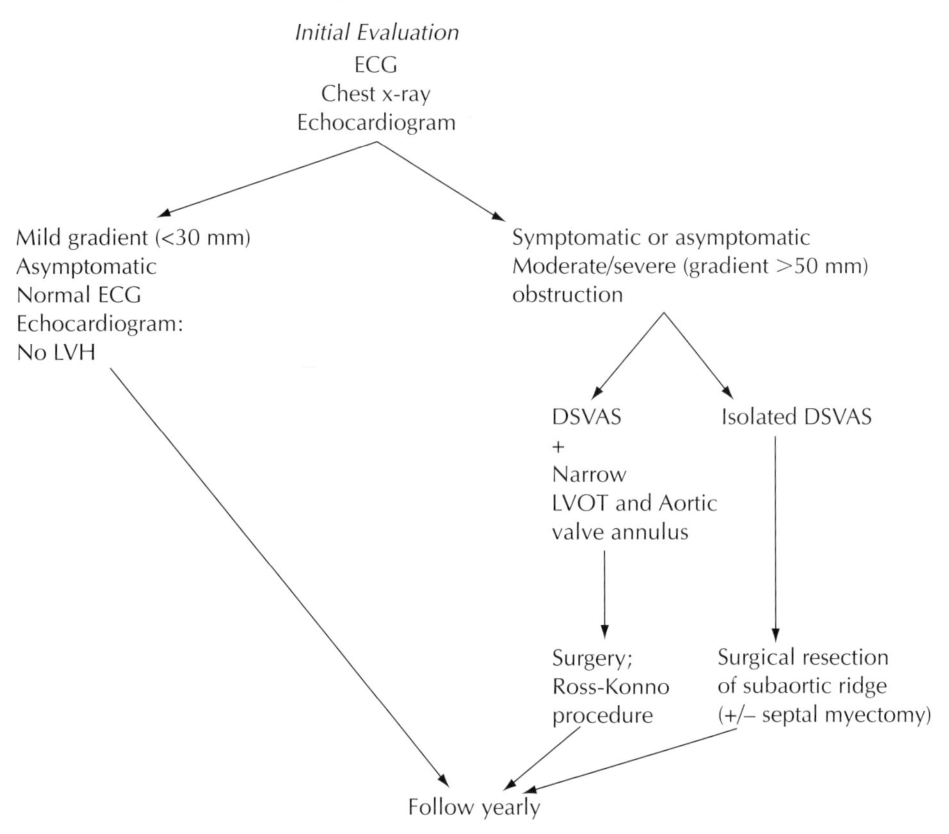

KEY: DSVAS, discrete subvalvar aortic stenosis; ECG, electrocardiogram; LVH, left ventricular hypertrophy.

BIBLIOGRAPHY

Valvar Aortic Stenosis

Beekman RH, Rocchini AP, Gillon JH, Mancini GB: Hemodynamic determinants of the peak systolic left ventricular-aortic pressure gradient in children with valvar aortic stenosis. *Am J Cardiol* 69:813, 1992.

Beppu S, Suzuki S, Matsuda H, et al: Rapidity of progression of aortic stenosis in patients with congenital bicuspid aortic valves. *Am J Cardiol* 71:322, 1993.

Borow KM, Colan SD, Neumann A: Altered left ventricular mechanics in patients with valvular aortic stenosis and coarctation of the aorta: Effects on systolic performance and late outcome. *Circulation* 72:515, 1985.

Campbell M: The natural history of congenital aortic stenosis. *Br Heart J* 30:514, 1968.

Carabello BA, Crawford FA Jr: Valvular heart disease. *N Engl J Med* 337:32, 1997.

Chizner MA, Pearle DL, deLeon AC. The natural history of aortic stenosis in adults. *Am Heart J* 99(4):419, 1980.

Cohen LS, Friedman WF, Braunwald E: Natural history of mild congenital aortic stenosis elucidated by serial hemodynamic studies. *Am J Cardiol* 30:1, 1972.

Donofrio MT, Engle MA, O'Loughlin JE, et al: Congenital aortic regurgitation: Natural history and management. *J Am Coll Cardiol* 20(2):366, 1992.

French JW, Guntheroth WG: An explanation of asymmetric upper extremity blood pressures in supravalvular aortic stenosis: The Goanda effect. *Circulation* 42:31, 1970.

Giddens NG, Finley JP, Nanton MA, Roy DL: The natural course of supravalvar aortic stenosis and peripheral pulmonary artery stenosis in William's syndrome. *Br Heart J* 62:315, 1989.

Gula G, Wain WH, Ross DN: Ten years' experience with pulmonary autograft replacements for aortic valve disease. *Ann Thorac Surg* 28:392, 1979.

Hsieh KS, Keane JF, Nadas AS, et al: Long-term follow-up of valvotomy before 1968 for congenital aortic stenosis. *Am J Cardiol* 58:338, 1986.

Keane JF, Driscoll DJ, Gersony WM, et al: Second natural history of congenital heart defects: Results of treatment of patients with aortic valvar stenosis. *Circulation* 87(2):I-16, 1996.

Keane JF, Perry B, Lock JE: Balloon dilation of congenital valvular aortic stenosis [editorial.] *J Am Coll Cardiol* 16:457, 1990.

Kelly TA, Rothbart RM, Cooper CM, et al: Comparison of outcome of asymptomatic to symptomatic patients older than 20 years of age with valvular aortic stenosis. *Am J Cardiol* 61:123, 1988.

Kirklin JW, Barratt-Boyes BG. *Cardiac Surgery*, 2d ed. New York, Churchill Livingstone, 1993; p 1231.

Kitchiner D, Jackson M, Walsh K, et al: The progression of mild congenital aortic valve stenosis from childhood into adult life. *Int J Cardiol* 42:217, 1993.

Lababidi Z, Wu JR, Walls JT: Percutaneous balloon aortic valvuloplasty: Results in 23 patients. *Am J Cardiol* 53:194, 1984.

Marino BS, Wernovsky G, Rychik J, et al: Early results of the Ross procedure in simple and complex left heart disease. *Circulation* 100(Suppl 19):II162, 1999.

Meliones JN, Beekman RH, Rocchini AP, Lacina SJ: Balloon valvuloplasty for recurrent aortic stenosis after surgical valvotomy in childhood: Immediate and follow-up studies. *J Am Coll Cardiol* 13:1106, 1989.

Nishimura RA, Pieroni DR, Bierman FZ, et al: Second natural history study of congenital heart defects: Aortic stenosis: Echocardiography. *Circulation* 87(Suppl):166, 1993.

Otto CM, Pearlman AS, Comes KA, et al: Determination of the stenotic aortic valve area in adults using Doppler echocardiography. *J Am Coll Cardiol* 7:509, 1986.

Pellikka PA, Nishimura RA, Bailey KR, Tajik AJ: The natural history of adults with asymptomatic, hemodynamically significant aortic stenosis. *J Am Coll Cardiol* 15:1012, 1990.

Roberts WC: The congenitally bicuspid aortic valve: A study of 85 autopsy cases. *Am J Cardiol* 26:72, 1970.

Rocchini AP, Beekman RH, Ben Shachar G, et al: Balloon aortic valvuloplasty: Results of the Valvuloplasty and Angioplasty of Congenital Anomalies Registry. *Am J Cardiol* 65:784, 1990.

Rosenfeld HM, Landzberg MJ, Perry SB, et al: Balloon aortic valvuloplasty in the young adult with congenital aortic stenosis. *Am J Cardiol* 73:1112, 1994.

Ross JJ, Braunwald E: Aortic stenosis. *Circulation* 38(Suppl):V61, 1968.

Shaddy RE, Boucek MM, Sturtevant JE, et al: Gradient reduction, aortic valve regurgitation and prolapse after balloon aortic valvuloplasty in 32 consecutive patients with congenital aortic stenosis. *J Am Coll Cardiol* 16:451, 1990.

Skjaerpe T, Hegrenaes L, Hatle L: Noninvasive estimation of valve area in patients with aortic stenosis by Doppler ultrasound and two-dimensional echocardiography. *Circulation* 72:810, 1985.

Vincent WR, Buckberg GD, Hoffman JI: Left ventricular subendocardial ischemia in severe valvar and supravalvar aortic stenosis: A common mechanism. *Circulation* 49:326, 1974.

Von Son JA, Danielson GK, Puga FJ, et al: Supravalvular aortic stenosis: Long-term results of surgical treatment. *J Thorac Cardiovasc Surg* 107:103, 1994.

Wagner HR, Ellison RC, Keane JF, et al: Clinical course in aortic stenosis. *Circulation* 56:I-47, 1977.

Williams JCP, Barrat-Boyes BG, Lowe JB: Supravalvular aortic stenosis. *Circulation* 24:1311, 1961.

Yeager M, Yock PG, Popp RL: Comparison of Doppler-derived pressure gradient to that determined at cardiac catheterization in adults with aortic valve stenosis: Implications for management. *Am J Cardiol* 57:644, 1986.

Nonvalvar Left Ventricular Outflow Tract Obstruction

Borow KM, Glagov S: Discrete subvalvular aortic stenosis: Is the presence of upstream complex blood flow disturbances an important pathogenic factor? *J Am Coll Cardiol* 19(4):825, 1992.

Brauner R, Laks H, Drinkwater DC Jr, et al: Benefits of early surgical repair in fixed subaortic stenosis. *J Am Coll Cardiol* 30(7):1835, 1997.

Bruce CJ, Nishimura RA, Tajik AJ, et al: Fixed left ventricular outflow tract obstruction in presumed hypertrophic obstructive cardiomyopathy: Implications for therapy. *Ann Thorac Surg* 68:100, 1999.

Cape EG, Vanauker MD, Sigfusson G, et al: Potential role of mechanical stress in the etiology of pediatric heart disease: Septal shear stress in subaortic stenosis. *J Am Coll Cardiol* 30:247, 1997.

Choi JY, Sullivan ID: Fixed subaortic stenosis: Anatomical spectrum and nature of progression. *Br Heart J* 65:280, 1991.

Chung KJ, Fulton DR, Kreidberg MB, et al: Combined discrete subaortic stenosis and ventricular septal defect in infants and children. *Am J Cardiol* 1429, 1984.

Coleman DM, Smallhorn JS, McCrindle BW, et al: Postoperative follow up of fibromuscular subaortic stenosis. *J Am Coll Cardiol* 24(5):1558, 1994.

De Vries AG, Hess J, Witsenberg M, et al: Management of fixed subaortic stenosis: A retrospective study of 57 cases. *J Am Coll Cardiol* 19(5):1013, 1992.

Essop MR, Skudicky D, Sareli P: Diagnostic value of transesophageal versus transthoracic echocardiography in discrete subaortic stenosis. *Am J Cardiol* 70:962, 1992.

Freedom RM, Pelech A, Brand A, et al: The progressive nature of subaortic stenosis in congenital heart disease. *Int J Cardiol* 8:137, 1985.

Frommelt MA, Snider AR, Bove EL, Lupinetti FM: Echocardiographic assessment of subvalvular aortic stenosis before and after operation. *J Am Coll Cardiol* 19:1018, 1992.

Geva T, Hornberger LK, Sanders SP, et al: Echocardiographic predictors of left ventricular outflow tract obstruction after repair of interrupted aortic arch. *J Am Coll Cardiol* 22:1953, 1993.

Gewillig M, Daenen W, Dumoulin M, Van der Hauwaert L: Rheologic genesis of discrete subvalvular aortic stenosis: A Doppler echocardiographic study. *J Am Coll Cardiol* 19:818, 1992.

Kleinert S, Geva T: Echocardiographic morphometry and geometry of the left ventricular outflow tract in fixed subaortic stenosis. *J Am Coll Cardiol* 22:1501, 1993.

Leichter DA, Sullivan I, Gersony WM: "Acquired" discrete subvalvar aortic stenosis: Natural history and hemodynamics. *J Am Coll Cardiol* 14:1539, 1989.

Maron BJ, Redwood DR, Roberts WC, et al: Tunnel subaortic stenosis: Left ventricular outflow tract obstruction produced by fibromuscular narrowing. *Circulation* 54:504, 1976.

Oliver JM, Gonzalez A, Gallego P, Sanchez-Recalde A, Benito F, Mesa JM: Discrete subaortic stenosis in adults: increased prevalence and slow rate of progression of the obstruction and aortic regurgitation. *JACC,* 2001, in press.

Sung C, Price EC, Cooley DA: Discrete subaortic stenosis in adults. *Am J Cardiol* 42:283, 1978.

Van Arsdell GS, Williams WG, Boutin C, et al: Subaortic stenosis in the spectrum of atrioventricular septal defects: Solutions may be complex and palliative. *J Thorac Cardiovasc Surg* 110(5): 1534, 1995.

Van Son JA, Schaff HV, Danielson GK, et al: Surgical treatment of discrete and tunnel subaortic stenosis: Late survival and risk of reoperation. *Circulation* 88(5, part 2):II159, 1993.

Vogt J, Dische R, Rupprath G, et al: Fixed subaortic stenosis: An acquired secondary obstruction? A twenty-seven year experience with 168 patients. *Thorac Cardiovasc Surg* 37:199, 1989.

Wright GB, Keane JF, Nadas AS, et al: Fixed subaortic stenosis in the young: Medical and surgical course in 83 patients. *Am J Cardiol* 52:830, 1983.

CHAPTER 7

COARCTATION OF THE AORTA

Coarctation of the aorta results from a discrete or long segment constriction of the aorta at the junction of the ductus arteriosus and the aortic arch. The defect is often associated with other congenital heart defects, most often a bicuspid aortic valve, as well as ventricular septal defect, subaortic obstruction, and mitral valve anomalies. Coarctation of the aorta is among the most common congenital cardiac abnormalities.

Anatomically, coarctation occurs in a juxtaductal position, but in neonates when the ductus arteriosus is patent, blood flow to the lower body may flow from the pulmonary artery across the ductus arteriosus to the descending aorta. This results in systemic pulmonary artery pressure and, in the presence of a significant ventricular septal defect, increased pulmonary blood flow. A large left-to-right shunt may also be present across the foramen ovale, creating right ventricular overload. Infants with long segment coarctation of the aorta, usually associated with a ventricular septal defect, often present during the neonatal period with congestive heart failure. Although a biscuspid aortic valve occurs in over 70% of cases, frank aortic stenosis is unusual during infancy.

Older children and adults with coarctation of the aorta may present with no symptoms and a history of normal growth and development. The diagnosis can be made easily by determining the difference between the upper and lower extremity blood pressures; varying degrees of hypertension are present in the upper extremities.

The genesis of coarctation of the aorta is best explained on the basis of hemodynamics. It is postulated that even a mild intracardiac left heart obstructive abnormality will cause decreased antegrade aortic blood flow and proportionately increased flow through the pulmonary artery and patent ductus arteriosus. This results in relatively less flow across the aortic isthmus. A contraductal shelf-like structure forms at the juxtaductal region, which bifurcates ductal blood flow retrograde into the left subclavian artery and antegrade to the descending aorta. Decreased blood flow across the aortic isthmus often results in tubular hypoplasia of this structure, most often seen in infants with the most severe coarctation. In extreme cases, interruption of the aortic arch may occur. However, the classic "adult-type" coarctation is the result of an isolated discrete shelf in the ductal region.

The hemodynamics very nicely account for numerous features of the coarctation syndrome (e.g., isthmal narrowing, persistent contraductal shelf, and increased frequency of associated lesions that can decrease antegrade aortic blood flow during fetal life). There also may be a role for ectopic ductal elements within the aorta and, indeed, such tissue has been identified within the aorta in patients with coarctation.

CLINICAL FEATURES

The spectrum of presentation of aortic coarctation is broad: a critically ill newborn with severe obstruction and heart failure, often with associated lesions; an asymptomatic young adult with a cardiac murmur, hypertension in the upper extremities, and decreased femoral and pedal pulses; an older adult who is found to have an aneurysm proximal to a relatively mild coarctation, with no significant differences in upper and lower extremity blood pressures.

Coarctation of the Aorta in Infancy

Symptomatic infants with coarctation of the aorta often have significant associated lesions, including patent ductus arteriosus and ventricular septal defect. Only occasionally do infants present with heart failure in the presence of an isolated coarctation. Infants often have a malalignment-type ventricular septal defect. The upper portion of the ventricular septum (conal septum) is displaced posteriorly, where it may partially obstruct the anterior portion of the left ventricular outflow tract, leading to decreased aortic blood flow. This is the hemodynamic basis for the malalignment ventricular septal defect–coarctation relationship.

It is often difficult to diagnose coarctation of the aorta by fetal echocardiography or during the neonatal period. The ductus arteriosus is open, allowing blood flow from the aortic arch to reach the descending aorta without obstruction, masking the potential for obstruction when the ductus closes after birth. When the ductus closes, a shelf that impinges on the juxtaductal region as well as constriction of ductal tissue in this area may further contribute to obstruction. Surgically closing a patent ductus arteriosus in the neonatal period may unmask coarctation of the aorta; thus, this potential diagnosis must be considered carefully in any newborn in whom a ductus must be ligated.

The infant with severe coarctation of the aorta presents to the neonatalogist and pediatric cardiologist in severe heart failure. The presence of a ventricular septal defect is common, and the combination of left ventricular outflow obstruction with a left-to-right shunt at the ventricular level as well as across the foramen ovale results in severe hemodynamic derangement and an extremely symptomatic newborn. In addition, associated mitral valve and aortic valve abnormalities may compound the problem. Physical examination reveals an infant in severe respiratory distress with poor pulses throughout and only nonspecific murmurs. The difference in blood pressures between the upper and lower extremities is masked by low cardiac output and right-to-left blood flow from the high-pressure right ventricle into the pulmonary artery, ductus arteriosus, and descending aorta. Thus, if the descending aorta is supplied by the right ventricle, there will be little difference in blood pressures between the arms and legs. However, if the flow to the lower extremity is dependent on the left ventricle with a closed or left-to-right shunting ductus arteriosus, blood pressure differences will emerge as cardiac output is improved by medical management. The latter patients, in general, have the best prognosis with appropriate management because, by definition, the left ventricle is adequately supplying the entire systemic cardiac output. In addition, there is less chance of associated lesions that might impair left ventricular dynamics.

Coarctation of the Aorta in Older Children and Adults

Coarctation of the aorta that is recognized after infancy is rarely associated with significant symptomatology. The diagnosis can be made from a combination of physical findings that include a left sternal border systolic ejection murmur, the murmurs of collateral blood vessels heard over the axillae and back, difference in blood pressure between the upper and lower extremities, and absent or decreased lower extremity pulses. Nevertheless, the identification of coarctation of the aorta is often delayed due to lack of recognition by primary physicians. In older patients, coarctation of the aorta is usually isolated—the only associated lesion being bicuspid aortic valve, which occurs in approximately 70% of all patients and is rarely significantly obstructive or regurgitant in children. However, in adults coarctation is occasionally diagnosed during the evaluation of symptomatic aortic valve disease, such as aortic regurgitation secondary to a bicuspid aortic valve. Included among other lesions that also are often of mild severity are mitral valve abnormalities, subvalvular aortic stenosis, and small ventricular septal defects.

Associated lesions and the long-term effects of hypertension may lead to late complications. Chronic elevated blood pressure in the upper body with coarctation of the aorta is associated with a small but significant incidence of cerebral vascular accidents. This may be in part due to an association of aneurysmal disease in the cerebral circulation. Later in life, calcific aortic stenosis or aortic regurgitation, or both, may accompany coarctation based on the usual presence of a bicuspid aortic valve. Progressive mitral valve disease and subaortic stenosis are also potential late problems.

Physical Examination

The abnormal physical findings in a patient with coarctation of the aorta are usually limited to the cardiovascular system. The patient is acyanotic, and there are no signs of congestive heart failure. The upper extremity pulses are brisk, but the femoral and pedal pulses are usually markedly diminished or occasionally absent. However, significant coarctation of the aorta can be present with relatively normal lower extremity pulses. Elevated blood pressure will be noted in the right arm and, usually, in the left arm; lower extremity blood pressures will be decreased and, often, difficult to auscultate. If the left subclavian artery is involved in the narrowed segment, coarctation could be overlooked if the blood pressure is taken in the left arm only. A rare patient with an aberrant right subclavian artery will have low blood pressure in the right arm. The degree of difference in blood pressure between the arms and legs may be influenced not only by the severity of the coarctation, but also by the degree of development of collateral blood vessels. When massive collateral vessels are present, the blood pressure differences between the arms and legs may be minimal despite severe narrowing at the site of the coarctation.

Cardiac examination reveals a left ventricular impulse and a normal first heart sound. Physiologic splitting of the second sound may be difficult to detect, especially in the presence of a bicuspid aortic valve. A systolic ejection click that is a reflection of the bicuspid aortic valve anatomy may be appreciated at the apex. A systolic ejection murmur of moderate intensity is usually heard along the left sternal border, radiating to the left and right base and to the neck. In addition, continuous bruits may be noted in the axillae and over the back. With a bicuspid aortic valve, a high-pitched protodiastolic murmur may be audible, indicating the presence of mild aortic insufficiency.

Noninvasive Evaluation

Electrocardiogram

The electrocardiogram (ECG) often meets voltage criteria for left ventricular hypertrophy, although moderate obstruction can be associated with a normal electrocardiogram.

Chest X-Ray

The heart has a left ventricular configuration with a prominent aortic knob. A reverse "3" sign may be noted with an indentation of the distal portion of the aortic arch at the site of the coarctation. The descending aorta may appear to be dilated. In long-standing severe coarctation with collateral formation, rib notching may be observed (Fig. 7-1).

Echocardiogram

The transthoracic echocardiogram can be very useful in visualizing coarctation in adult patients but requires suprasternal views to identify the site of narrowing (Figs. 7-2*A* and 7-2*B*). Doppler evaluation of the descending aorta typically reveals an abnormal flow pattern, which is suggestive of a significant coarctation of the aorta. Although a gradient may be predicted, blood pressure measurements of upper and lower extremities are far more reliable. The echocardiogram will also indicate the presence of a bicuspid aortic

FIGURE 7-1

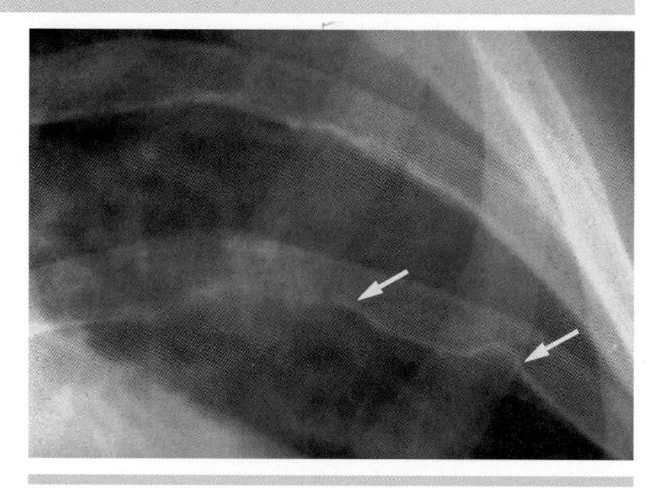

Prominent rib notching (arrows) in a patient with long-standing, severe coarctation of the aorta.

FIGURE 7-2

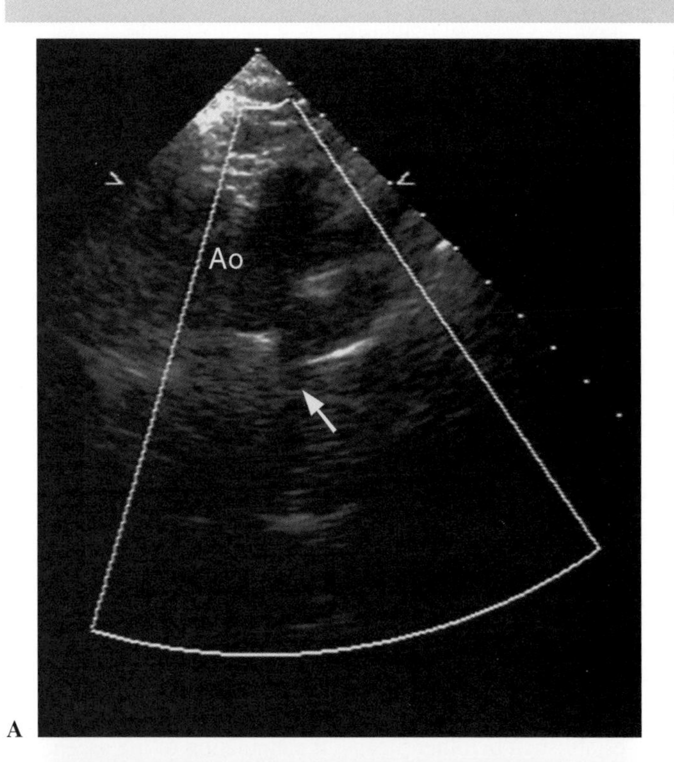

A

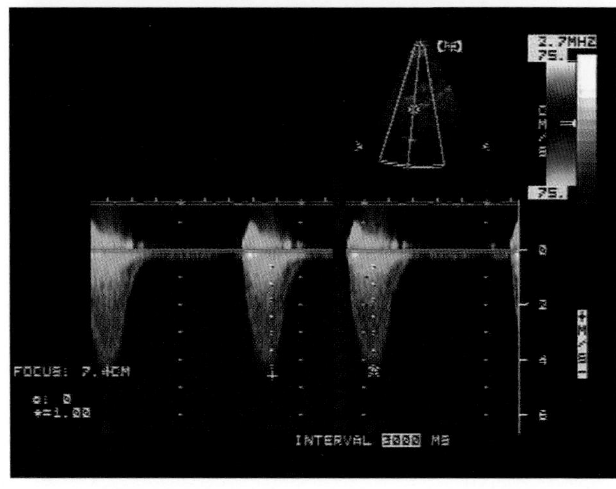

B

A. Suprasternal long-axis view from an adult with severe coarctation of the aorta. There is narrowing just distal to the origin of the left subclavian artery (arrow). Ao, aorta. *B*. Continuous-wave doppler imaging from the suprasternal view in the same patient demonstrates a peak gradient across the coarctation of 84 mm Hg.

valve as well as possible abnormalities of the mitral valve and subaortic region. Transesophageal echocardiography can be useful in depicting the anatomy of the coarctation when transthoracic imaging is inadequate.

Magnetic Resonance Imaging

Magnetic resonance imaging (MRI) has become an important modality for the diagnosis and follow-up of adults with coarctation of the aorta. These studies provide excellent imaging of the thoracic aorta, site of coarctation, and associated collateral vessels. In general, MRI and other noninvasive imaging techniques have replaced cardiac catheterization and angiography for patients with coarctation of the aorta.

Cardiac Catheterization

Cardiac catheterization is usually reserved for patients with complex coarctation of the aorta and associated lesions. Assessment of collateral blood flow may be assessed by angiography. Coronary angiography is generally indicated in the preoperative assessment of older patients. The gradient across the coarctation may be measured with pressure above and below the obstruction. An angiogram in the distal aortic arch provides excellent visualization of the coarctation and provides information about the ascending aorta and aortic valve.

Retrograde aortography in patients with severe coarctation of the aorta can be associated with significant complications. Attempts at manipulation across a severe coarctation have resulted in perforation of collateral vessels. Such attempts may not be necessary if the diagnosis has been established by other means. If cannulation of the ascending aorta or coronary artery is required, then a right brachial approach may be preferred.

Angiography may also show so-called pseudo-coarctation of the aorta. In this condition, the aorta is kinked or buckled, with only a small ridge distal to the left subclavian artery (Fig. 7-3). Usually little or no systolic hypertension or differences between upper and lower extremity blood pressures are noted. Collateral circulation is not increased. Such cases are most often recognized in older adults on the basis of an appearance of an aneurysm of the aortic arch. Rupture of this region has been reported. An occasional patient with long-standing, unrecognized mild coarctation of the aorta, especially when associated with a bicuspid aortic valve, will have findings of this type at late presentation. Surgical repair may be required on the basis of aortic dilatation rather than obstruction at the site of coarctation, as is present in most cases.

Cardiac catheterization and angiography are also important in patients with abdominal coarctation—a condition associated with neurofibromatosis. Angiography will also diagnose renal and mesenteric artery involvement. Abdominal or low thoracic long segment coarctation has also been reported as an acquired lesion in patients with an inflammatory type of aortitis similar to Takayasu disease.

Natural History

Unoperated coarctation of the aorta in infancy, which is often associated with ventricular septal defect and other obstructive left heart lesions, has an extremely poor prognosis. Few

FIGURE 7-3

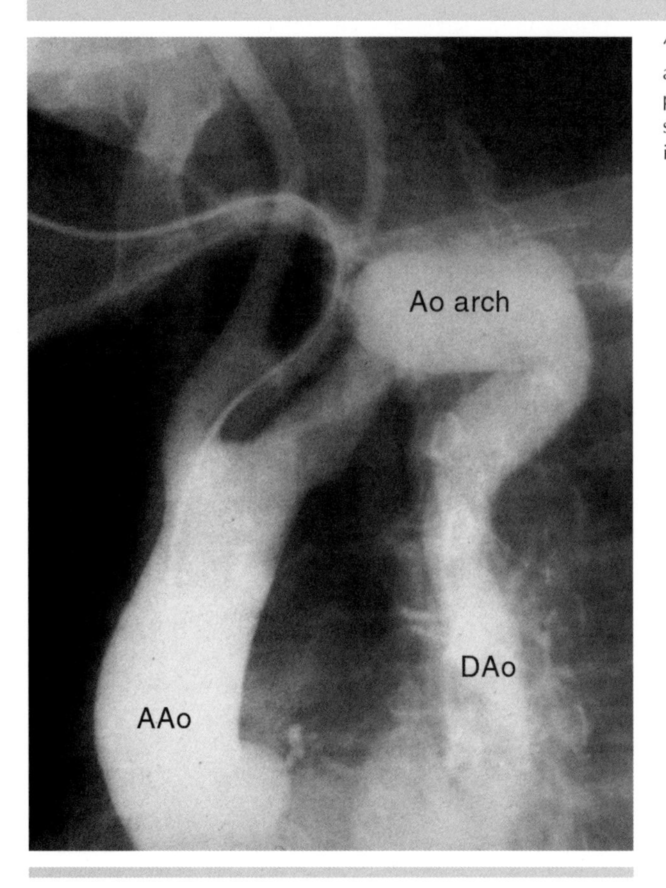

"Pseudo coarctation" demonstrating marked dilation and distortion of the aortic arch. There is no blood pressure gradient between the ascending and descending aorta. AAo, ascending aorta; DAo, descending aorta; Ao arch, aortic arch.

patients live beyond the neonatal period without urgent surgical intervention. Milder and usually isolated coarctation in older patients is not associated with symptoms for many years or decades. However, chronic hypertension leads to left ventricular hypertrophy and an increased incidence of heart failure in early to mid-adulthood, associated with ischemic heart disease in many patients. There is an increased incidence of cerebral vascular accidents. The average life expectancy of a patient with significant unoperated coarctation of the aorta has been reported to be approximately 30 years, although survival is much better in those with milder forms of coarctation. Twenty percent of untreated patients succumb between the first and second decades of life, and 80% die before the age of 50 years.

MANAGEMENT

Patients with significant coarctation of the aorta usually have had surgical repair during childhood, although in many cases lack of recognition delays the operation for many years. Historically, it was thought that the optimal timing of surgery was during the second decade of life, when the size of the aorta would definitely be adequate, in order to prevent the development of a napkin ring deformity at the site of the anastomosis. However, with improvement in surgical techniques, repair in infancy—although occasionally associated with the necessity for later revision—became a more definitive operation. Furthermore, a number of reports indicated that patients whose coarctation repair was delayed until young adulthood had frequent, late cardiovascular complications, including chronic hypertension, heart failure, and early coronary disease. Other studies indicated that repair in the first years of life was not associated with hypertension in adolescence, although long-term data regarding these patients later in adulthood are not available. It is reasonable to conclude that early surgery is advantageous for this group of patients to avoid long-standing hypertension and other late complications. Nevertheless, some patients with significant coarctation remain unrecognized until adolescence or adulthood, and individuals may be encountered whose original surgery or interventional procedure was incomplete, necessitating reoperation or interventional procedures.

Patients with extremely mild coarctation (upper–lower extremity gradients of less than 20 to 30 mm) may be followed without intervention, but increasing gradient, associated aneurysm formation, or severe narrowing at the coarctation site with marked collateral formation eventually lead to interventional or surgical correction in most cases.

Surgical Repair

Resection of the coarctation with end-to-end anastomosis of the proximal and distal aorta is the surgical treatment of choice for the majority of patients. In young patients an oblique repair, including the narrowed segment of the aortic arch, is possible when necessary (Fig. 7-4*A*). Among infants, at the time coarctation is repaired, other significant intracardiac lesions such as ventricular septal defect also are corrected during a single procedure.

In an occasional patient in whom the length of the coarctation is too great or previous surgery has created technical difficulties, a Dacron bypass graft from the ascending aorta or subclavian artery to the descending aorta may be effectively utilized (Fig. 7-5). Patients may be encountered who had repair in infancy by means of a subclavian turndown procedure in which the proximal left subclavian artery was utilized to augment the narrowed segment, thus avoiding an end-to-end anastomosis (Fig. 7-4*B*). This procedure is now performed infrequently. Patch aortoplasty is a surgical procedure that avoids complete transection of the aorta, eliminating a circumferential scar that would have the potential to contract and cause recoarctation (Fig. 7-4*C*). However, aneurysm formation at the site of the repair has occurred with some frequency, and this operation is rarely used today.

Surgical risk associated with coarctation repair is low. Of most concern is spinal cord ischemia and paresis, which has been reported to occur in a few cases. Fortunately, this devastating complication is rarely seen in recent years.

Balloon Angioplasty or Stenting

Surgery continues to be generally accepted as treatment for coarctation, although catheter techniques are increasingly used. Early reports of aneurysm formation limited the en-

FIGURE 7-4

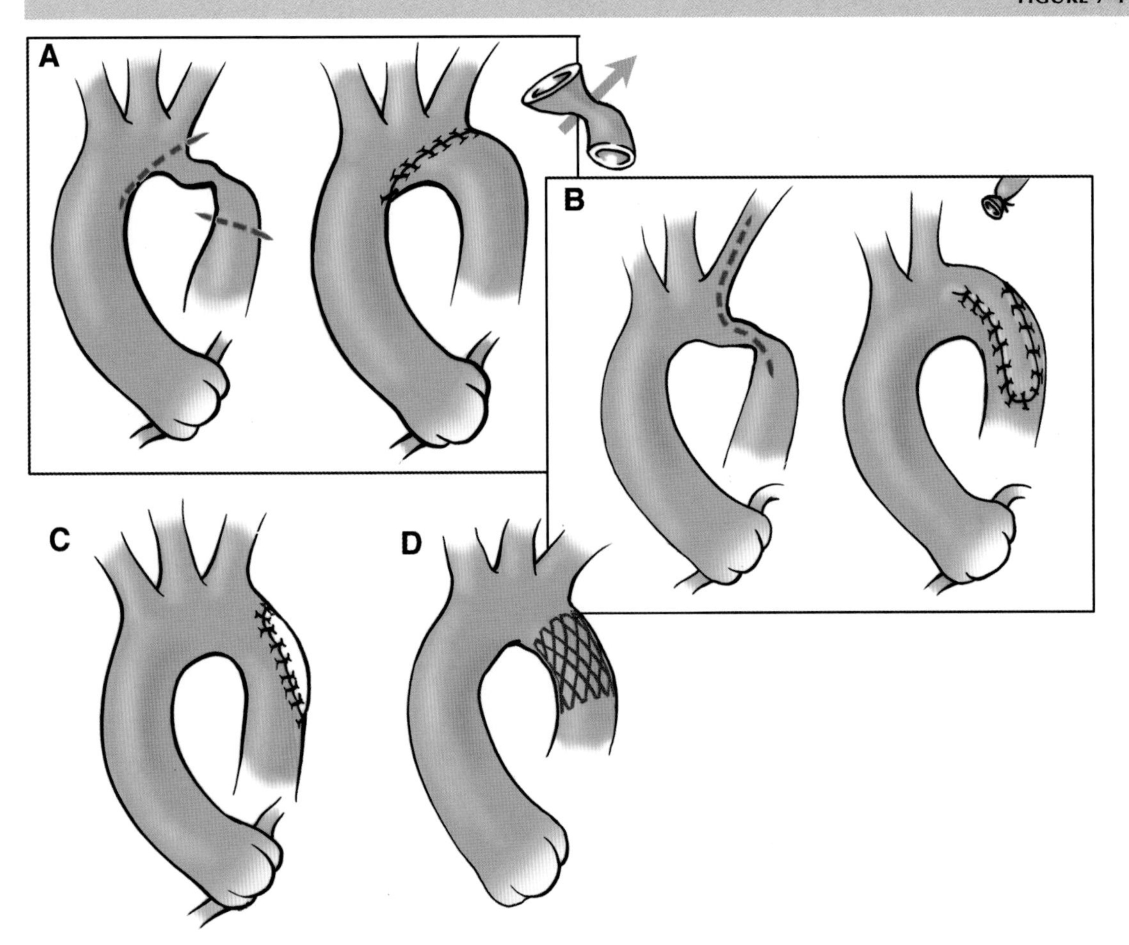

Various methods used to repair coarctation of the aorta: *A*. In the end-to-end anastomosis, the coarcted region is removed and the ascending and descending aorta are directly anastomosed. *B*. In the subclavian flap procedure, the wall of the subclavian artery is utilized to enlarge the coarcted region. Panel *C* shows the patch angioplasty procedure to relieve the obstruction at the coarcted area. A stent repair is shown in Panel *D*.

thusiasm for balloon angioplasty at many centers, but technical improvements have led to its use for native coarctation at some hospitals. More recently, stenting of the coarctation has been utilized for both native and recurrent coarctation with a high degree of success; the risk of aneurysm formation appears to be markedly decreased using this approach (Figs. 7-4*D*, 7-6*A* and *B*). In older patients, stenting for recoarctation is now commonly used to relieve residual obstruction.

FIGURE 7-5

Aortogram showing a bypass graft (arrow) from the ascending aorta to the descending aorta in a patient with persistent severe obstruction who had had multiple procedures for coarctation of the aorta. AAo, aorta, DAo, descending aorta.

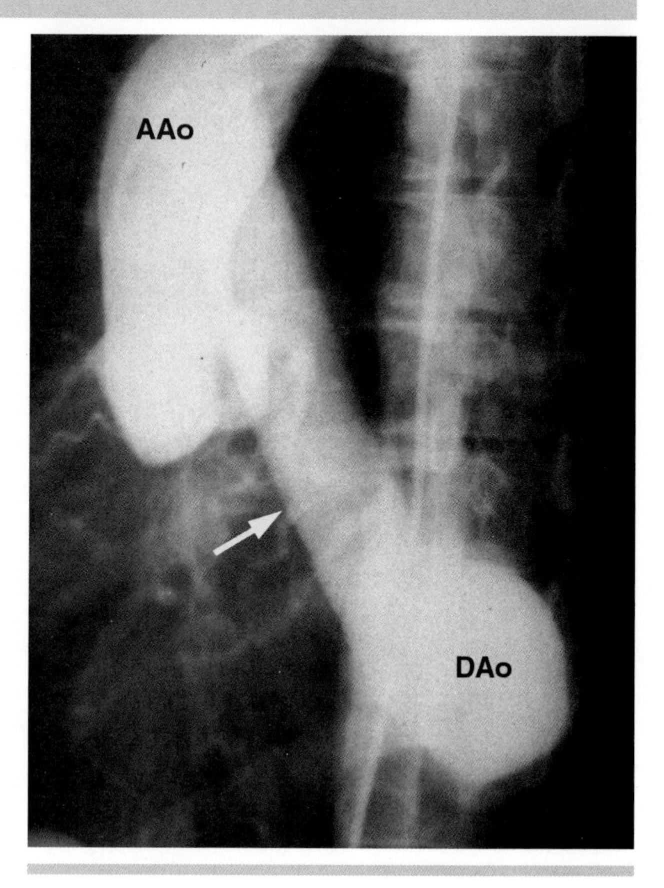

LONG-TERM FOLLOW-UP

The prognosis after repair of isolated coarctation of the aorta is usually excellent. Routine antibiotic prophylaxis for prevention of endocarditis is continued. Frequent assessment of blood pressure is important; hypertension may persist in the absence of obstruction. This finding is apparent in patients in whom upper-extremity hypertension was severe, and relief of obstruction was in late childhood or adult life. In the absence of recurrent coarctation, such patients are managed similarly to any patient with essential hypertension. However, it is important to determine that there is no evidence of residual or recurrent coarctation to explain elevated upper-extremity blood pressure. Exercise studies with upper- and lower-extremity blood pressure determinations may be useful but are often difficult to interpret in this regard because even patients with well-repaired coarctation may display upper–lower extremity gradients during high cardiac output states.

Patients who have had coarctation repair should be followed closely for the development or progression of associated cardiac defects such as aortic valve stenosis or

FIGURE 7-6

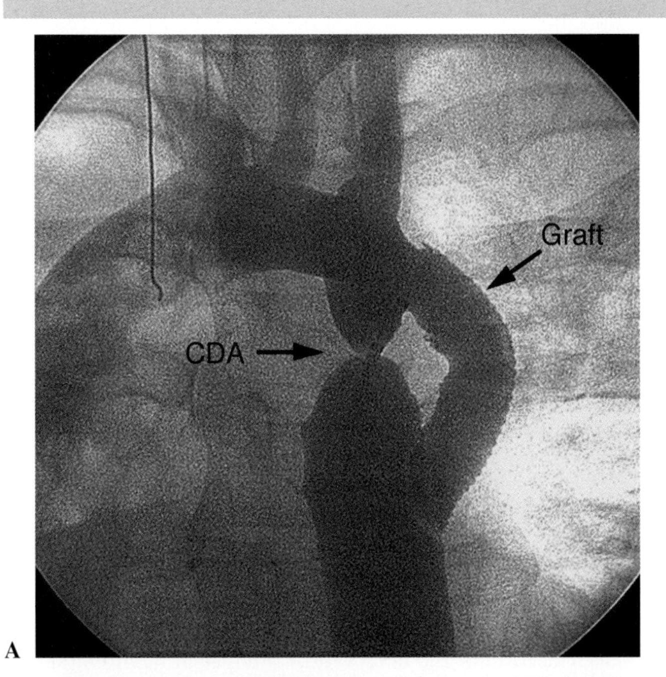

A

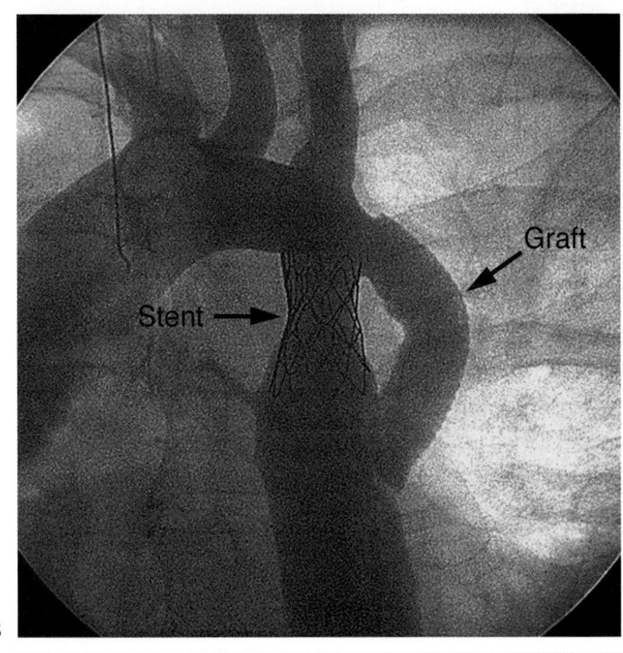

B

A. An aortogram in an adult woman with severe coarctation of the aorta (COA) previously treated with a bypass graft from the distal transverse arch to the descending aorta. She presented with severe hypertension secondary to recurrent obstruction at the graft anastomosis. The angiogram shows the native COA and opacification of the bypass with a 70-mm gradient between the upper and lower extremities. *B*. An aortogram in the same patient as *A* following stent placement at the site of the native coarctation of the aorta. The gradient between the upper and lower extremities was eliminated.

regurgitation, dilation of the ascending aorta, or subvalvar aortic stenosis. The incidence of aortic dissection is rare, but is increased in coarctation patients with a bicuspid aortic valve compared with the general population. Such individuals should be watched carefully for aortic root dilation as well as aortic valve calcification and the late development of aortic stenosis.

Aneurysm formation at the site of a coarctation repair may be an issue in some patients. This finding is most often described after patch aortoplasty, and may be associated with rupture. The risk may be increased during pregnancy. Coarctation should be repaired prior to pregnancy, but if this is not possible, careful follow-up with frequent blood pressure measurements and serial, noninvasive assessments is required. Cardiac MRI is the most useful modality to monitor patients who have aneurysms. Operative intervention may be necessary to eliminate large or progressively expanding aortic aneurysms.

Coarctation patients also should be followed closely in terms of prevention of early coronary disease by monitoring of lipids, ECGs, echocardiograms, and exercise studies. An active lifestyle should be recommended with restrictions based on the presence and severity of residual heart disease.

SUMMARY

Coarctation of the aorta results from a narrowing of a segment of aorta juxtaposed to the entrance of the ductus arteriosus. The form of the defect most often seen in childhood involves a long segment narrowing that includes the isthmus of the aortic arch. In the presence of patent ductus arteriosus or ventricular septal defect, or both, patients present in the neonatal period with congestive heart failure. This requires urgent repair of the coarctation and, if necessary, of the intracardiac defect. Patients with isolated coarctation may not present until later in childhood, adolescence, or even during adult life. In mild cases, upper extremity hypertension may not be prominent, and without upper and lower extremity blood pressure determinations, the presence and source of mild hypertension may not be appreciated. Without surgery, coarctation of the aorta leads to hypertension, coronary artery disease, and left ventricular dysfunction. Early repair is thought to prevent long-standing hypertension, but significant coarctation must be corrected when discovered at any age. Patients are usually asymptomatic, but physical examination indicates a left sternal border systolic ejection murmur, and the murmurs of collateral blood vessels may be heard over the entire precordium and back. Femoral and pedal pulses are often absent or markedly diminished, but some patients with significant coarctation may have palpable lower extremity pulses.

A bicuspid aortic valve occurs in 70% of patients with coarctation of aorta. When a bicuspid valve is present, a systolic ejection click at the apex and the murmur of mild aortic insufficiency may also be present. Measurements of blood pressure in the right arm and one leg will make the diagnosis of coarctation of the aorta unless there is an aberrant right subclavian artery or peripheral vascular disease in older patients. Echocardiography is useful to define the coarctation of the aorta, rule out associated congenital heart defects, and evaluate left ventricular hypertrophy and function. The coarctation is best visualized by MRI examination, and in the present era, angiography is rarely necessary.

Surgical repair is definitive, but adult patients may be encountered who had incomplete correction earlier in life and now require reintervention. Balloon angioplasty of native coarctation remains controversial because of the possibility of aneurysm formation. Balloon angioplasty or stenting is now well accepted for patients who have had early surgery and in whom significant recoarctation has occurred. Many centers now advocate primary stenting of coarctation of the aorta, and this approach is becoming more accepted in adults. However, there is not yet long-term follow-up.

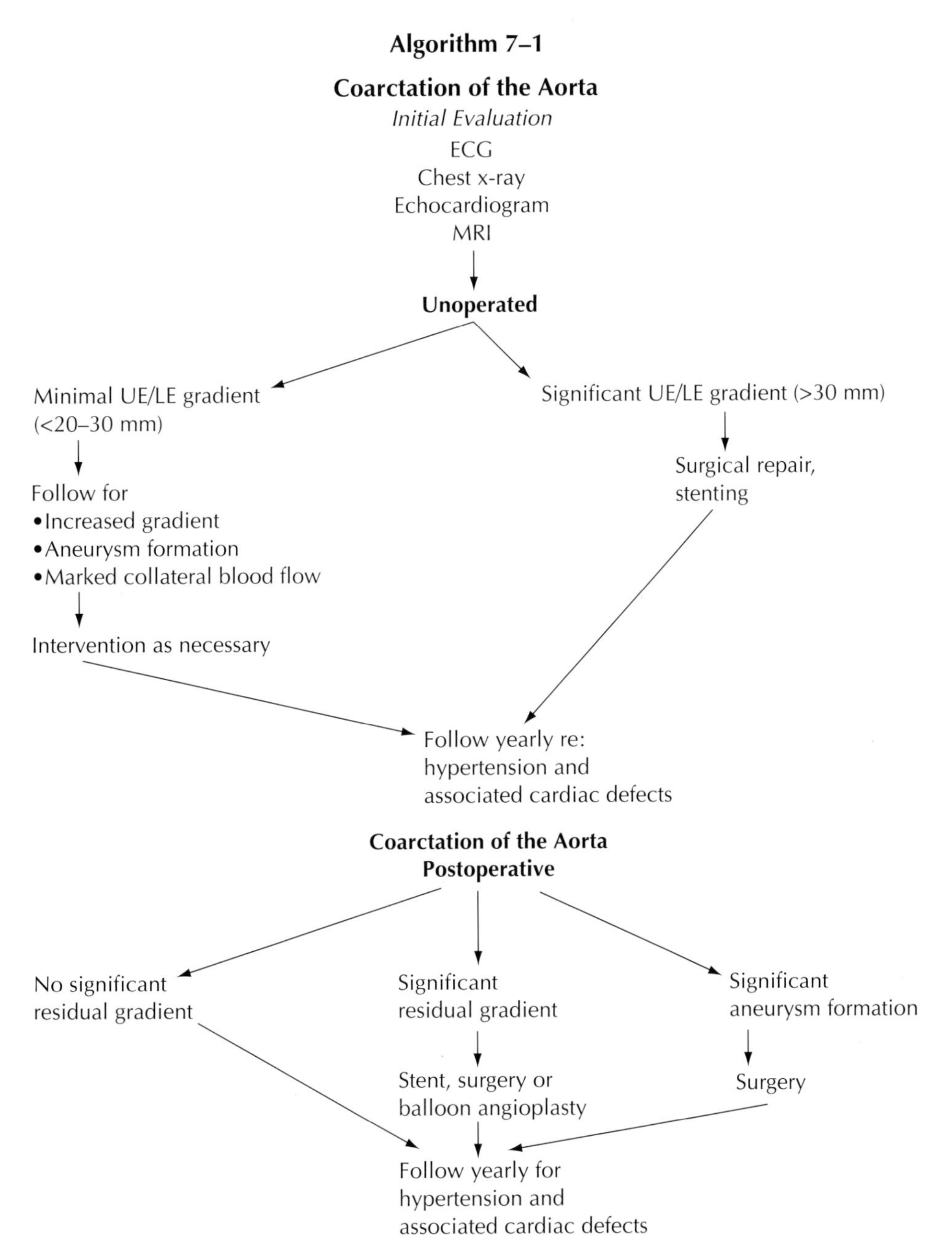

KEY: ECG, electrocardiogram; LE, lower extremity; MRI, magnetic resonance imaging; UE, upper extremity.

Patients who have had coarctation repair should be followed for the development of coronary artery disease and other cardiovascular complications. Late hypertension in the absence of residual obstruction is well documented in many patients, and pharmacologic management of hypertension may be required. The status of an associated bicuspid aortic valve also must be monitored.

BIBLIOGRAPHY

Arenas J, Myers J, Gleason M, et al: End-to-end repair of aortic coarctation using absorbable polydioxanone suture. *Ann Thorac Surg* 51:413, 1991.

Brewer L, Fosbeg R, Mulder G: Spinal cord complications following surgery for coarctation of the aorta. *J Thorac Cardiovasc Surg* 64:368, 1972.

Bromberg B, Beekman RH, Rocchini A, et al: Aortic aneurysm after patch aortoplasty repair of coarctation: A prospective analysis of prevalence, screening tests and risks. *J Am Coll Cardiol* 14:734, 1989.

Campbell M: Natural history of coarctation of the aorta. *Br Heart J* 32:633, 1970.

Clarckson P, Nicholson M, Barratt-Boyes B, et al: Results after repair of coarctation of the aorta beyond infancy. A 10 to 28 year follow-up with particular reference to late systemic hypertension. *Am J Cardiol* 51:1481, 1983.

Cohen M, Fuster V, Steele PM, et al: Coarctation of the aorta: Long-term follow-up and prediction of outcome after surgical correction. *Circulation* 80:840, 1989.

Ebeid MR, Prieto LR, Latson LA: Use of balloon-expandable stents for coarctation of the aorta: Initial results and intermediate-term follow-up. *J Am Coll Cardiol* 30:1853, 1997.

Freed M, Rocchini A, Rosenthal A, et al: Exercise-induced hypertension after surgical repair of coarctation of the aorta. *Am J Cardiol* 43:253, 1979.

Gardiner H, Celermajer D, Sorenson K, et al: Arterial reactivity is significantly impaired in normotensive young adults after successful repair of aortic coarctation in childhood. *Circulation* 89:1745, 1994.

Gersony WM: Coarctation of the aorta, in *Heart Disease in Infants, Children and Adolescents*, 3d ed, AJ Moss et al (eds). Baltimore, Williams & Wilkins, 1990.

Hellenbrand WE, Allen HD, Golinko RJ, et al: Balloon angioplasty for aortic recoarctation: Results of Valvuloplasty and Angioplasty of Congenital Anomalies Registry. *Am J Cardiol* 65:793, 1990.

Ing F, Starc T, Griffiths S, Gersony W: Early diagnosis of coarctation of the aorta in children: A continuing dilemma. *Pediatrics* 93:378, 1996.

Kaemmerer H, Theissen P, Konig U, et al: Follow-up using magnetic resonance imaging in adult patients after surgery for aortic coarctation. *J Thorac Cardiovasc Surg* 41:107, 1993.

Kan J, White R, Mitchell S, et al: Treatment of restenosis of coarctation by percutaneous transluminal angioplasty. *Circulation* 68:1087, 1983.

Kappetein A, Zwinderman A, Bogers A, et al: More than thirty-five years of coarctation repair. An unexpected high relapse rate. *J Thorac Cardiovasc Surg* 107:87, 1994.

Kino K, Sano S, Sugawara E, et al: Later aneurysm after subclavian flap aortoplasty for coarctation of the aorta. *Ann Thorac Surg* 61:1262, 1996.

Knyshov G, Sitar L, Glagola M, Atamanyuk M: Aortic aneurysms at the site of the repair of coarctation of the aorta: A review of 48 patients. *Ann Thorac Surg* 61:935, 1996.

Lock J, Castaneda-Zuniga W, Bass J, et al: Balloon dilatation of excised aortic coarctation. *Radiology* 143:689, 1982.

Marrion B, Humphries J, Rowe R, Mellits E: Prognosis of surgically corrected coarctation of the aorta. A 20 year postoperative appraisal. *Circulation* 47:119, 1973.

Rao PS, Najjar HN, Mardini MK et al: Balloon angioplasty for coarctation of the aorta: Immediate and long-term results (review). *Am Heart J* 115:657, 1988.

Rocchini A, Rosenthal A, Barger A, et al: Pathogenesis of paradoxical hypertension after coarctation resection. *Circulation* 54:382, 1976.

Rudolph A, Heymann M, Spitznas U: Hemodynamic considerations in the development of narrowing of the aorta. *Am J Cardiol* 30:514, 1972.

Salazar O, Steinberger J, Carpenter B, et al: Predictors of hypertension in long term survivors of repaired coarctation of the aorta. *J Am Coll Cardiol* 27(suppl A):35A, 1996.

Shaddy R, Boucek MM, Sturtevant JE, et al: Comparison of angioplasty and surgery for unoperated coarctation of the aorta. *Circulation* 87:793, 1993.

Snider AR, Silverman N: Suprasternal notch echocardiography: A two-dimensional technique for evaluation of congenital heart disease. *Circulation* 63:165, 1981.

Sohn S, Rothman A, Shiota T, et al: Acute and follow-up intravascular ultrasound findings after balloon dilation of coarctation of the aorta. *Circulation* 90:340, 1994.

Stafford M, Griffiths S, Gersony W: Coarctation of the aorta: A study in delayed detection. *Pediatrics* 69:159, 1982.

Stewart A, Ahmed R, Travill C, Newman C: Coarctation of the aorta life and health 20–44 years after surgical repair. *Br Heart J* 69:65, 1993.

Suzrez de Lezo J, Pan M, Romero M, et al: Balloon-expandable stent repair of severe coarctation of the aorta. *Am Heart J* 129:1002, 1995.

Tynan M, Finley J, Fontes V, et al: Balloon angioplasty for the treatment of native coarctation: Results of Valvuloplasty and Angioplasty of Congenital Anomalies Registry. *Am J Cardiol* 65:790, 1990.

Waldhausen J, Nahrwold D: Repair of coarctation of the aorta with a subclavian flat. *J Thorac Cardiovasc Surg* 51:532, 1966.

CHAPTER 8

CONGENITALLY CORRECTED TRANSPOSITION OF THE GREAT ARTERIES

Congenitally corrected transposition of the great arteries, commonly known as L-TGA, is an uncommon defect that occurs in 0.5% of all patients born with congenital heart disease. The lesion is characterized by discordance between the atria and ventricles, as well as between the ventricles and the great arteries. The embryologic defect results in the formation of a ventricular L-loop rather than a D-loop, which is present in the normal (situs solitus) heart. As a result, the morphologic right ventricle lies to the left of the morphologic left ventricle and becomes the systemic ventricle. The morphologic right ventricle gives rise to the aorta, which is anterior and to the left of the pulmonary artery. These abnormalities result in the flow of desaturated blood from the right atrium through a right-sided mitral valve and morphologic left ventricle into a posteriorly placed pulmonary artery. Pulmonary venous blood returns to the left atrium, passes through a left-sided tricuspid valve and morphologic right ventricle, and exits via an anteriorly positioned aorta (Figs. 8-1*A* and 8-2).

As a result of the discordance at both the atrioventricular (AV) and great vessel level, physiologic blood flow remains normal. Thus, the abnormal blood flow from the atriae to the ventricles is anatomically "corrected" by the transposed great arteries. However, only 3% of patients with L-TGA have no additional cardiac lesions. The remainder have one or more associated defects, including ventricular septal defect (VSD), pulmonary stenosis, tricuspid valve (the systemic AV valve) abnormalities, and heart block. A large VSD is present in 80% of patients with L-TGA. Pulmonary stenosis coexists in 80% of patients with a VSD and exists as an isolated lesion in 20%. In addition, left AV valve (tricuspid) deformities are common. They are often but not always of the Ebstein type. Left AV valve insufficiency may be progressive and is poorly tolerated in L-TGA patients who have sys-

FIGURE 8-1

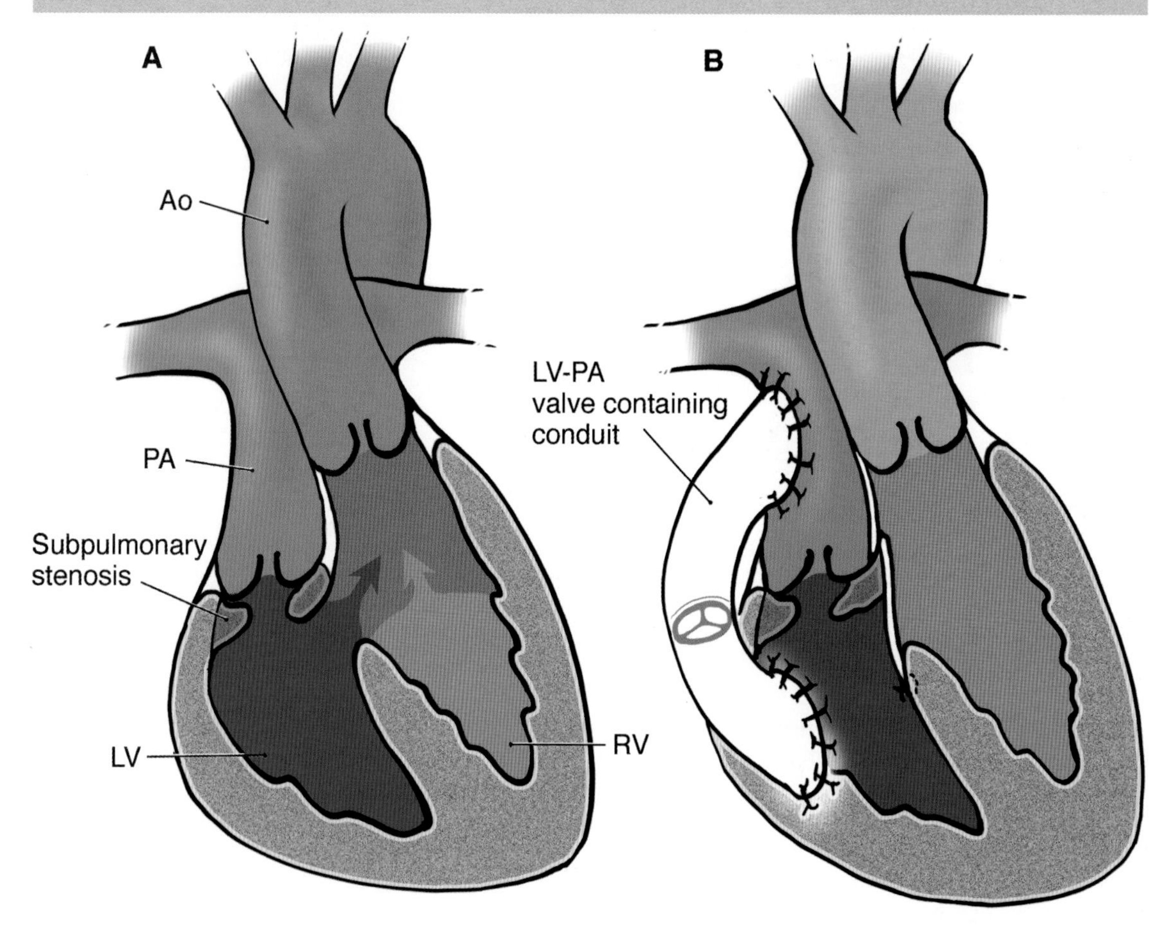

A. LTGA with ventricular septal defect and subpulmonary stenosis. *B.* At surgery, the ventricular septal defect is closed and the left ventricle is connected to the pulmonary artery by use of the homograft or valve-containing conduit. Resection of the subpulmonary stenosis is avoided because of the high risk of complete heart block.

temic right ventricles. Finally, AV conduction abnormalities, including complete heart block, are common in the presence of L-TGA.

CLINICAL FEATURES

The rare patient with L-TGA and no other structural cardiac lesions is asymptomatic. In this case, an abnormality of a routine chest x-ray or electrocardiogram (ECG) may lead to the diagnosis, but older adults without known congenital heart disease have had the defect first recognized at autopsy.

FIGURE 8-2

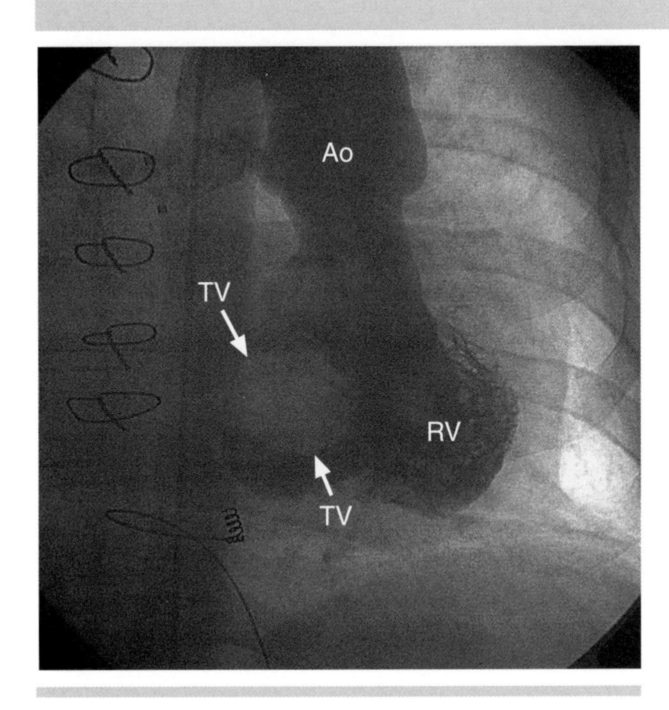

A right ventriculogram in a patient with congenitally corrected transposition of the great vessels. The morphologic right ventricle is the systemic ventricle and is situated to the left of the right-sided left ventricle. The aorta is anterior and arises from an infundibulum off of the right ventricle. RV, right ventricle; Ao, aorta; TV, tricuspid valve.

The age and clinical presentation for the great majority of patients depend on the associated lesions. If a large VSD is present without pulmonary outflow obstruction, patients can present in early infancy with congestive heart failure as a result of pulmonary overcirculation from a large left-to-right shunt. The hemodynamic consequences are similar to those for patients with normal intracardiac anatomy and an unrestricted VSD.

When a VSD is associated with pulmonary stenosis, pulmonary blood flow is restricted and the physiology is similar to that of tetralogy of Fallot (see Chap. 10). When severe subpulmonary obstruction is present, cyanosis will be severe. When milder degrees of pulmonary stenosis are present, the circulation may be balanced with bidirectional shunting or trivial shunting in either direction. The direction of shunting in these cases depends on the difference between resistance at the site of the pulmonary outflow tract obstruction and the systemic vascular resistance.

Young adults with L-TGA may develop symptoms related to the presence of left AV valve regurgitation, failure of the systemic right ventricle, or rhythm disturbances. The incidence of left AV valve regurgitation increases with age and is thought to be related to the geometry of a tricuspid valve in the systemic circulation or, in many cases, Ebstein-like abnormalities of the left AV valve. When significant left AV valve regurgitation is present, volume overload of the systemic right ventricle can lead to right ventricular dysfunction.

The question has been raised as to whether intrinsic significant ventricular failure of the systemic right ventricle causes progressive tricuspid insufficiency, or whether it is tricuspid regurgitation that leads to right ventricular failure. Recent reports suggest that the latter is most important for the great majority of cases, although right ventricular failure also has been recognized in older adults with L-TGA in the absence of valvar regurgitation.

The potential for both primary and secondary failure of the systemic right ventricle leads to difficult management problems when significant left AV valve insufficiency is present in conjunction with advanced ventricular dysfunction. In patients who come to medical attention at this stage, regardless of whether ventricular failure is the result of AV valve insufficiency or primary myocardial failure, outcome is often poor, even if AV valve surgery is performed.

Physical Examination

Physical examination findings for patients with L-TGA will vary according to the presence or absence of associated cardiac lesions. A loud second heart sound is uniformly noted in the second left intercostal space, secondary to the anterior position of the aortic valve. The accentuated second heart sound may be mistaken for pulmonary hypertension. The pulmonary component of S_2 is frequently obscured by its posterior position and makes splitting of the second heart sound difficult to appreciate. If no other cardiac lesions are present, the remainder of the examination may be unremarkable.

In patients with a VSD, a holosystolic murmur is audible along the left lower sternal border, comparable in location to a VSD in patients with normal cardiac anatomy. If pulmonary stenosis is present, the systolic murmur is usually maximal at the third left intercostal space.

When the patient has left AV valve regurgitation, the holosystolic murmur usually radiates toward the left lower sternal border and may be confused with the murmur of a VSD. The murmur is less well heard at the apex than is mitral regurgitation in a normal heart.

Noninvasive Evaluation

Electrocardiography

The diagnosis of L-TGA may be suspected on the ECG by (1) the absence of septal Q waves in leads I, aVL, and V_4–V_6, (2) Q waves in V_1/V_{3R}, and/or (3) the presence of unexplained heart block in a young patient (Fig. 8-3). First-degree AV block is present in 50% of patients in normal sinus rhythm. The incidence of complete heart block increases with age, possibly related to fibrosis along the unusually long AV conduction system in patients with AV discordance. Prior to the identification of the bundle of His superior to the VSD, ECG evidence of complete heart block almost always developed after open heart surgical repair.

Disturbances of AV conduction are common in patients with L-TGA. The bundle of His is anomalous relative to the normal heart and is located in a position just superior to the site of a typical subaortic VSD. In the normal heart, the conduction bundle is along the inferior portion of the VSD. The location of the AV conduction system in patients with L-TGA was established during early intraoperative mapping studies. Currently VSD closure can be achieved with a low incidence of heart block by surgeons who accurately identify the site of the AV conduction system in this anomaly. Nevertheless, AV conduction is

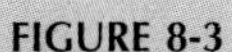

FIGURE 8-3

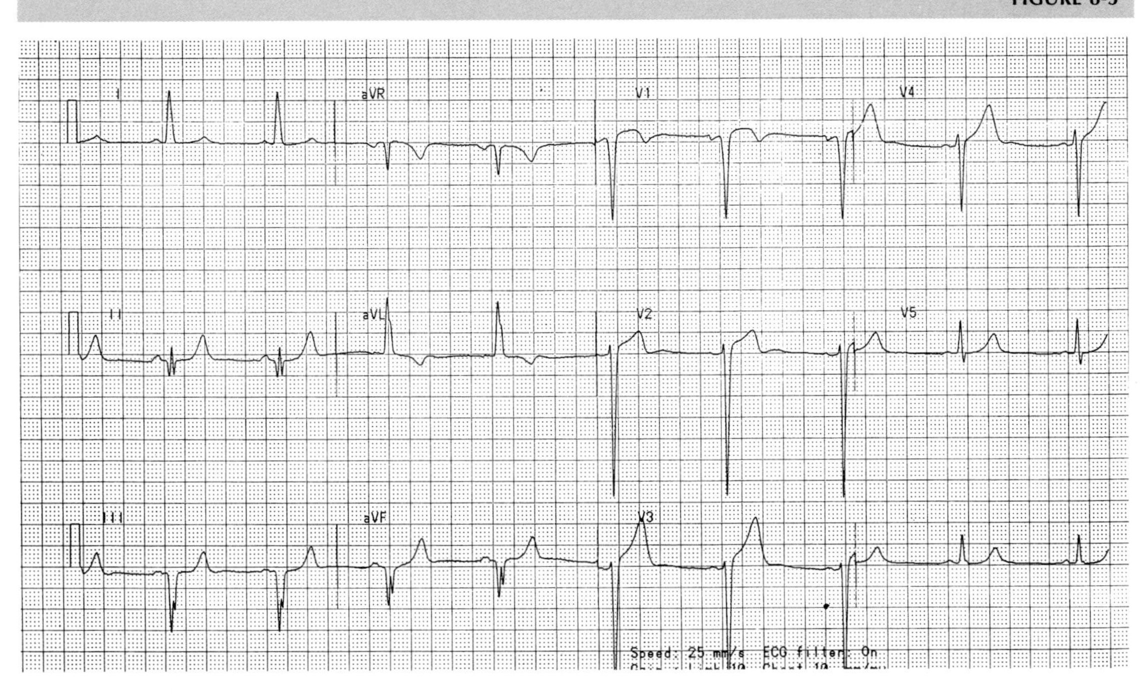

An electrocardiogram from a patient with L-TGA and no associated lesions. The QRS shows absence of septal q waves in leads 1 and avL and a Q wave in V1. Since the left and right ventricle are reversed, the normal left-to-right septal activation produces an R wave in leads 1 and avL.

always tenuous in patients with L-TGA. AV block has been described prior to surgical manipulation and may occur spontaneously. In some cases, complete heart block may have been present since birth.

Chest X-Ray

The chest x-ray in a patient with L-TGA has a characteristic profile characterized by a straight left superior border as a result of the levo-positioned aorta (Fig. 8-4). When severe pulmonic obstruction and a VSD result in a right-to-left shunt, the dilated ascending aorta may be even more prominent, and the pulmonary vascularity is decreased. When a VSD is present without pulmonic obstruction, the heart will be large with increased pulmonary vascular markings. Prominence of the right pulmonary artery may produce a "waterfall" appearance in the right hilum.

Echocardiography

The diagnosis of L-TGA can be readily established by echocardiography (Fig. 8-5). These features include (1) a posteriorly placed pulmonary artery and an anterior aorta that is to the left of the pulmonary artery, (2) the presence of two papillary muscles and a mitral

FIGURE 8-4

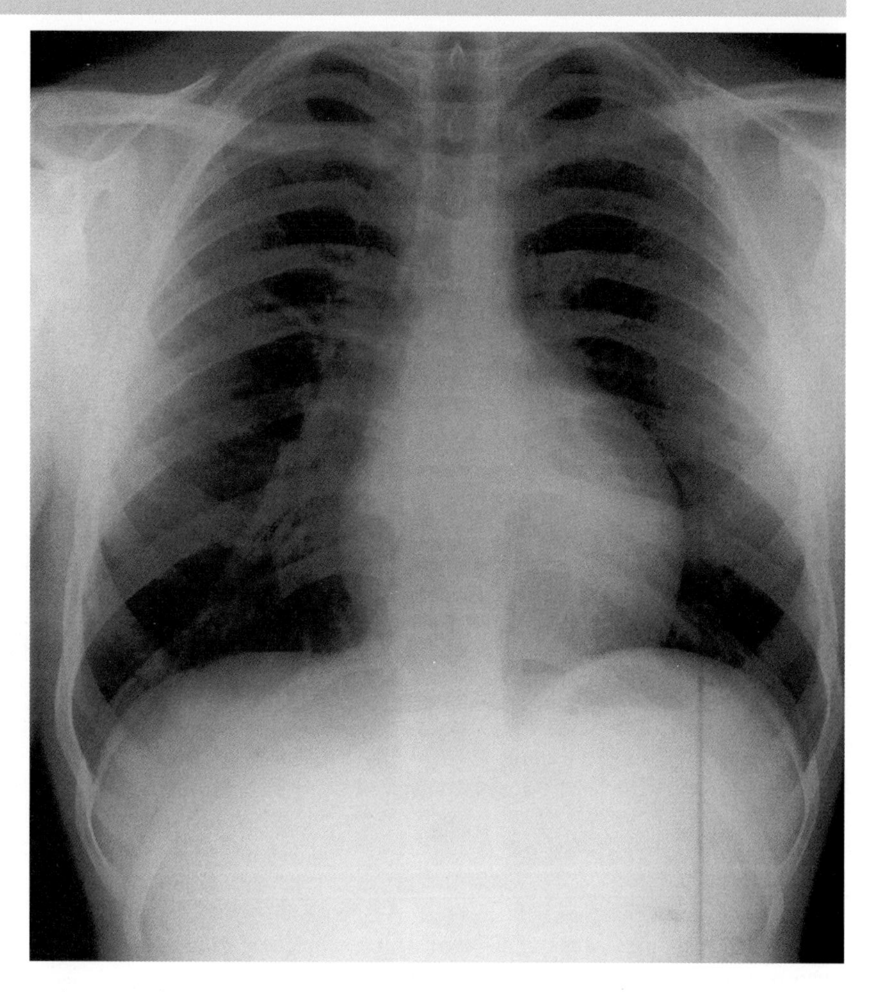

A chest x-ray from a patient with congenitally corrected transposition of the great vessels without associated lesions. The left heart border is abnormal due to the absence of the main pulmonary artery segment in this region.

valve in the right-sided left ventricle, (3) inferior attachment of the left-sided tricuspid valve as compared with the right AV valve (opposite of normal), (4) absence of continuity between the aorta and the left AV valve as a result of a subaortic infundibulum, (5) right ventricular morphology of the systemic ventricle, and (6) abnormal orientation and dynamics of the ventricular septum.

Echocardiography is particularly useful in delineating the presence of a VSD, the gradient across the left ventricular (pulmonary) outflow tract, and the degree of AV valve insufficiency (Fig. 8-6*A* and *B*).

FIGURE 8-5

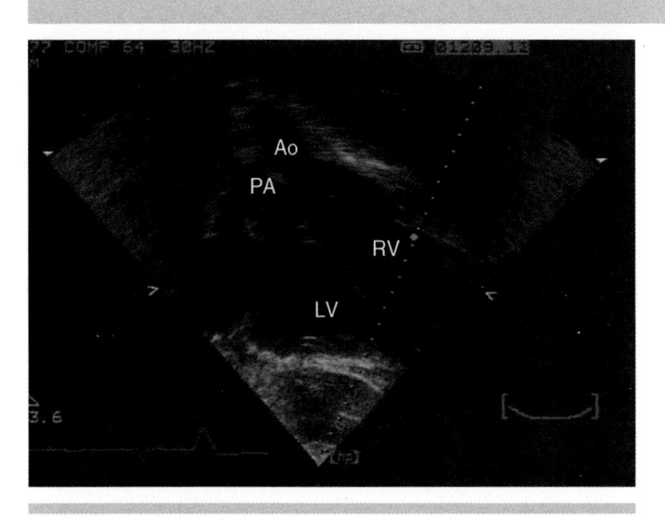

Subcostal long-axis view in a patient with congenitally corrected transposition of the great vessels. Note the pulmonary artery (PA), which arises from the right-sided morphologic left ventricle (LV) and the leftward aorta (Ao), which arises from the morphologic right ventricle (RV).

MANAGEMENT

The management of the patient with L-TGA depends on the associated cardiac defects. In the unusual patient with no other lesions, normal development during childhood and adolescence is expected. Cardiac symptoms may appear in adulthood when left AV valve regurgitation, heart block, or failure of the right (systemic) ventricle may develop.

When significant left AV valve regurgitation is present, valve repair or replacement should be performed before ventricular dysfunction ensues. In contrast to the patient with chronic mitral valve insufficiency in whom medical therapy may forestall surgery for many years, the patient with L-TGA and left AV valve regurgitation appears to be more prone to develop early irreversible ventricular dysfunction. When surgery for left AV valve regurgitation is performed, the abnormalities of the valve (such as Ebstein-like attachment) are less amenable to repair; valve replacement is often required, and the overall results are less satisfactory when compared with mitral valve replacement in patients with normal ventricular anatomy.

Patients with primary failure of the morphologic right ventricle, or those with advanced ventricular dysfunction secondary to AV valve insufficiency, are managed with digitalis, diuretics, and angiotensin-converting enzyme (ACE) inhibitors. A recent surgical approach for such patients is the "double switch" operation consisting of an arterial switch and an intra-arterial Senning or Mustard procedure (Chapter 12). Normal pulmonary and aortic valves and a "prepared" high pressure left ventricle are required. However, for most severely ill patients, cardiac transplantation may be the only feasible option.

The incidence of heart block increases with the age of the patient with L-TGA. The onset is unpredictable and is sometimes preceded by abnormalities of the AV conduction system such as second-degree AV block. Occurrence after surgery has been frequent in the past. The onset of complete heart block warrants insertion of a permanent pacemaker. Patients with concomitant AV valve regurgitation especially benefit from dual-chambered pacing to maintain AV synchrony.

FIGURE 8-6*A*

Apical four-chamber view in an adult with congenitally corrected transposition of the great arteries, showing an enlarged systemic morphologic RV (MRV) on the left side. The tricuspid valve is attached to the large left atrium. The small morphologic left ventricle (MLV) is on the right and connects to the right atrium through a mitral valve. MRV, morphologic right ventricle; MLV, morphologic left ventricle; RA, right atrium; LA, left atrium.

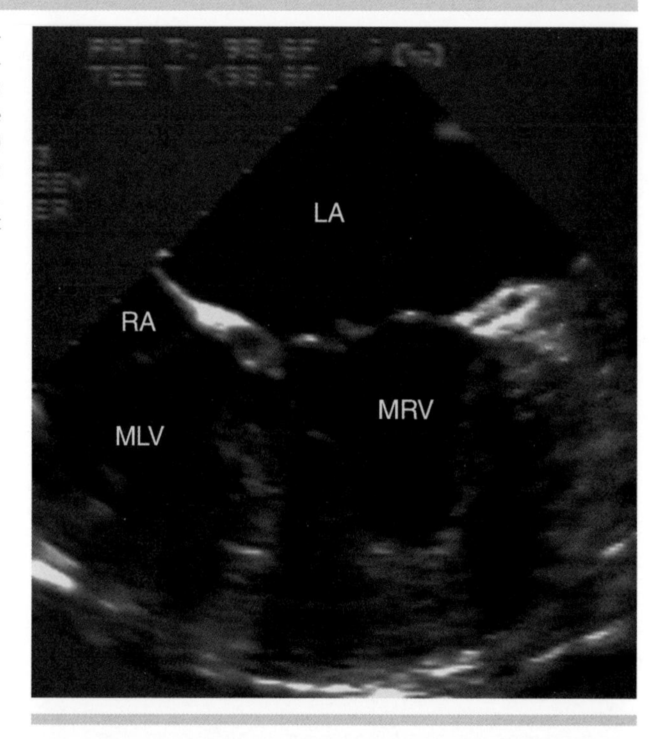

FIGURE 8-6*B*

Color Doppler from an apical four-chamber view in the same patient as in Fig. 8-6*A*, showing severe left AV valve regurgitation from the systemic right ventricle into the left atrium. MLV, morphologic left ventricle; MRV, morphologic right ventricle.

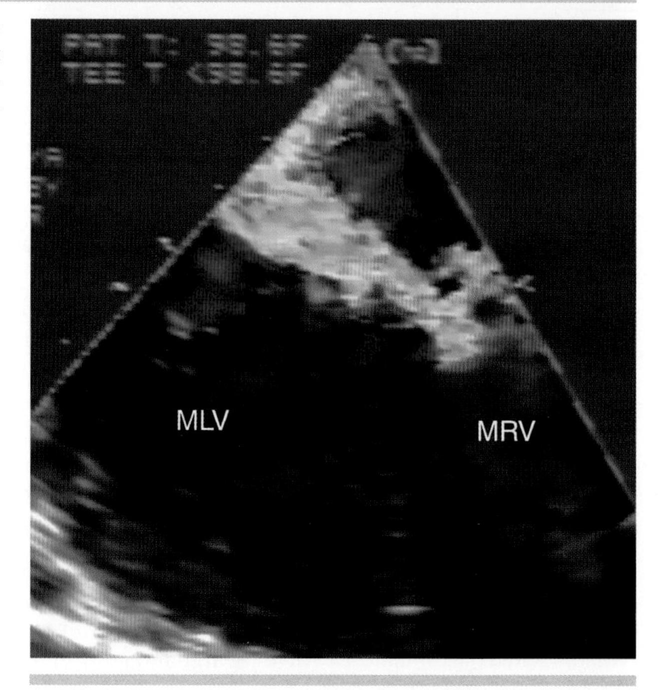

L-TGA with a Ventricular Septal Defect

Patients with L-TGA, a large unrestricted VSD, and pulmonary hypertension develop heart failure during infancy. The defect will require urgent surgical closure, if congestive heart failure cannot be adequately controlled, but as with any large VSD, surgery should be done within the first two years to prevent pulmonary vascular obstructive disease. Because of the operative risk for heart block, some patients may have undergone pulmonary artery banding initially and VSD closure later in life. Nevertheless, some of these patients may have developed heart block as a result of the VSD closure.

Patients with a large unrestricted VSD who were not treated by either pulmonary artery banding or VSD closure early in life usually develop pulmonary vascular obstructive disease. As this progresses, the magnitude of the left-to-right shunt across the VSD decreases. Further increases in pulmonary vascular resistance ultimately result in reversal of the shunt through the VSD whereby a proportion of the desaturated systemic venous blood contributes to systemic cardiac output. This is the same process that occurs with Eisenmenger's disease in non–L-TGA patients.

The patient who has significant pulmonary hypertension with a Q_p/Q_s of 1.5 to 2.0 and mild to moderately elevated pulmonary vascular resistance may still be a candidate for VSD closure. However, once the Q_p/Q_s is less than 1.5, VSD closure is contraindicated because elimination of the defect prevents right-to-left shunting which is necessary to maintain systemic cardiac output in the presence of fixed pulmonary vascular resistance. The approach to management of such patients is similar to that for other forms of Eisenmenger's syndrome (see Chap. 16).

L-TGA with a Ventricular Septal Defect and Pulmonary Stenosis

When both a VSD and pulmonic stenosis coexist in patients with L-TGA, management depends on the degree of pulmonary outflow obstruction. If stenosis is severe, pulmonary blood flow is diminished and patients are cyanotic as a result of right-to-left shunting across the VSD into the aorta. By adulthood, most of these patients have already undergone either a systemic-to-pulmonary-artery shunt to increase pulmonary blood flow, or open heart repair with VSD closure and relief of pulmonary obstruction. The latter almost invariably would have required a valved or nonvalved conduit or homograft from the pulmonary ventricle to the pulmonary artery (see Fig. 8-1*B*). Surgical relief of pulmonary obstruction without a conduit is usually not feasible because obstruction is most often subpulmonic and wedged between the right and left AV valves. Not only is the repair technically difficult, but complete heart block is almost inevitable. In recent years, the atrial switch–Rastelli procedure (see Chap. 11) has been utilized at some centers. This allows the anatomic left ventricle to become the systemic ventricle. In rare instances, the pulmonary outflow obstruction is valvar and can be managed by surgical valvotomy without a conduit.

Patients in whom the degree of pulmonary obstruction is moderate may have enough pulmonary stenosis to prevent either extremes of right-to-left shunting with cyanosis and polycythemia, or significant left-to-right shunting with pulmonary hypertension and volume overload of the systemic ventricle. These "well-balanced" patients are often asymptomatic without surgery. Examination usually reveals no cyanosis, with a grade III to IV systemic murmur across the precordium. The murmur reflects both pulmonary obstruction and left-to-right shunting across the VSD.

The clinical course in patients who underwent a modified Blalock-Taussig shunt for severe pulmonary obstruction and a VSD is variable. Although the shunt permits normal growth and development during infancy and early childhood, its palliative effect may be limited by the subsequent development of obstruction at the anastomotic site, causing inadequate pulmonary blood flow, anatomic distortion of one of the pulmonary arteries, or a relative decrease in the shunt secondary to growth of the patient. The development of pulmonary vascular obstructive disease from excessive pulmonary blood flow is rare, because the larger, less well-controlled shunts (Pott's or Waterston procedures) were abandoned many years ago. Once satisfactory palliation has been achieved by an early systemic-to-pulmonary-artery shunt, the next stage in management consists of intracardiac repair of the lesion and takedown of the shunt. The ideal surgical candidates have adequate-sized pulmonary arteries with normal pulmonary vascular resistance and satisfactory ventricular function. Older patients who received shunts during childhood may have subsequently developed pulmonary artery abnormalities, which include preferential flow to one of the pulmonary arteries, pulmonary artery obstruction or hypoplasia at the site of the anastomosis, or pulmonary vascular obstructive disease in one or both of the pulmonary arteries. These complications increase the risk of the open heart repair and, in some cases, preclude further surgical options.

When cardiac surgery is considered for L-TGA with VSD and pulmonary stenosis, a cardiac catheterization is performed to assess ventricular function, the degree of left AV valve regurgitation, pulmonary artery anatomy and pressure, and pulmonary vascular resistance. Biplane ventriculography should be performed with careful attention to catheter placement to avoid artifactual AV valve regurgitation. This may occur because of the vertical orientation of the ventricular septum and its relationship to the left AV valve. A ventriculogram in the pulmonary ventricle is useful to assess the right AV valve, site of pulmonary outflow obstruction, and pulmonary artery anatomy. The latter is especially important if a previous systemic-to-pulmonary artery shunt has distorted the pulmonary artery. Transient and even permanent complete heart block have been reported during cardiac catheterization.

The decision to proceed with intracardiac repair of this lesion requires careful consideration of the relative risks and benefits of the operation. Surgery is invariably necessary in the presence of either a large left-to-right shunt with volume overload of the left heart or, with associated pulmonary stenosis, a right-to-left shunt with cyanosis and polycythemia. The indications for surgery are less well established in "well-balanced" acyanotic patients with sufficient pulmonary obstruction to maintain normal pulmonary artery pressure and prevent volume overload of the left heart. Because these patients are usually asymptomatic, the rationale for surgical repair should be based on long-term benefit. Although surgery eliminates the potential complications of a right-to-left shunt and normalizes the pressure in the systemic venous ventricle, late development of left AV valve insufficiency, dysfunction of the systemic ventricle, and/or conduction abnormalities remain of concern. These problems may be related to changes in ventricular geometry caused by surgical repair, or they may be part of the natural history of the lesion. Thus, the decision to recommend elective surgical repair for the asymptomatic patient with "balanced" hemodynamics remains difficult.

Regardless of treatment, the follow-up of the adult patient with L-TGA should include periodic assessment of systemic ventricular function, status of the left AV valve, and AV conduction system. Assessment of right ventricular function by echocardiography may be difficult and, more recently, cardiac magnetic resonance imaging (MRI) has become an important imaging modality. Antibiotic prophylaxis to prevent bacterial endocarditis is required for all of these patients.

The Postoperative Patient with a Conduit or Homograft

The patient who has undergone a conduit for repair of L-TGA with VSD and pulmonary obstruction should be followed for the future development of obstruction within the conduit or homograft. The surgical repair may have included a left ventricular–pulmonary artery porcine-valved conduit, valveless conduit, or homograft (aortic or pulmonary).

The majority of patients who have had a porcine-valved conduit inserted develop significant obstruction at an average of 10 years following insertion. Reoperation will be required. Although the incidence of obstruction may be lower when a nonvalved conduit is used, this advantage must be weighed against the effects of chronic pulmonary insufficiency. The latter is usually well tolerated for many years in the absence of pulmonary hypertension, especially in L-TGA, where pulmonary regurgitation relates to the low-pressure morphologic left ventricle. Problems with conduit obstruction subsequently led to the use of a pulmonary or aortic homograft to connect the morphologic left ventricle to the pulmonary artery. Although it was hoped that the development of obstruction would be less likely than for the porcine-valved conduit, the reoperation rates and timing may well be similar.

Obstruction in the conduit or homograft is a progressive lesion that usually occurs after many years. Patients are usually asymptomatic or report only exertional fatigue as long as ventricular function is preserved and there is no right-sided AV valve regurgitation. Signs of conduit obstruction are readily detectable by examination. The typical grade 2 systolic ejection murmur, which is uniformly present across the conduit or homograft, gradually increases in intensity and length to grades 3 and 4. Although echocardiography may be useful in assessing the gradient across the conduit or homograft in younger patients, it is less effective in older patients because of imaging problems. An estimate of the pressure in the right-sided ventricle can be calculated by the regurgitant jet, if present, across the right AV valve.

Conduit gradients are referred to as mild (less than 50 mm Hg), moderate (50 to 75 mm Hg), or severe (more than 75 mm Hg). These gradients assume a normal resting cardiac output. Reoperation is indicated in any patient with severe obstruction or in the symptomatic patient with moderate obstruction. Earlier reoperation should also be recommended if ventricular function is depressed or if right-sided AV valve regurgitation is present. Because the right-sided ventricle is the morphologic left ventricle, it is unusual to see ventricular dysfunction as a consequence of conduit obstruction.

When conduit obstruction is suspected, a right-sided cardiac catheterization should be performed to confirm the location and degree of obstruction, and to assess ventricular function. Left heart catheterization and angiography is also indicated. The risk of reoperation for isolated conduit obstruction should be very low if carried out by an experienced congenital heart disease surgeon. Cardiopulmonary bypass is frequently initiated from the iliac vessels prior to the median sternotomy to avoid entering the conduit, which is frequently adherent to the sternum.

SUMMARY

Adult patients with L-TGA may present to the cardiologist or internist as (1) an asymptomatic individual who has had no previous surgical procedures; (2) a postoperative patient following operations for pulmonary stenosis, ventricular septal defect, and/or left AV valve (tricuspid) insufficiency; (3) an asymptomatic patient with left AV valve regurgitation or ventricular dysfunction; or (4) an asymptomatic patient with a rhythm disturbance, usually AV block.

A patient with L-TGA and no associated lesions or AV block may be asymptomatic, and have no significant cardiac findings on physical examination. Thus, such patients may not be recognized until late in life. In some cases, a routine physical examination, chest x-ray, or ECG reveals the L-TGA anatomy. Such patients should be followed regularly. Late manifestations, including acquired heart block, AV valve insufficiency, and/or right ventricular (systemic) ventricular dysfunction have been seen in adults who have been asymptomatic for decades. Yearly evaluations with an ECG and echocardiogram as well as a Holter recording, as indicated, are prudent for such patients. No physical restrictions are required. Women who become pregnant can carry an infant to term. However, the obstetrician and cardiologist must be aware of potential issues related to heart block, AV valve regurgitation, and right ventricular dysfunction.

Postoperative Ventricular Septal Defect and/or Pulmonary Stenosis

Postoperative patients who have no significant residual left-to-right shunt or pulmonary outflow tract obstruction should be followed periodically. Observation for the development of heart block is required. Patients with conduits generally require reoperation, most often within 10 to 12 years. A progressive increase in systolic ejection murmur along the left sternal border and base is an indication of increased conduit obstruction. Echocardiography may be helpful in determining the degree of obstruction, and cardiac catheterization may be necessary. Severe obstruction may ensue prior to symptoms, emphasizing the need for frequent evaluations.

Left Atrioventricular Valve Insufficiency

Left AV valve insufficiency may be part of the natural history of a patient with L-TGA. In addition, abnormalities may be exacerbated by surgery for other associated defects. Valve replacement may be necessary earlier than for patients who have mitral insufficiency with normal ventricular anatomy because systemic right ventricular performance appears to be more adversely affected by tricuspid valve disease.

Algorithm 8–1
L-TGA Unoperated

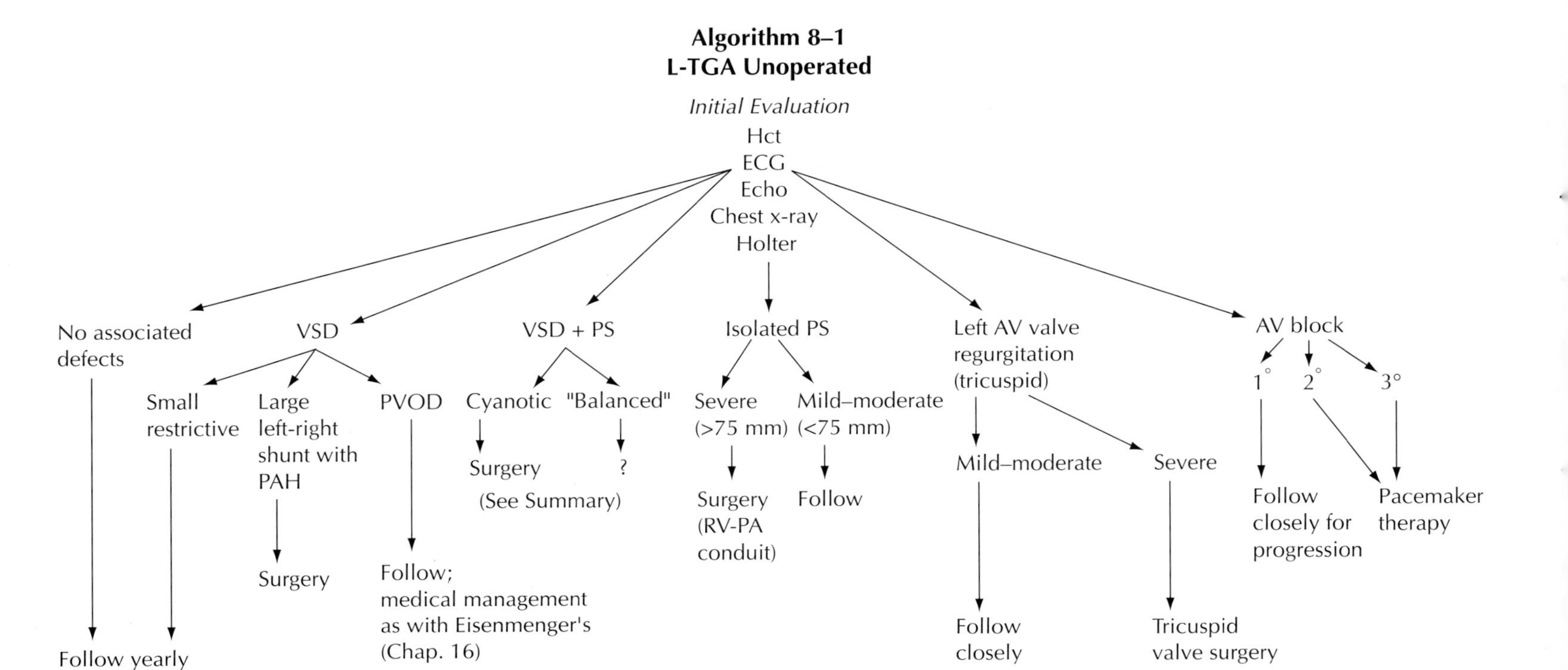

KEY: AV, atrioventricular; ECG, electrocardiogram; Echo, echocardiogram; PA, pulmonary artery; PAH, pulmonary artery hypertension; PS, pulmonary stenosis; PVOD, pulmonary vascular obstructive disease; RV, right ventricle; VSD, ventricular septal defect.

Cardiac Arrhythmias

Patients with L-TGA and various degrees of heart block or tachyarrhythmias should be treated similarly to other patients with these findings. If complete heart block occurs immediately after cardiac surgery, pacemaker therapy should be instituted immediately. In patients who have not undergone surgery, complete heart block is also an indication for a pacemaker. Other types of AV conduction abnormalities may also require pacemaker placement, depending on their type and severity.

Algorithm 8–2
L-TGA Operated

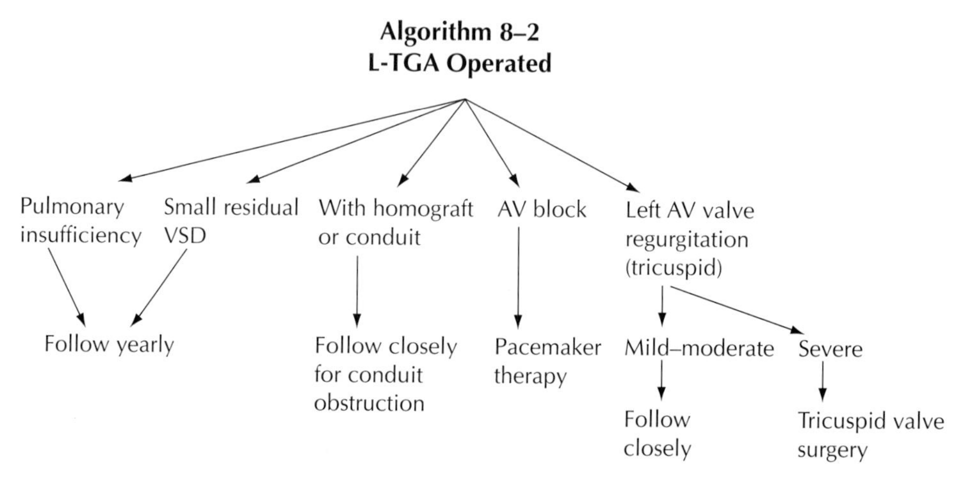

KEY: AV, atrioventricular; VSD, ventricular septal defect.

BIBLIOGRAPHY

Anderson KR, Danielson GK, McGoon DW, Lie JT: Ebstein's anomaly of the left-sided tricuspid valve. Pathological anatomy of the valvular malformation. *Circulation* 58:87, 1978.

Anderson RH, Becker AE, Arnold R, Wilkinson JL: The conducting tissues in congenitally corrected transposition. *Circulation* 50:911, 1974.

Anderson RH, Becker AE, Losekoot TG, Gerlis LM: Anatomically corrected malposition of great arteries. *Br Heart J* 37:993, 1975.

Connelly MS, Liu PP, Williams WG, et al: Congenitally corrected transposition in the adult. Functional status and complications. *J Am Coll Cardiol* 27:1238, 1996.

de Laval MR, Bastons P, Stark J, et al: Surgical technique to reduce the risks of heart block following closure of ventricular septal defect in atrioventricular discordance. *J Thorac Cardiovasc Surg* 78:515, 1979.

Di Donato R, Troconis CJ, Marino B, et al: Combined Mustard and Rastelli operations. An alternative approach for repair of associated anomalies in congenitally corrected transposition in situs inversus [I,D,D]. *J Thorac Cardiovasc Surg* 104:1246, 1992.

Geva T, Sanders SP, Ayres NA, et al: Two-dimensional echocardiographic anatomy of atrioventricular alignment discordance with situs concordance. *Am Heart J* 125:459, 1993.

Graham TP Jr, Bernard YD, Mellen BG, et al: Long-term outcome in congenitally corrected transposition of the great arteries: A multi-institutional study. *J Am Coll Cardiol* 36:255, 2000.

Horvath P, Szufladowicz M, de Leval MR, et al: Tricuspid valve abnormalities in patients with atrioventricular discordance: Surgical implications. *Ann Thorac Surg* 57:941, 1994.

Huhta JC, Maloney JD, Ritter DG et al: Complete atrioventricular block in patients with atrioventricular discordance. *Circulation* 67:1374, 1983.

Ikeda U, Furuse M, Suzuki I, et al: Long-term survival in aged patients with corrected transposition of the great arteries. *Chest* 101:1382, 1992.

Ikeda U, Kimura K, Suzuki O, et al: Long-term survival in "corrected transposition." *Lancet* 337:180, 1991.

Imai Y, Sawatari K, Hoshino S, et al: Ventricular function after anatomic repair in patients with atrioventricular discordance. *J Thorac Cardiovasc Surg* 107:1272, 1994.

Krongrad E, Ellis K, Steeg CN, et al: Subpulmonary obstruction in congenitally corrected transposition of the great arteries due to ventricular membranous septal aneurysms. *Circulation* 54:679, 1976.

Lundstrom U, Bull C, Wyse RK, Somerville J: The natural and "unnatural" history of congenitally corrected transposition. *Am J Cardiol* 65:1222, 1990.

Melero-Pita A, Alonso-Pardo F, Bardaji-Mayer JL, Higueras J: Corrected transposition of the great arteries. *N Engl J Med* 334:866, 1996.

Presbitero P, Sommerville J, Rabajoli F, et al: Corrected transposition of the great arteries without associated defects in adult patients: Clinical profile and follow up. *Br Heart J* 74:57, 1995.

Prieto LR, Hordof AJ, Secic M, et al: Progressive tricuspid valve disease in patients with congenitally corrected transposition of the great arteries. *Circulation* 98:997–1005.

Van Praagh R, Durnin R, Jockin H, et al: Anatomically corrected malposition of the great arteries (S, D, L). *Circulation* 51:20, 1975.

van Son JA, Danielson GK, Huhta JC, et al: Late results of systemic atrioventricular valve replacement in corrected transposition. *J Thorac Cardiovasc Surg* 109(4):642–52, 1995.

Westerman GR, Lang P, Castaneda AR, Norwood WI: Corrected transposition and repair of associated intracardiac defects. *Circulation* 66:1197, 1982.

Williams WG, Suri R, Shindo G, et al: Repair of major intracardiac anomalies associated with atrioventricular discordance. *Ann Thorac Surg* 31:527, 1981.

Yagihara T, Kishimoto H, Isobe F, et al: Double switch operation in cardiac anomalies with atrioventricular and ventriculoarterial discordance. *J Thorac Cardiovasc Surg* 107:351, 1994.

CHAPTER 9

CONGENITAL ANOMALIES OF THE CORONARY CIRCULATION

There are several important forms of congenital coronary artery anomalies, as follows: (1) anomalies associated with abnormal origin of the coronary arteries, (2) anomalous origin of a coronary artery from the pulmonary artery, (3) coronary artery fistula, and (4) coronary artery abnormalities associated with specific forms of congenital heart disease.

I. ANOMALIES ASSOCIATED WITH ABNORMAL ORIGIN OF THE CORONARY ARTERIES FROM THE AORTIC SINUSES

The normal coronary artery consists of a left main coronary artery (LMCA), which originates from the left aortic sinus and runs posterior to the pulmonary root before dividing into the left anterior descending and circumflex coronary arteries. The right coronary artery (RCA) originates from the right aortic sinus and runs posteriorly in the right atrioventricular groove. It supplies blood flow to the right ventricle and, when the artery is dominant, the inferior portion of the ventricular septum and variable portions of the inferoposterior left ventricle.

Although there are a number of different anomalies involving the origin of the coronary arteries from the aortic sinuses, only two appear to be clinically important because of their association with acute coronary artery ischemia and sudden death: (1) origin of the LMCA from the right coronary sinus, and (2) origin of the RCA from the left aortic sinus.

ANOMALOUS ORIGIN OF THE LEFT MAIN CORONARY ARTERY FROM THE RIGHT CORONARY SINUS

When the LMCA originates from the right coronary sinus, the artery may reach the left ventricle by coursing either anteriorly or posteriorly between the aortic and pulmonary roots. An anterior course of the left coronary artery is not associated with clinical manifestations. However, when the LMCA courses posteriorly (Fig. 9-1*A* and *B*), the abnormality has been associated with coronary ischemia and sudden death in young athletes. In one study involving 43 patients with this abnormality, 34 of the deaths were cardiac in origin, 76% occurred in patients who were younger than 20 years of age, and all but one of the patients died during or immediately after vigorous exertion.

Although the exact mechanism of sudden death in these patients has not been conclusively determined, the problem is considered to be related to the abnormal takeoff of the LMCA from the right coronary sinus. Ischemia results from inadequate blood flow through a slit-like opening in the LMCA or from compression of the coronary artery by the expanding aorta during exercise against the stationary pulmonary trunk, or both.

Clinical Features

Patients with anomalies of the coronary arteries are most often asymptomatic. Therefore, the diagnosis of this entity can be difficult, especially if there are no clinical indications. The *physical examination* is unrevealing, and the resting *electrocardiogram* (ECG) is often normal. Although exercise testing with or without thallium is commonly used to evaluate young patients who have symptoms of chest pain, unexplained dyspnea, and exertional syncope, these studies most often are not sufficiently sensitive to detect patients with this form of anomaly, and this may be the case even in symptomatic patients.

Echocardiography can be useful in patients in whom the proximal course of the coronary arteries can be mapped; both transthoracic and transesophageal techniques are required. The diagnosis can be suspected by failure to demonstrate the LMCA from its usual location in the left coronary sinus and by visualization of the ostia and proximal segment of two coronary arteries from the right sinus. In addition, it is possible to trace an anomalous LMCA on short-axis views as it courses between the aortic and pulmonary roots. Exercise echocardiographic studies may or may not be useful. *Cardiac catheterization* with angiography defines the anatomy.

Management

Once the diagnosis has been made, surgery is indicated to prevent sudden death or myocardial ischemia. Several surgical approaches have been utilized, including (1) coronary

FIGURE 9-1

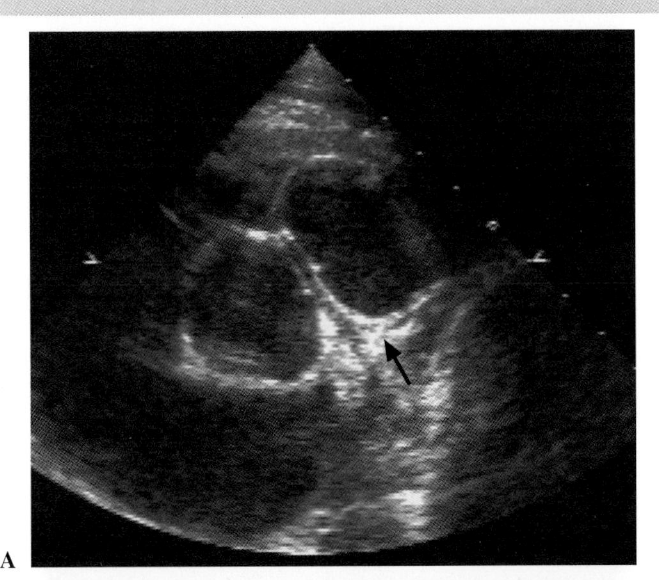

A

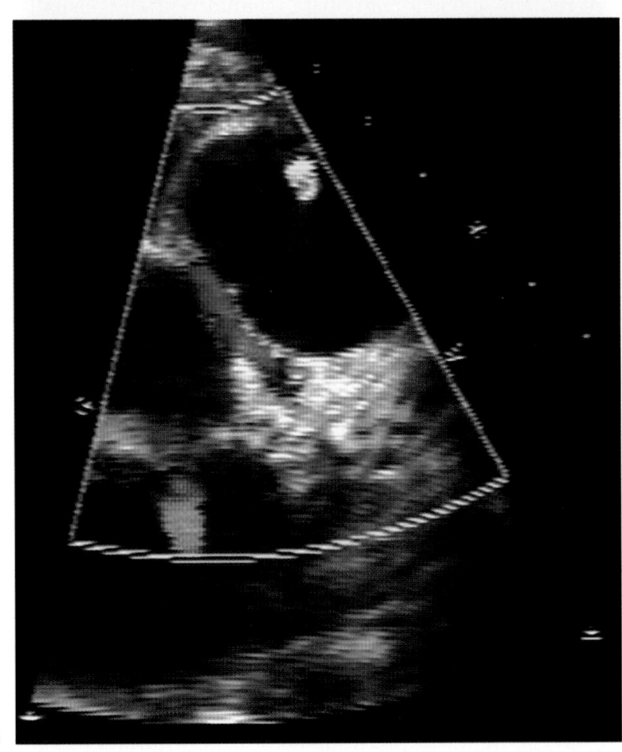

B

Parasternal short-axis view from an adolescent with chest pain. The left main coronary artery arises from the right coronary sinus and traverses posteriorly between the aorta and the pulmonary artery. *A*. Two-dimensional image showing the left main coronary artery and bifurcation (arrow) into the left anterior descending and circumflex arteries. *B*. Color Doppler study showing the coronary artery in between the two great vessels.

artery bypass grafting to the left anterior descending and circumflex arteries, (2) enlargement of the narrowed left main coronary ostium by extending the incision from the ostium through the common wall of the aorta and the anomalous artery, and (3) incising the artery as it courses along the left sinus of Valsalva.

ANOMALOUS ORIGIN OF THE RIGHT CORONARY ARTERY FROM THE LEFT SINUS OF VALSALVA OR FROM THE LEFT MAIN CORONARY ARTERY

It is postulated that this entity may also be responsible for sudden cardiac death or acute myocardial ischemia in young patients. However, there is conflicting evidence about the risks of this anomaly. In an autopsy study of 26 patients, there was no evidence that death was related to this abnormality. However, in another study of 34 patients in whom the diagnosis was made during coronary angiography, symptoms of coronary artery ischemia were present in 12 patients in the absence of atherosclerosis.

The potential mechanism for coronary ischemia is compression of the RCA between the aortic and pulmonary root or the slit-like orifice of the anomalous right coronary artery, or both. Optimal treatment remains unclear, and operative intervention is usually reserved for patients in whom there are clinical signs of myocardial ischemia.

II. ANOMALOUS ORIGIN OF A CORONARY ARTERY FROM THE PULMONARY ARTERY

Anomalous origin of the left coronary artery from the pulmonary artery is an uncommon entity in which the LMCA originates from the pulmonary trunk. Fetal development is unaffected by this abnormality, because coronary artery perfusion pressure into the left coronary artery is maintained by the hypertensive pulmonary artery and there are no significant differences in oxygen saturation between the blood originating in the pulmonary artery and the aorta. The drop in pulmonary vascular resistance during early infancy sets the stage for the clinical manifestations of this defect.

The clinical manifestations are related to the left coronary artery perfusion pressure which, in turn, is determined by the pulmonary artery pressure and by the adequacy of the coronary artery collateral blood vessels from the right coronary artery.

Shortly after birth, antegrade flow into the left coronary artery is maintained from the hypertensive pulmonary artery. As the pulmonary vascular resistance normally declines and pulmonary artery pressure falls, coronary artery perfusion of the left coronary artery diminishes as a result of a gradual reversal in the direction of blood flow. Initially myocardial perfusion is from the pulmonary artery and, subsequently, from the RCA via collaterals into the left coronary artery. Once the perfusion pressure falls below that of the RCA, collateral flow from the RCA provides blood flow into the left coronary system with retrograde flow from the left coronary artery into the pulmonary artery. Despite the collateral flow, there is a decline in left coronary artery perfusion pressure and potential for a coronary artery "steal" via the left main trunk into the retrogradely filling pulmonary artery. This results in myocardial ischemia, myocardial infarction, and mitral regurgitation. If collateral vessels are not present, ischemia may occur earlier and is more severe.

Patients present with one of the following clinical patterns: (1) fatal intractable heart failure and/or ischemia during infancy in the absence of surgical intervention, (2) early heart failure with spontaneous improvement, or (3) few or no early symptoms and survival into adulthood.

Anomalous origin of the right coronary artery from the pulmonary artery is less often encountered. Patients with this anomaly are almost never recognized prior to adolescence or adulthood. They present with chest pain during exercise or stress.

CLINICAL FEATURES

Infancy and Childhood

Almost all patients with anomalous origin of the left coronary artery from the pulmonary artery are severely symptomatic during infancy. A 1-year mortality rate of 65 to 90% has been reported without surgical intervention. Symptoms are not usually seen before 2 months of age, presumably because pulmonary vascular resistance remains high enough to maintain adequate left coronary artery perfusion pressure. After this age, signs of severe congestive heart failure develop, with evidence of coronary ischemia, myocardial infarction, and mitral regurgitation secondary to papillary muscle infarction. Symptoms, which consist of dyspnea, irritability, wheezing, pallor, and sweating, are typically provoked by the stress of eating, bowel movements, or crying. Untreated, the patients will most often die within the first year of life. However, a small percentage of patients have early heart failure and improve spontaneously. It is hypothesized that these patients improve because collateral blood flow increases, and ventricular and mitral valve function improve.

Adult Patients

Approximately 10 to 15% of patients with this entity do not develop severe congestive heart failure during infancy and reach adolescence and young adulthood without major cardiac consequences. These patients typically come to medical attention because of symptoms of exertional angina, dyspnea, palpitations, or a murmur of mitral regurgitation. An occasional patient may present with sudden death. The patients who reach adulthood without surgical intervention presumably have the most well-developed collateral vessels from the RCA in this spectrum and possibly a more dominant RCA that supplies a greater portion of the left ventricle than is usually the case. Despite the left-to-right shunt from the aorta to the right and left coronaries into the pulmonary arteries, the myocardium is well perfused owing to rich collateralization. However, symptoms may occur during exercise when demand is greater. A significant, large left-to-right shunt is not present.

Physical Examination

The clinical findings are related to the clinical presentation. Patients who present during infancy invariably have severe congestive heart failure with severe left ventricular dysfunction and significant mitral regurgitation secondary to papillary muscle infarction or dysfunction from ischemia. A small percentage of patients have a continuous murmur resulting from left-to-right shunting from the coronary artery system into the pulmonary artery.

Adults may demonstrate a nonspecific systolic murmur with varying degrees of mitral regurgitation. A continuous murmur may be heard over the left upper sternal border, occasionally mimicking a patent ductus arteriosus.

Noninvasive Studies

In infants with congestive heart failure from anomalous origin of the left coronary artery, ECG typically shows prominent Q waves and T wave inversions in leads I and aVL. These abnormalities in an infant are often helpful in distinguishing this entity from cardiomyopathy. In an infant with congestive failure these ECG abnormalities are of sufficient concern to warrant additional studies to establish whether the diagnosis of an anomalous left coronary from the pulmonary artery is present.

In the adult, the ECG is nearly always abnormal and may range from nonspecific ST abnormalities to evidence of an old anterolateral myocardial infarction. An exercise thallium study is usually abnormal.

The diagnosis can usually be made with *echocardiography*, but these studies require considerable skill. Two-dimensional imaging alone may fail to detect 50% of these defects, but the addition of color flow mapping adds considerably to the diagnostic accuracy. Direct visualization of the anomalous connection can be limited by deficiencies in lateral resolution and may give the false impression that the LMCA is originating from the aortic sinus. Color flow mapping is helpful in establishing the diagnosis by demonstrating retrograde flow from the left coronary artery into the pulmonary artery (Fig. 9-2). In some cases, the diagnosis remains uncertain and angiography must be performed to establish the diagnosis.

Echocardiography may also show abnormalities of the left ventricle, including endocardial fibroelastosis, mitral annular dilation with mitral regurgitation, left ventricular aneurysm formation, and hypoplasia of the left coronary artery system. In addition, dilation of the RCA is often seen.

Cardiac Catheterization

Selective angiography of the RCA shows a dilated coronary artery with right-to-left collateral filling of the LMCA and retrograde filling of the pulmonary artery. Branch coro-

FIGURE 9-2

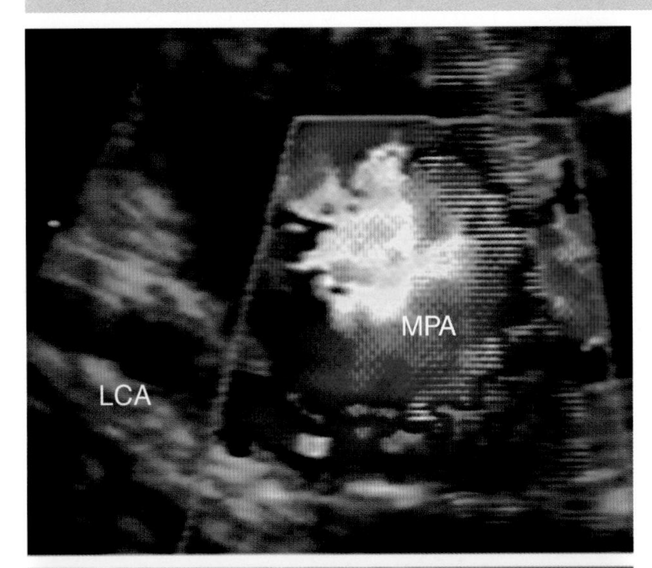

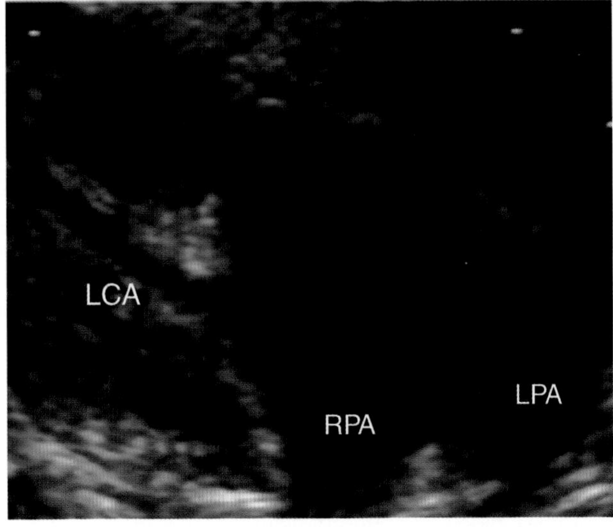

Parasternal short-axis view in a patient with anomalous origin of the left coronary artery from the pulmonary artery. (*Top*) In the color Doppler study, the red color represents retrograde flow from the left coronary artery into the pulmonary artery. (*Bottom*) The same view without color, showing the left coronary artery entering the main pulmonary artery. LCA, left coronary artery; LPA, left pulmonary artery; MPA, main pulmonary artery; RPA, right pulmonary artery.

nary filling is excellent. This produces a small-to-moderate left-to-right shunt into the pulmonary artery. The RCA is usually, but not always, dilated. In the distressed infant, the left ventricle is dilated and dysfunctional with significant mitral regurgitation. The adult who presents with an aberrant left coronary artery will have excellent collateral coronary blood flow (Fig. 9-3).

FIGURE 9-3

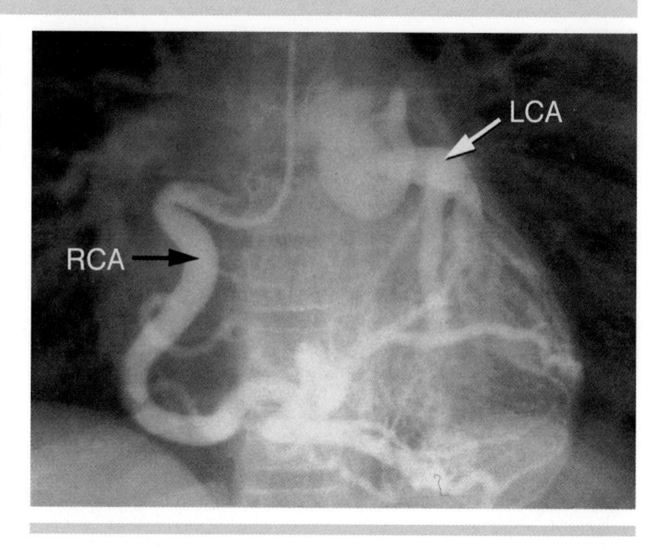

A right coronary artery injection in a patient with an "adult-type" anomalous left coronary artery from the pulmonary artery. The right coronary artery is massively dilated; there is a significant shunt from the right coronary artery into the pulmonary artery via collaterals to the left coronary artery. LCA, left coronary artery; RCA, right coronary artery.

MANAGEMENT

Infants with anomalous origin of the left coronary artery who present with left ventricular dysfunction and congestive heart failure require urgent surgery, and in experienced centers, survival rates are high. Early surgical techniques included several types of interventions to improve left coronary blood flow without attempting to reimplant the left coronary artery into the aorta. These included pulmonary artery banding to increase perfusion pressure into the left coronary artery; anastomosis of a turned-down left common carotid artery into the left coronary artery, which was detached from the pulmonary trunk; a left subclavian artery anastomosis to the left coronary artery; and coronary artery bypass to the left coronary artery after closing the proximal end to the pulmonary trunk.

Simple ligation of the left coronary artery at the origin of the pulmonary trunk with the purpose of eliminating the coronary artery "steal" into the low-pressure pulmonary artery was most often used in infants. This procedure usually resulted in survival and improvement of critically ill infants who had severe congestive heart failure and myocardial ischemia because of significant coronary blood flow into the pulmonary artery.

Surgical Repair

The current surgical approach is to reestablish a system of two coronary arteries by transferring the left coronary artery from the pulmonary root into the aortic sinus. Direct reimplantation of the anomalous left coronary artery from the pulmonary root to the native aortic sinus was first reported in 1972. Initially, this procedure was only available for older children and adults, but surgical techniques improved to the degree that reimplantation is now the procedure of choice in all patients, even the smallest infant. Rarely, when reimplantation is not considered feasible because of the distance from the pulmonary trunk to the aortic sinus, a technique has been employed that consists of an arterial graft tunnel within the main pulmonary artery to the ostium of the LMCA (Takeuchi procedure).

The early postoperative course in infants with advanced left ventricular dysfunction and mitral regurgitation is typically associated with low cardiac output with the need for significant inotropic support including, in some instances, the use of a ventricular assist device. Despite rather severe preoperative myocardial dysfunction and mitral regurgitation, successful surgery usually results in decreased mitral insufficiency and substantial improvement in left ventricular function. Occasionally, significant mitral regurgitation persists that may require late reoperation.

LONG-TERM FOLLOW-UP

The functional status of postoperative survivors is generally good. There is substantial improvement in the left ventricular function. Careful long-term follow-up is required in these patients to demonstrate the absence of coronary ischemia. Mitral insufficiency most often improves with time.

A tunnel repair can produce obstruction above the pulmonary valve, a fistula between the tunnel and the proximal pulmonary artery, and obstruction between the tunnel and the LMCA anastomosis. Surgical repair using an arterial or venous conduit may also be susceptible to anastomotic problems, and the potential for coronary artery ischemia will need to be assessed. However, a successful standard reimplantation procedure is rarely associated with late complications, although residual mitral insufficiency must be followed.

III. CORONARY ARTERY FISTULA

A coronary artery fistula is a communication between a coronary artery and another portion of the heart. Most coronary artery fistulas drain into the right side of the heart, including the right atrium, coronary sinus, right ventricle, and pulmonary artery. The left atrium and left ventricle are involved less frequently. The involved coronary artery typically shows marked dilation of the proximal segments.

CLINICAL FEATURES

The clinical manifestations of a coronary artery fistula are related to the size of the communication and may vary from negligible for the smallest fistulas to severe, in the case of the rare patient who has a large left-to-right shunt with volume overload. A communication between the coronary artery and the right side of the heart produces a left-to-right shunt of variable proportion. A fistula that enters the left atrium or left ventricle does not have increased pulmonary blood flow, but results in additional volume in the left heart. Multiple exit sites for the fistula have been described.

The detection of a coronary artery fistula is often related to the size of the defect. It may be an incidental finding having no clinical manifestations in patients with a small communication, or produce symptoms in patients with overt evidence of a hemodynamically significant arteriovenous connection. After childhood, the major concern is myocardial ischemia, secondary to a "steal" of coronary blood flow into a low resistance chamber or vessel. This may become manifest during exercise.

Physical Examination

The murmur is usually continuous and maximal at the left or right mid- or lower sternal border. This location helps to distinguish this anomaly from a patent ductus arteriosus, which can usually be heard best at the second left intercostal space and more lateral to the sternal border. Other types of anomalies that may produce a continuous murmur include ruptured sinus of Valsalva aneurysm into the right or left atrium, or right ventricle; collateral blood flow associated with an aortic coarctation; and a systemic arteriovenous fistula involving the chest or lung. Continuous murmurs must be differentiated from to-and-fro murmurs over the aortic or pulmonary valves.

Noninvasive Evaluation and Cardiac Catheterization

The diagnosis can often be established by echocardiography, which may show marked dilation of the involved coronary artery as well as abnormal color flow at the entrance of the fistula into the heart. Cardiac catheterization will assess the hemodynamics and magnitude of shunt. Coronary angiography will disclose specific anatomic details of the coronary artery and coronary branches and their relationship to the exit site of the fistula into the heart (Fig. 9-4). Often multiple sites are present, and this has surgical implications.

MANAGEMENT

When a coronary artery fistula has been diagnosed by the presence of a continuous murmur, closure of the fistula is usually advised. The arguments for closure include prevention of endocarditis, and to eliminate the potential for progressive enlargement, rupture, thromboembolic complications, and late myocardial ischemia. The operative results at specialized centers are good. Closure of the fistula may be accomplished with suture ligation; however, cardiopulmonary bypass may be required to close the defect at its insertion site within a cardiac chamber. Coronary artery bypass graft may be necessary to maintain viability of a vessel that has been compromised secondary to more proximal ligation.

Patients in whom extremely small coronary artery fistulae are recognized as an incidental finding during coronary angiography or with improved sensitivity of echocardiography likely have a more favorable natural history that may not require intervention. In some patients, interventional techniques during cardiac catheterization have been used successfully without compromising important coronary vessels to close the fistula.

FIGURE 9-4

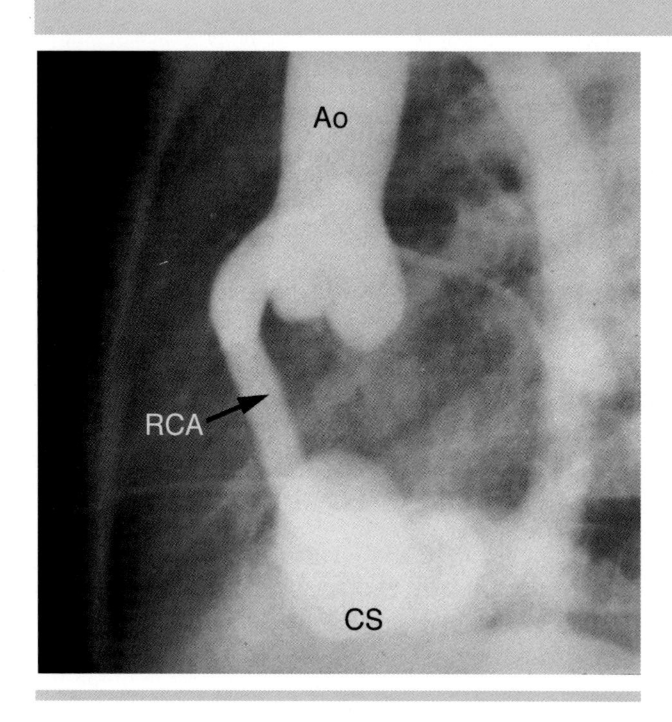

Ascending aortogram demonstrating a coronary artery fistula from the right coronary artery to the coronary sinus. Note the massive dilatation of the right coronary artery. Ao, aorta; CS, coronary sinus; RCA, right coronary artery.

IV. CORONARY ARTERY ABNORMALITIES ASSOCIATED WITH CONGENITAL HEART DISEASE

Several important forms of congenital heart disease are associated with coronary artery anomalies which can have major implications on the surgical repair. These abnormalities are particularly important in patients with tetralogy of Fallot, D-transposition of the great arteries (D-TGA), and pulmonary atresia with an intact ventricular septum.

TETRALOGY OF FALLOT

Coronary artery anomalies have been reported in 18 to 31% of patients with tetralogy of Fallot, and there may be important surgical implications associated with these abnormalities. All of the anomalies involve the presence of a large coronary artery crossing the right ventricular outflow tract just below the pulmonary valve. These include the takeoff of the left anterior descending artery from the right coronary artery, the presence of a large conus branch across the right ventricular outflow tract, a paired anterior descending coronary artery off the right coronary artery, and origin of both coronary arteries from a single left ostium. In all of these situations, the potential exists that the coronary artery can be damaged or severed during a right ventriculotomy to correct right ventricular outflow tract obstruction.

This complication is rarely encountered today because the majority of tetralogy of Fallot repairs are performed using a transatrial approach, or a limited right ventriculotomy. In patients operated on during the 1960s and 1970s who had these coronary artery anomalies, the surgical approach included the use of a conduit from the anterior right ventricle to the pulmonary artery to avoid damaging the coronary artery.

PULMONARY ATRESIA WITH AN INTACT VENTRICULAR SEPTUM

In this lesion, embryonic sinusoids within the right ventricle may persist and communicate with the epicardial coronary arteries in a variety of ways. Usually this occurs in patients with tiny right ventricular chambers and severe right ventricular hypertrophy (see Chap. 5). The communications may feed one or both of the coronary arteries and may be associated with coronary stenosis either proximal or distal to the insertion site of the fistulous communications, or both. In some patients with coronary stenosis, the coronary fistulous connections are sufficiently well developed to produce a right ventricular–dependent coronary circulation. An angiogram in the right ventricular cavity is required to demonstrate retrograde filling of one or more coronary arteries via the fistulous connection. Coronary angiography is carried out to determine if the left ventricular myocardium is normally perfused, or whether significant segments are perfused from the right ventricle through myocardial sinusoids. It is essential to identify this abnormality prior to surgical repair because decompression of the right ventricle to relieve right ventricular outflow tract obstruction reduces right ventricular pressure and coronary artery perfusion, which may result in major coronary artery ischemia and infarction at the time of surgery.

Patients who have pulmonary atresia with an intact ventricular septum usually require an early systemic-pulmonary shunt and, if the tricuspid valve and right ventricular chamber have growth potential, surgical relief of pulmonary atresia. If the right ventricle is minuscule, a Fontan procedure is the ultimate treatment. However, if the myocardium is perfused via the right ventricle through sinusoids because of stenotic coronary arteries, then a systemic right ventricle must be preserved as part of the Fontan operation. Cardiac transplantation may be the only option for some of these patients.

D-TRANSPOSITION OF THE GREAT ARTERIES

The current management for patients with a simple D-TGA or a D-TGA with a ventricular septal defect is an arterial switch operation during the neonatal period (see Chap. 11). In this anomaly, the aorta arises from the right ventricle and the pulmonary artery from the left ventricle. During the arterial switch procedure, the coronary arteries are transferred from the anterior semilunar root to the posterior root to reestablish an anatomic connection between the left ventricle and the aorta. The success of the operation relies on coronary artery transfer without compromising the blood supply of the coronary circulation.

Seven different coronary artery patterns have been recognized in patients with D-TGA, but normal anatomy is most often present. Early studies identified certain unusual coronary artery patterns that were associated with increased mortality. However, the specific coronary artery pattern has assumed less importance today as surgical experience with this operation has advanced. The presence of an intramural coronary artery remains a difficult challenge for the surgeon. An intramural coronary artery refers to a segment of coronary artery that courses within the wall of the aorta without a separate layer of adventitial tissue between the coronary artery and the aorta. Although follow-up angiograms after the arterial switch operation have shown varying coronary artery abnormalities in approximately 10% of patients, the vast majority of the patients are asymptomatic. However, patients have yet to be followed beyond early adulthood.

SUMMARY

Congenital anomalies of the coronary circulation may be isolated or associated with other forms of congenital heart disease. The most important anomaly related to the origin of the LMCA is when the left coronary artery originates from the right coronary sinus and courses posteriorly between the aortic and pulmonary roots. The vessel may be impinged upon, and acute myocardial ischemia and death may occur suddenly without a history of earlier symptoms. The defect is difficult to discover either by physical examination or by noninvasive studies, including exercise testing. The risk of other forms of abnormal origin of the coronary artery or single coronary arteries appears to be less.

Anomalous origin of the left coronary artery from the pulmonary artery is an important congenital abnormality. It is most often manifested in early infancy by myocardial infarction because of poor perfusion of the myocardium when pulmonary artery pressure falls shortly after birth. When rich collateral blood flow is present, a "steal" from the coronary circulation into the pulmonary artery may result in myocardial ischemia. However, some patients have an extremely well-developed collateral system that allows excellent myocardial blood flow despite the left-to-right shunt from the RCA to the pulmonary artery. These individuals may present later in adolescence or young adulthood with coronary symptoms or an adverse event following exercise. Anomalous origin of the RCA from the pulmonary artery is less often encountered. Adults with this anomaly also have presented with symptoms of myocardial ischemia, usually during exercise.

Surgical repositioning of the coronary arteries is successful in repairing anomalous coronary artery defects, and even among infants with severe manifestations, reversal of myocardial ischemic findings has been well described with improvement of previously impaired myocardial function. Some patients have significant mitral valve insufficiency resulting from papillary muscle ischemia or infarction earlier in life.

Coronary artery fistulas most often drain to the right ventricle or right atrium, but occasionally to the left heart chambers and pulmonary artery. Patients with these fistulas are usually identified on the basis of a cardiac murmur with virtually no incidence of ischemic symptoms in infancy or childhood. However, when significant coronary blood flow is diverted to a chamber in an adult, there is concern about late coronary manifestations. Thus, surgical or catheter-based closure of the fistula is recommended. There may be multiple sites of entry to the cardiac chamber; the operative procedure is usually carried out under cardiopulmonary bypass to be certain that all components of the fistula are eliminated.

Abnormal coronary arteries are frequently encountered in patients with other forms of congenital heart disease. Coronary anomalies associated with tetralogy of Fallot are frequent, but the most important abnormality is when a large coronary artery crosses a right ventricular outflow tract. If a right ventriculotomy is carried out, there is a risk of interference with the vessel and a resultant myocardial infarction. This complication occurred to a greater degree in past years than in the modern era, when transatrial repair of tetralogy of Fallot is usual. Among patients with pulmonary atresia and an intact ventricular septum, abnormalities of the coronary arteries are frequent, and these may be anatomic findings which could prevent repair of this defect in infancy. If coronary blood flow is dependent on right ventricular blood flow via myocardial sinusoids, decompression of the right ventricle as part of a surgical procedure to relieve right ventricular outflow tract obstruction may produce catastrophic myocardial ischemia and infarction. Even among the great majority of patients in whom coronary flow appears to be entirely normal, coronary abnormalities may lead to segmental left ventricular abnormalities.

A variety of coronary abnormalities are encountered in patients with D-transposition of the great arteries, and it is important that surgical techniques of coronary reimplanta-

Algorithm 9–1
Congenital Anomalies of the Coronary Circulation

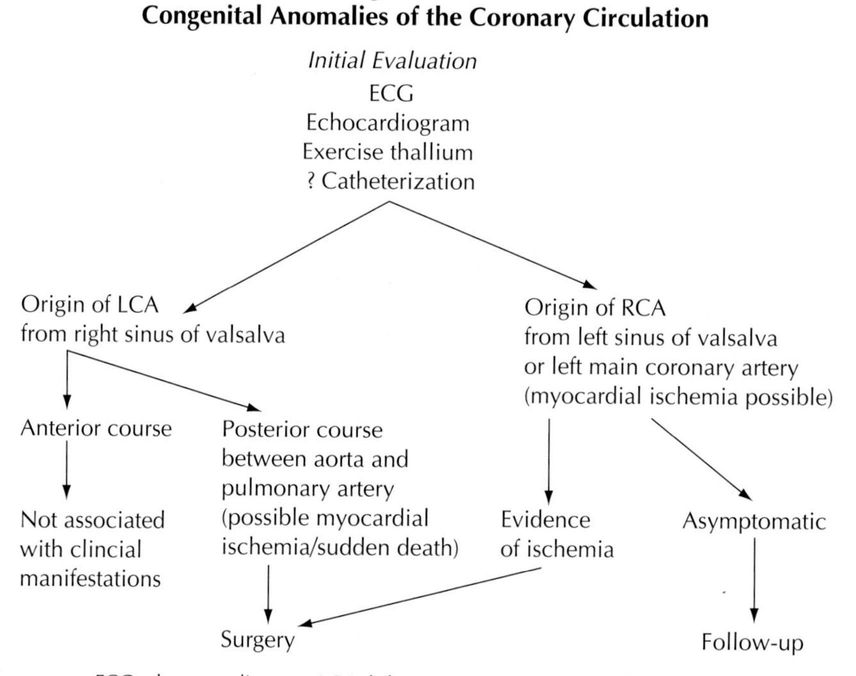

KEY: ECG, electrocardiogram; LCA, left coronary artery; RCA, right coronary artery.

Algorithm 9–2
Anomalous Coronary Artery from Pulmonary Artery

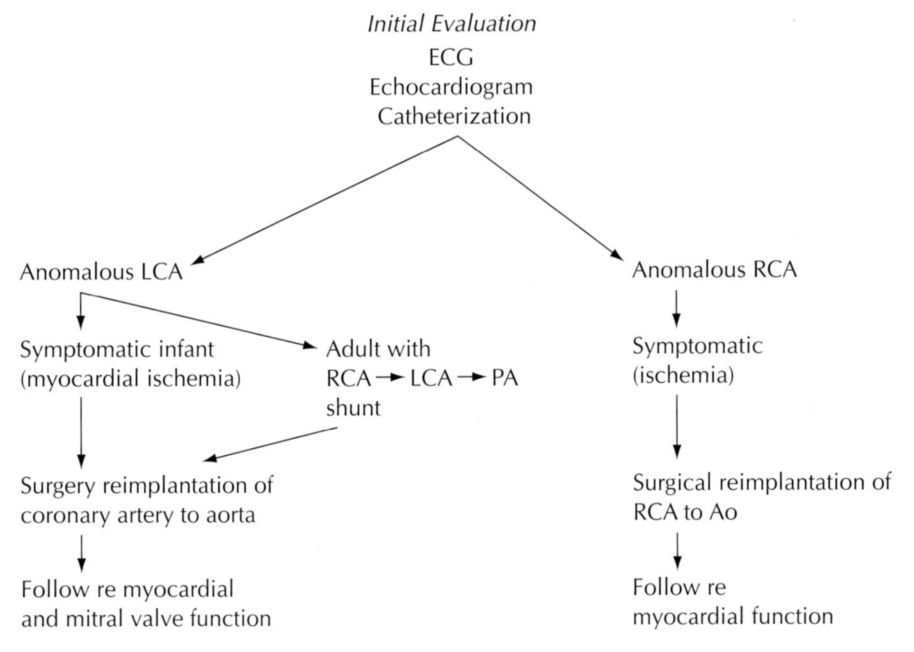

KEY: Ao, aorta; ECG, electrocardiogram; LCA, left coronary artery; PA, pulmonary artery; RCA, right coronary artery.

Algorithm 9–3
Coronary AV Fistula

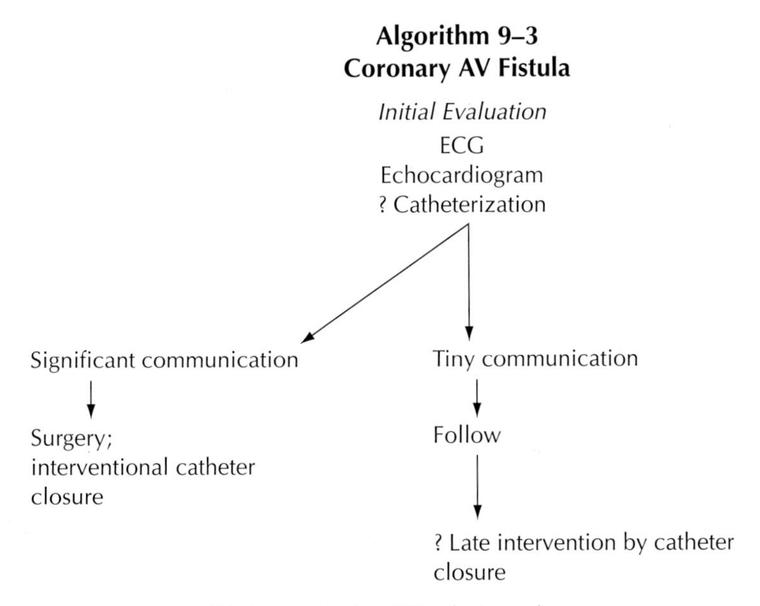

KEY: AV, atrioventricular; ECG, electrocardiogram.

Algorithm 9–4
Coronary Artery Anomalies,
Association with Congenital Heart Disease

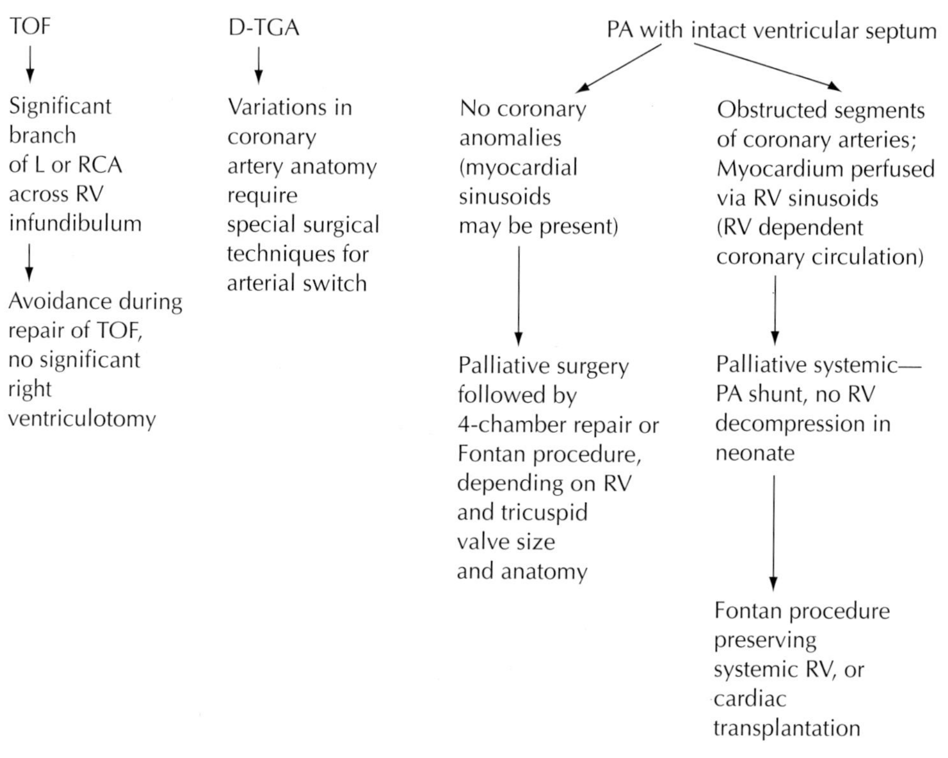

KEY: D-TGA, D-transposition of the great arteries; PA, pulmonary atresia; RV, right ventricle; TOF, tetralogy of Fallot.

tion reflect the anatomy of these vessels. The most difficult challenge for the surgeon who is carrying out an arterial switch operation is the presence of intramural coronary arteries. These vessels require special techniques when reimplantation to the neoaorta is made during the infant switch operation. Results of the arterial switch are usually excellent. Rarely coronary abnormalities may be discovered later in life in asymptomatic patients who have had successful arterial switch operations.

BIBLIOGRAPHY

Ahmed S et al: Silent left coronary artery-cameral fistula: Probable cause of myocardial ischemia. *Am Heart J* 104:869, 1982.

Alexi-Meskishvili V et al: Anomalous origin of the left coronary artery from the pulmonary artery in adults. *J Cardiol Surg* 10:309, 1995.

Augustsson MN et al: Anomalous origin of the left coronary artery from the pulmonary artery (adult type). *Pediatrics* 29:274, 1962.

Backer CL et al: Anomalous origin of the left coronary artery: A twenty-year review of surgical management. *J Thorac Cardiovasc Surg* 103:1049, 1992.

Barth C III et al: Sudden death in infancy associated with origin of both left main and right coronary arteries from a common ostium above the left sinus of Valsalva. *Am J Cardiol* 57:365, 1986.

Basso C et al: Clinical profile of congenital coronary artery anomalies with origin from the wrong aortic sinus leading to sudden death in young competitive athletes. *J Am Coll Cardiol* 35:1493, 2000.

Bland EF et al: Congenital anomalies of coronary arteries: Report of unusual case associated with cardiac hypertrophy. *Am Heart J* 8:787, 1933.

Bregman D et al: Anomalous origin of right coronary artery from pulmonary artery. *J Thorac Cardiovasc Surg* 72:626, 1976.

Click RL et al: Anomalous coronary arteries: Location, degree of atherosclerosis and effect on survival—A report from a coronary artery study. *J Am Coll Cardiol* 13:531, 1989.

Fang BR et al: Two dimensional and Doppler-echocardiographic features of coronary arteriovenous fistula. *J Ultrasound Med* 9:39, 1990.

Foster JH et al: Mitral insufficiency due to anomalous origin of the left coronary artery from the pulmonary artery. *Pediatrics* 34:649, 1964.

Gaither NS et al: Anomalous origin and course of coronary arteries in adults: Identification and improved imaging utilizing transesophageal echocardiography. *Am Heart J* 122:69, 1991.

Griffiths SP et al: Spontaneous complete closure of a congenital coronary artery fistula. *J Am Coll Cardiol* 2:1169, 1983.

Hobbs RE et al: Coronary artery fistulae: A ten-year review. *Clev Clin Q* 49:191, 1982.

Hoffman JIE: Coronary arterial abnormalities and congenital anomalies of the aortic root, in *Pediatric Cardiovascular Medicine*, JH Moller, IE Hoffman (eds). New York, Churchill Livingstone, 2000.

Kragel AH, Roberts WC: Anomalous origin of either the right or left main coronary artery from the aorta with subsequent coursing between aorta and pulmonary trunk: Analysis of 32 necropsy cases. *Am J Cardiol* 62:771, 1988.

Laks H, Ardehali A, Grant PW, Allada V: Aortic implantation of anomalous left coronary artery. An improved surgical approach. *J Thorac Cardiovasc Surg* 109:519, 1995.

Liberthson RR, Dinsmore RE, Fallon JT: Aberrant coronary artery origin from the aorta. Report of 18 patients, review of literature and delineation of natural history and management. *Circulation* 59:748, 1979.

Liberthson RR, Sagar K, Berkoben JP et al: Congenital coronary arteriovenous fistula. Report of 13 patients, review of literature and delineation of management. *Circulation* 59:849, 1979.

Maron BJ, Roberts WC, McAllister HA, et al: Sudden death in young athletes. *Circulation* 62:218, 1980.

Moodie DS, Fyfe D, Gill CC, et al: Anomalous origin of the left coronary artery from the pulmonary artery (Bland-White-Garland syndrome) in adult patients: Long-term follow-up after surgery. *Am Heart J* 106:381, 1983.

Roberts WC: Major anomalies of coronary arterial origin seen in adulthood. *Am Heart J* 111:941, 1986.

Roberts WC, Shirani J: The four subtypes of anomalous origin of the left main coronary artery from the right aortic sinus (or from the right coronary artery). *Am J Cardiol* 70:119, 1992.

Roberts WC, Siegel RJ, Zipes DP: Origin of the right coronary artery from the left sinus of Valsalva and its functional consequences: Analysis of 10 necropsy patients. *Am J Cardiol* 49:863, 1982.

Schmidt KG, Cooper MJ, Silverman NH, Stanger P: Pulmonary artery origin of the left coronary artery: Diagnosis by two-dimensional echocardiography, pulsed Doppler ultrasound and color flow mapping. *J Am Coll Cardiol* 11:396, 1988.

Sherwood MC, Rockenmacher S, Colan SD, Geva T: Prognostic significance of clinically silent coronary artery fistulas. *Am J Cardiol* 83:407, 1999.

Starc TJ, Bowman FO, Hordof AJ: Congestive heart failure in a newborn secondary to coronary artery–left ventricular fistula. *Am J Cardiol* 58:366, 1986.

Strunk BL, Hieshima GB, Shafton EP: Treatment of congenital coronary arteriovenous malformations with micro-particle embolization. *Cathet Cardiovasc Diagn* 22:133, 1991.

Taylor AJ, Rogan KM, Virmani R: Sudden cardiac death associated with isolated congenital coronary artery anomalies. *J Am Coll Cardiol* 20:640, 1992.

Thomas CS Jr, Campbell WB, Alford WC, et al: Complete repair of anomalous origin of the left coronary artery in the adult. *J Thorac Cardiovasc Surg* 66:439, 1973.

Virmani R, Chun PKC, Goldstein RE, et al: Acute takeoffs of the coronary arteries along the aortic wall and congenital ostial valvelike ridges: Association with sudden death. *J Am Coll Cardiol* 3:766, 1984.

PART II

CYANOTIC HEART DISEASE

CHAPTER 10

TETRALOGY OF FALLOT

Tetralogy of Fallot is the most common form of cyanotic congenital heart disease, constituting 10% of all congenital heart defects. This lesion is classically defined as (1) obstruction of right ventricular outflow (pulmonic stenosis), (2) ventricular septal defect (VSD), (3) overriding aorta, and (4) right ventricular hypertrophy (Fig. 10-1). The developmental abnormality involves anterior and cranial displacement of the infundibular septum, producing obstruction of the right ventricular outflow tract and a malalignment VSD. As a consequence, right ventricular hypertrophy and varying degrees of aortic override are present.

Obstruction to pulmonary blood flow is most often at both the infundibular and valvar levels. The pulmonary valve is frequently bicuspid, and the pulmonary annulus is typically small. Depending on the severity of right ventricular outflow obstruction, hypoplasia of the pulmonary arteries may be present, and branch stenoses are not uncommon. In some cases, collateral pulmonary arterial vessels of varying number and size arise from the aorta.

CLINICAL FEATURES

The basic physiology of tetralogy of Fallot is restriction of pulmonary blood flow as a result of pulmonary stenosis with a right-to-left shunt across a large VSD. The timing of presentation and degree of cyanosis vary with the anatomy of the right ventricular outflow tract. If pulmonary stenosis is severe, pulmonary blood flow is markedly reduced and right ventricular blood is ejected through the VSD into the ascending aorta, resulting in significant cyanosis. If pulmonary stenosis is less severe, shunting through the VSD is "balanced" and cyanosis is minimal.

Infancy and Childhood

Tetralogy of Fallot is usually recognized in early infancy by a prominent systolic murmur or cyanosis, or both. Because the degree of pulmonary stenosis varies from patient to patient, the clinical presentation may range from severe cyanosis to near-normal arterial oxy-

FIGURE 10-1

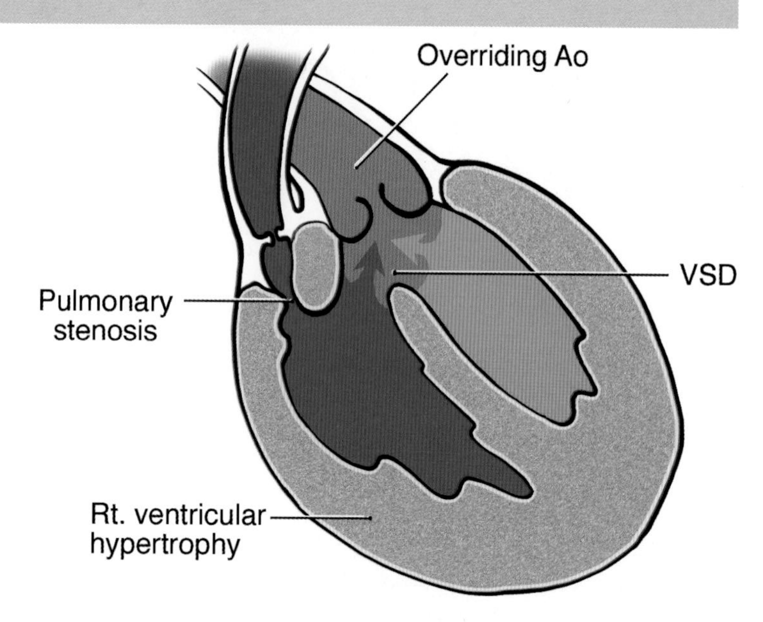

Schematic showing the typical features of tetralogy of Fallot: ventricular septal defect (VSD), pulmonary stenosis, overriding aorta, and right ventricular hypertrophy. The defect results from an anterior displacement of the outlet ventricular septum, resulting in infundibular stenosis as well as the VSD and overriding aorta. The pulmonary valve annulus is also small.

gen saturation with minimally decreased pulmonary blood flow. An occasional infant with only mild pulmonary stenosis may even present initially with congestive heart failure secondary to left-to-right shunting through the VSD. However, with the development of progressive infundibular stenosis over time, right-to-left shunting and cyanosis increase as pulmonary blood flow diminishes.

The classic symptoms of severe disease in infancy include (1) exertional dyspnea, (2) cyanosis, and (3) hypercyanotic spells. In the infant, exertional dyspnea may be manifested during activities such as feeding and crying. Young cyanotic children typically assume a squatting position following activity to help relieve dyspnea. This maneuver relieves dyspnea by increasing systemic vascular resistance, thereby decreasing right-to-left shunting, and by pooling highly desaturated blood in the lower extremities, reducing the proportion of desaturated blood returning to the heart.

Hypercyanotic spells frequently occur during the first two years of life and typically are seen in patients with only mild resting cyanosis. Although usually self-limiting, "tetralogy" spells may lead to severe hypoxemia, hypercapnia, and acidosis. The infant may become unconscious, and seizures and hemiparesis can occur. Hypercyanotic spells appear to be the result of a decrease in systemic vascular resistance, which produces a dramatic fall in pulmonary blood flow with increased right-to-left shunting and severe cyanosis.

Natural History

Natural history studies of patients with unoperated severe tetralogy of Fallot have demonstrated a 50% survival rate to age 5, 25% to age 10, and only 3 to 5% survival to age 25. Death has been attributed to severe hypoxemia, hypercyanotic spells, cerebrovascular accident, brain abscess, and infective endocarditis. In one series, sudden death constituted a substantial proportion of the deaths.

Unoperated adults with tetralogy of Fallot, therefore, represent a highly selected group of patients whose anatomy is compatible with late survival. These patients usually have less severe pulmonary stenosis and adequate-sized pulmonary arteries. The gradual deterioration of these patients may be the result of progressive infundibular hypertrophy, which increases right ventricular outflow tract obstruction and results in greater cyanosis, or complications of chronic polycythemia. Occasionally, cyanotic adults will be encountered who have severe pulmonary stenosis or atresia with small pulmonary arteries, but enough pulmonary collateral blood flow to allow long-term survival.

Physical Examination

The clinical findings in unoperated patients with tetralogy of Fallot vary according to the degree of pulmonary stenosis and right-to-left shunting. The cardiac examination reveals a normal first heart sound and a single second heart sound caused by closure of the aortic valve. An early aortic ejection sound may be present in severe tetralogy secondary to a dilated aortic root.

A systolic ejection murmur is present at the left upper and middle sternal border, resulting from turbulent blood flow across the right ventricular outflow tract. The intensity of the murmur is inversely related to the severity of the pulmonary stenosis. When pulmonary stenosis is severe, pulmonary blood flow is greatly reduced and only a low-intensity systolic ejection murmur may be present. In patients with mild-to-moderate pulmonary stenosis, blood flow is greater and the murmur is louder. During a hypercyanotic spell in an infant, a previously loud murmur may disappear as pulmonary blood flow is severely reduced. Right-to-left shunting of blood across the large VSD does not produce a murmur because the pressure is equal in both ventricles, allowing direct, nonturbulent flow from the right ventricle to the overriding aorta.

When pulmonary atresia is present, the systolic murmur is absent because there is no continuity between the right ventricle and the pulmonary arteries. In these patients, continuous murmurs may be present, reflecting blood flow from aortic collateral vessels to various segments of the lungs. A more common cause of a continuous murmur in tetralogy of Fallot is the patient who has undergone a palliative systemic-pulmonary artery shunt (e.g., Blalock-Taussig, Potts, and Waterston shunts).

The inverse relationship between the systolic murmur and the degree of pulmonary stenosis in tetralogy of Fallot differs from isolated valvar pulmonary stenosis in which the grade and late-peaking quality of the murmur is directly related to the severity of the stenosis.

Noninvasive Evaluation

The *chest x-ray* in patients with classic tetralogy of Fallot shows a normal heart size, which has been described as boot-shaped or "couer on Sabot" (Dutch shoe) owing to right ventricular hypertrophy and the diminished size of the main pulmonary artery shadow. The ascending aorta is frequently large and the aortic arch is on the right in 20% of patients with tetralogy of Fallot. The *electrocardiogram* (ECG) reveals sinus rhythm with right axis deviation and right ventricular hypertrophy.

Echocardiography provides excellent detail of the anteriorly displaced infundibular septum, malalignment VSD, and the anatomy of the right ventricular outflow tract obstruction (Fig. 10-2). In patients with pulmonary atresia, the absence of continuity between the right ventricular outflow tract and the pulmonary arteries can also be demonstrated. In small patients, the proximal course of the coronary arteries can frequently be visualized.

FIGURE 10-2

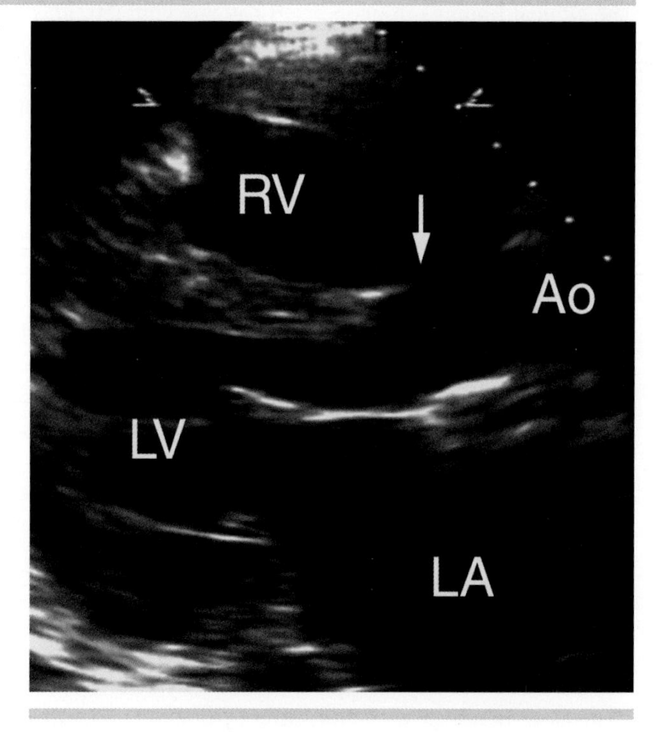

Parasternal long-axis view in a patient with tetralogy of Fallot. There is a large malalignment ventricular septal defect (VSD) with an overriding aorta. RV, right ventricle; LV, left ventricle; LA, left atrium; Ao, aorta. The arrow points to the large VSD.

Cardiac Catheterization

Although considerable information may be obtained from echocardiography, cardiac catheterization may be necessary to assess the pulmonary artery anatomy prior to complete repair. Demonstration of pulmonary artery anatomy is important, especially if a palliative shunt had been carried out in childhood, which may result in distortion and/or stenosis of the vessels. In addition, anomalies of the coronary arteries can be identified.

The salient hemodynamic features of tetralogy of Fallot include equalization of systolic pressures in the right and left ventricles and ascending aorta secondary to the large VSD. The pulmonary artery pressure is low; however, it is not routinely measured in children who have not undergone a shunt procedure because of the risk of inducing a hypercyanotic spell by catheter obstruction or spasm of the right ventricular outflow tract.

The direction of shunting depends on the degree of right ventricular outflow obstruction. Oximetry usually shows a stepdown in oxygen saturation from the left ventricle to the aorta caused by ejection of right ventricular blood into the ascending aorta.

Angiograms are usually performed in the right ventricle, left ventricle, and ascending aorta. The right ventriculogram demonstrates the level of right ventricular outflow tract obstruction as well as the details of the pulmonary artery anatomy (Fig. 10-3). In

FIGURE 10-3

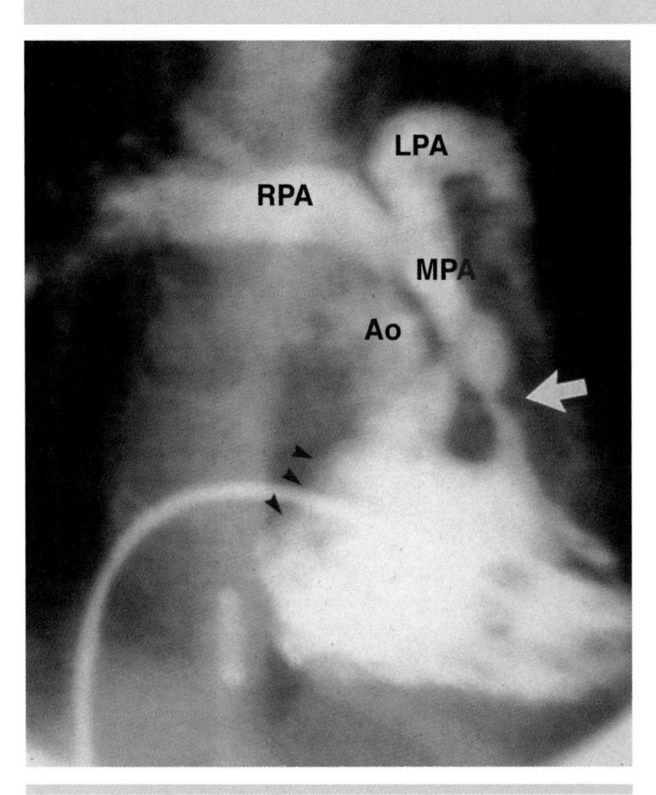

Right ventricular angiogram in a patient with tetralogy of Fallot. Contrast fills both the pulmonary artery and aorta, and there is marked overriding of the aorta, allowing unencumbered blood flow from the right ventricle. There is no significant tricuspid insufficiency. Small arrows outline the tricuspid annulus. The large white arrow indicates the region of severe infundibular stenosis. Ao = aorta, MPA = main pulmonary artery, LPA = left pulmonary artery, RPA = right pulmonary artery.

some cases, the left pulmonary artery is not visualized because it became isolated when the ductus closed in early infancy or as a complication of an early palliative shunt procedure. When this occurs, blood flow to the left pulmonary artery may be supplied by collateral vessels from the thoracic aorta.

The left ventriculogram is useful to delineate an additional VSD, which may be difficult to detect by echocardiography. An aortogram is performed to exclude an aberrant coronary artery that may cross the right ventricular outflow tract, the presence and location of major collateral pulmonary vessels (MAPCAs) from the aorta, and/or a patent ductus arteriosus. Selective coronary arteriography may be required if a coronary artery anomaly is suspected, or in older adults if acquired coronary artery disease might be present.

Coronary artery anomalies occur in 5% of patients with tetralogy of Fallot. The most important anomaly is origin of the left anterior descending artery from the right coronary artery, in which the left anterior descending artery crosses the right ventricular outflow tract. This anomaly could interfere with surgical repair among patients who require a right ventriculotomy. In such cases, a conduit or homograft from the right ventricle to the pulmonary artery may have been needed to avoid damaging the coronary artery when a limited right ventriculotomy is deemed inadequate to relieve obstruction. However, in recent years this has been rarely done, since repair is carried out through an atriotomy without a ventriculotomy. In rare instances, a single right coronary artery or single left coronary artery occurs in tetralogy of Fallot.

The pulmonary artery pressure should be measured if there is concern that pulmonary hypertension may be present. This must be considered in older patients who have had a Potts or Waterston shunt as well as in the occasional patient with large aortopulmonary collateral vessels and high pulmonary blood flow. When a shunt is present, the pulmonary artery may be entered by passing a catheter either retrograde from the aorta through the shunt or antegrade from the right ventricle into the pulmonary artery. A pulmonary angiogram is performed to visualize the pulmonary arteries and to assess for significant branch stenoses that would require surgical repair.

MANAGEMENT

Tetralogy of Fallot is treated surgically. Prior to the era of open-heart surgery, palliation of this disease was achieved with a shunt from the subclavian artery or aorta to the pulmonary artery. Once cardiopulmonary bypass techniques became available, open-heart definitive repair consisted of VSD closure and relief of right ventricular outflow tract obstruction. In the early years, correction was carried out in late childhood, often after an initial shunt in infancy. Total correction can now be offered during the first year of life if the pulmonary arteries are of adequate size, so that an early shunt procedure can be avoided in most cases.

Palliative Surgery

The most effective palliative treatment for tetralogy of Fallot was established in 1944 by Drs. Blalock and Taussig at Johns Hopkins Hospital by means of subclavian artery to ipsilateral pulmonary artery anastomosis. The procedure, known as the Blalock-Taussig shunt, results in excellent palliation for tetralogy of Fallot by increasing pulmonary blood flow in a controlled manner, reducing cyanosis and improving exercise capacity. In neonates, a modified Blalock shunt consisting of a graft between the subclavian artery and the pulmonary artery is now most often used. The advantage of the modified Blalock shunt is that an acceptable systemic-pulmonary artery shunt can be produced, without pulmonary hypertension or distortion of the pulmonary arteries, and the anastomosis is easier to eliminate at the time of definitive open-heart repair.

In addition to the Blalock-Taussig shunt, two other shunts, the Potts and the Waterston, were also used, but have been abandoned because of complications relating to excessive pulmonary blood flow, pulmonary hypertension, distortion of the pulmonary arteries, and unequal flow to the left and right lungs (Fig. 10-4*A* through *C*). The Potts shunt is a side-by-side anastomosis between the descending aorta and the left pulmonary artery. In addition to problems relating to excessive pulmonary blood flow and pressure (e.g., early congestive heart failure and late pulmonary vascular disease), this shunt frequently causes distortion of the left pulmonary artery, and is difficult to take down at the time of open heart repair. The Waterston shunt is a side-by-side anastomosis between the ascending aorta and the right pulmonary artery. It is also associated with excessive pulmonary blood

FIGURE 10-4

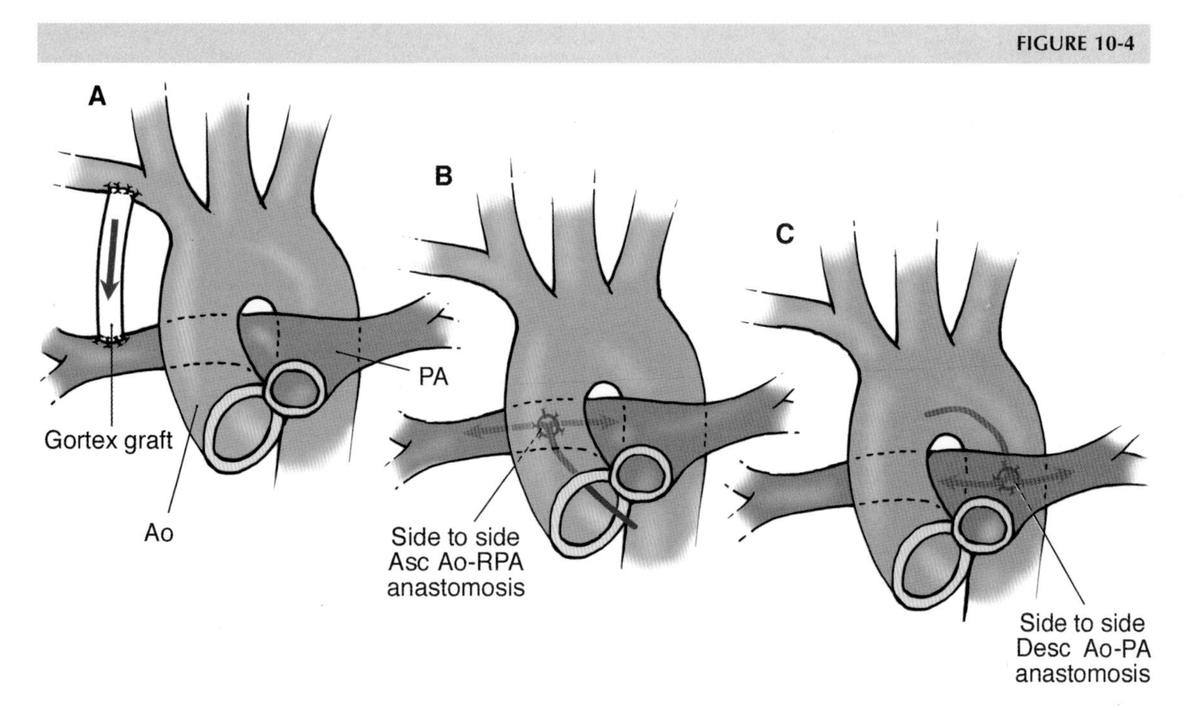

Systemic to pulmonary artery shunts are demonstrated. The modified Blalock shunt is shown in panel *A* with a Gortex conduit placed from the right subclavian to the right pulmonary artery. (*B*) The Waterston shunt is a side-to-side anastomosis of the right pulmonary artery to the posterior wall of the ascending aorta, and (*C*) the Potts anastomosis is a surgical connection between the anterior wall of the descending aorta and the left pulmonary artery.

flow and pressure and may result in distortion of the right pulmonary artery, obstruction to left pulmonary artery flow, or both.

Palliative shunts were used as the primary treatment of tetralogy of Fallot until open-heart surgery became available. Most of these patients subsequently underwent open-heart repair of this defect with takedown of the shunt. Today it is unusual to encounter an adult with tetralogy of Fallot who has had a Blalock-Taussig shunt and no subsequent open heart repair. Complete repair should be recommended for these patients if the pulmonary artery anatomy is suitable and pulmonary resistance is not elevated. The presence of normal pulmonary artery pressure can be inferred by the presence of a continuous murmur and diminished pulmonary vascularity on the chest x-ray. Absence of a continuous murmur suggests either a diminutive or absent shunt or the presence of pulmonary vascular disease.

The incidence of complications after palliative shunts relates to the type of procedure performed. Excessive pulmonary blood flow and pulmonary hypertension are rarely seen in patients after a Blalock-Taussig shunt, whereas older patients with a prior Potts or Waterston shunt are occasionally seen who have major distortion of the left or right pulmonary artery or pulmonary vascular obstructive disease. These complications may substantially increase the risks of open-heart repair or even render the patient inoperable. Reappearance of cyanosis after a successful Blalock shunt suggests either that the patient has "outgrown" the shunt or that a stenosis has developed at the anastomosis. However, adults occasionally are seen with adequate pulmonary blood flow several decades after creation of a Blalock shunt during childhood, without having had a more definitive operation.

Despite the beneficial effects of a shunt on survival and symptoms, the long-term consequences argue for early definitive repair. These include (1) an increased risk for bacterial endocarditis, (2) anatomic distortion of the pulmonary arteries at the anastomotic site, (3) sequelae of chronic arterial desaturation and polycythemia when the shunt is small, (4) development of pulmonary hypertension and pulmonary vascular obstructive disease from excessive pulmonary blood flow when the shunt is large, and (5) long-standing volume overload of the left ventricle, even when shunt size is ideal.

Surgical Repair

Most present-day adults who had correction of tetralogy of Fallot in childhood underwent repair through a right ventriculotomy, which exposes the VSD and permits resection of excess right ventricular muscle and enlargement of the right ventricular outflow tract. The right ventricular outlet is enlarged with an outflow tract patch, which is extended across the pulmonary annulus if the pulmonary valve is involved in the obstruction, and even across the bifurcation of the left and right pulmonary arteries. When a transannular patch is required, significant pulmonary insufficiency results. In recent years, the surgical approach has changed at many institutions, in that the repair is carried out using a transatrial approach. The VSD closure and infundibular resection are performed through the tricuspid valve and, if necessary, a small incision is made across the annulus to insert a transannular patch (Fig. 10-5). This approach avoids an extensive right ventriculotomy, which may contribute to decreased right ventricular function, late right ventricular fail-

FIGURE 10-5

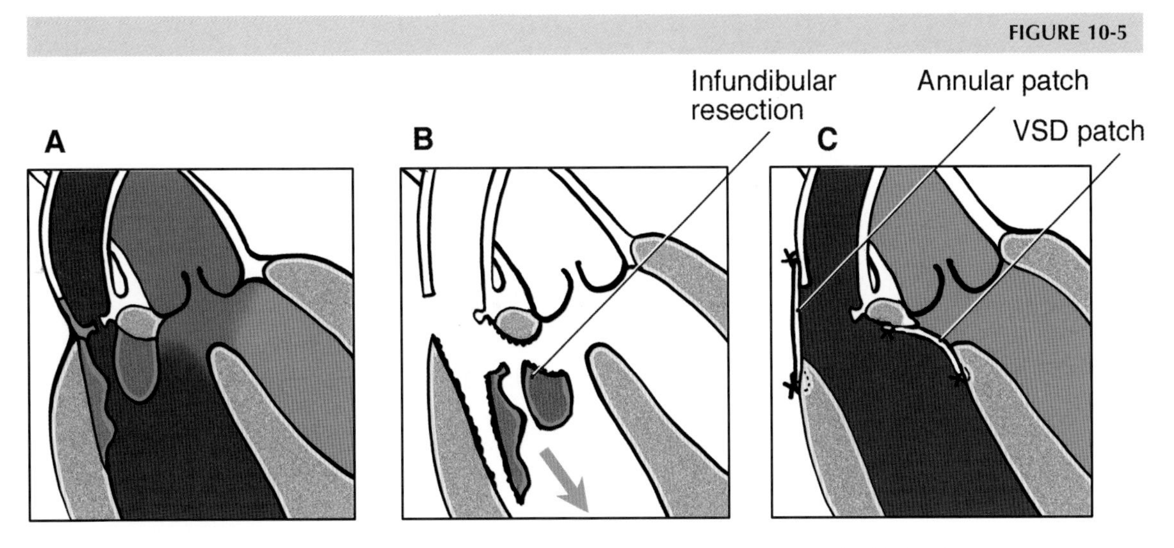

Surgical repair of tetralogy of Fallot: (*A*) preoperatively; (*B*) resection of the obstructive infundibular tissue; (*C*) patch closure of the ventricular septal defect; and, when enlargement of the annulus is necessary, an annular patch from the right ventricular outflow tract to the main pulmonary artery.

ure, and arrhythmias. The possibility of incising an unsuspected large coronary artery is also eliminated.

A number of associated lesions may occur with tetralogy of Fallot. Many of these are eliminated at the time of open-heart repair, including patent ductus arteriosus, previous surgical systemic to pulmonary arterial shunts, and atrial septal defect. Although uncommon, multiple VSDs may occur and should be identified prior to surgery.

In patients with tetralogy of Fallot and pulmonary atresia, there is no continuity between the right ventricle and pulmonary artery. In these patients, continuity is established with a homograft or conduit, which is placed from the body of the right ventricle to the main pulmonary artery.

If symptoms of increasing cyanosis or hypercyanotic spells develop in the first 3 to 4 months of life, definitive repair is usually carried out provided the pulmonary arteries are large enough to support right ventricular output. If the pulmonary artery size is inadequate, a shunt is performed as a first stage to enhance growth of the pulmonary arteries and relieve cyanosis. Complete repair with takedown of the shunt is subsequently performed if and when adequate size of the pulmonary arteries is established. In marginal cases, the risk of primary open heart correction during infancy must be balanced against the combined risks of a shunt with ongoing cyanosis, the need for a second operation with the potential problems of pulmonary artery distortion, and a period of left ventricular volume overload induced by a shunt.

Although most adults with tetralogy of Fallot have undergone complete repair earlier in life, the cardiologist must also be familiar with the evaluation of a patient who has had either no surgery or only a palliative shunt.

THE ADULT WITHOUT PRIOR SURGERY

In the current era, it is unusual to encounter an adult with tetralogy of Fallot who has not had palliative or corrective surgery. Most such patients are from countries where cardiac surgery is not performed on a regular basis. Many adults with uncorrected tetralogy may have already experienced one or more of the complications associated with cyanotic heart disease, such as brain abscess, cerebrovascular accident, bacterial endocarditis, and paradoxical embolism. Long-term survival without surgery suggests that pulmonary stenosis was only mild to moderate during childhood or large-sized collateral vessels have permitted adequate pulmonary blood flow.

Preoperative cardiac catheterization and angiography is indicated to determine the level of right ventricular outflow tract obstruction, the pulmonary artery anatomy, and the status of the coronary arteries. Unoperated adults who have tetralogy of Fallot with favorable anatomy are candidates for complete repair, which can be performed with a low operative mortality. Surgery results in a marked improvement in exercise capacity and eliminates cyanosis and the complications associated with a right-to-left shunt.

THE PATIENT AFTER COMPLETE REPAIR

In the modern era, most adults with tetralogy of Fallot have undergone complete repair during childhood. Although many of these patients have been closely followed by a pediatric cardiologist, an occasional patient is seen who has not sought medical care for many years and presents now with late problems related to this anomaly. Thus, the adult cardiologist must be familiar with the typical examination of the postoperative patient, be able to recognize significant residual hemodynamic abnormalities, and be familiar with the late postoperative problems that may occur among patients with this disease.

The stable postoperative patient with tetralogy is acyanotic and should display no evidence of a residual VSD or significant right ventricular outflow tract obstruction. The first heart sound is normal. The second heart sound is usually single, because the pulmonary valve is most often abnormal. A systolic ejection murmur that does not usually exceed grade II to III, accompanied by an early diastolic murmur of varying intensity, is audible along the left upper and mid-sternal border in most patients. These murmurs are typical of mild right ventricular outlfow tract obstruction and pulmonary regurgitation. The presence of a harsh systolic murmur at the base with an associated thrill suggests significant residual right ventricular outflow tract obstruction. A systolic murmur that is maximal at the lower left sternal border is abnormal and suggests either a residual VSD or tricuspid insufficiency.

Pulmonary insufficiency is usually present postoperatively, and may be more marked if a transannular patch was required to enlarge a small pulmonary annulus or if distal pulmonary artery obstruction is present. The early diastolic murmur related to pulmonary insufficiency is of low frequency and maximal along the left upper and mid-sternal border. The presence of a continuous murmur is abnormal and implies a persistent communication between a systemic artery and a lower pressure pulmonary artery. This may occur if there is a residual palliative shunt or if there are significant aortic collateral vessels to the pulmonary arteries.

The chest x-ray of an uncomplicated postoperative patient usually shows a mildly enlarged heart with normal pulmonary vascularity. The ECG usually demonstrates a right bundle branch block, which may be secondary to the right ventriculotomy, VSD repair, and/or infundibular resection. In some patients there is marked prolongation of QRS duration, which may have implications related to risk for ventricular tachycardia. In some patients, left axis deviation is also present. This finding has no prognostic significance.

The major issues in the adult patient postrepair of tetralogy of Fallot include: (1) the effect of long-standing pulmonary insufficiency on right ventricular function as a possible indication for reoperation, (2) management of patients with other significant residual hemodynamic abnormalities, and (3) the management of both atrial and ventricular tachyarrhythmias.

Pulmonary Insufficiency

A transannular patch is most often required when surgical repair of tetralogy of Fallot is carried out in severely cyanotic infants. These patients will have the most prominent pulmonary insufficiency. Whereas even relatively severe pulmonary insufficiency is well tolerated in the vast majority of tetralogy patients with normal pulmonary artery pressure, in some patients right ventricular dilatation is quite marked, prompting reoperation for late pulmonary valve replacement. Most centers continue to treat isolated pulmonary insufficiency conservatively; however, the presence of significant associated tricuspid insufficiency or progressive right ventricular dysfunction, or both, are considered to be definite indications for intervention. Prior to contemplating pulmonary valve replacement in an individual patient, pulmonary artery anatomy must be evaluated.

The ability of the right ventricle to tolerate chronic pulmonary insufficiency appears to be most influenced by the presence of residual branch pulmonary artery obstruction. Many patients who appear to require late pulmonary valve replacement have had a first-stage palliative shunt prior to complete repair, which may have caused distortion of the left or right pulmonary artery. In such cases, balloon angioplasty or stent placement may be used to manage branch pulmonary stenosis before consideration of valve replacement.

In the vast majority of patients with normal pulmonary vascular resistance and no pulmonary artery obstruction, it is clear from three decades of observation that pulmonary insufficiency is well tolerated and does not usually require intervention. However, it remains to be seen whether this will continue to be the case as these patients become even older. It is also possible that conditions such as coronary artery disease or systemic hypertension could worsen the effects of pulmonary insufficiency due to abnormalities of ventricular compliance or systolic function.

When patients are encountered with significant pulmonary and tricuspid insufficiency, with severe right ventricular dilatation and dysfunction, it may be difficult to determine the exact cause of right ventricular decompensation. Multiple factors, such as inadequate myocardial preservation during surgery, extent of right ventricular myocardial resection and outflow patch, residual right ventricular outflow tract obstruction, and early combined tricuspid and pulmonary insufficiency may all contribute to right ventricular decompensation. Older patients who develop sustained atrial tachyarrhythmias also may present with signs of right heart failure, and tricuspid insufficiency may develop. The combination of pulmonary and tricuspid regurgitation is poorly tolerated by the right ventricle. In such patients, pulmonary valve replacement with tricuspid valve repair or replacement has been performed to improve symptoms and right heart function. Although the optimal timing of surgery may be difficult to determine, it is important to avoid the effects of long-standing volume overload from two regurgitant lesions on the right ventricle. If surgery has been deferred until severe cardiomegaly and irreversible right ventricular dysfunction have developed, then cardiac transplantation may be the only option. On the other hand, premature valve replacement in a patient who would be stable for many years should be avoided because there are limited data in this asymptomatic population and valve degeneration of a bioprosthesis or homograft will occur over time. If valve-containing stents or biomechanical valves become available, there would be many candidates among this group of patients.

Residual Right Ventricular Outflow Tract Obstruction

Right ventricular pressure is usually mildly elevated in most postoperative tetralogy patients. In those with significant right ventricular outflow obstruction, the site may be infundibular, valvar, and/or supravalvar. If noninvasive findings suggest severe obstruction with right ventricular pressure of 75 mm or more (lower if tricuspid regurgitation or right ventricular dysfunction are already present), cardiac catheterization should be performed to determine the site of obstruction. On occasion, significantly elevated right ventricular pressure may be caused by distal pulmonary artery stenoses, or pulmonary vascular obstructive disease from a previous Potts or Waterston shunt. Stenting has now become the procedure of choice to relieve isolated mechanical obstructions of the pulmonary arteries. Surgery is usually reserved for patients requiring additional procedures.

Residual Ventricular Septal Defect

A large residual VSD occurs infrequently in patients seen at experienced centers, but must always be considered in the postoperative tetralogy patient with persistent congestive heart failure. The defect is usually related to an inadequate VSD patch, but also may be secondary to an additional VSD that was not recognized during surgery. The presence of a significant ventricular communication is usually recognized early in the postoperative period, and reoperation is then necessary. Small residual VSDs are more common and usually do not require reoperation.

Aortic Insufficiency

Significant aortic insufficiency is an infrequent finding in postoperative tetralogy of Fallot and may be a result of marked dilation of the aortic root, bacterial endocarditis, or injury to the aortic valve at the time of surgery.

Subvalvar Aortic Stenosis

A few patients have developed subvalvar aortic stenosis many years after repair of tetralogy of Fallot. This type of obstruction is more common in patients who had correction of tetralogy with atrioventricular canal or double outlet right ventricle. Subaortic stenosis should be suspected by the late finding of a harsh systolic ejection murmur along the left mid-sternal border. Surgical revision is generally recommended for gradients greater than 50 mm Hg.

Ventricular Arrhythmias

Late sudden death is an uncommon but well-recognized sequelae of tetralogy of Fallot repair. Early studies during the 1980s focused on the presence of ventricular arrhythmias and residual hemodynamic abnormalities as risk factors for this devastating complication. At some centers, aggressive treatment of PVCs with dilantin and β-blockers was advocated, although data to support drug efficacy was limited. Current studies show an 85% actuarial survival at 32 to 36 years postrepair, with an increased risk of late sudden death in later years. The mechanism of sudden death is felt to be ventricular tachyarrhythmias, which may be related to hemodynamic and/or electrical abnormalities.

Efforts to identify patients at risk for sudden death have included both electrophysiologic (EP) study as well as noninvasive ECG markers. EP studies have yielded mixed results in this population. In one study designed to determine outcome of inducible VT post tetralogy repair, there was no difference in subsequent mortality between patients with and without inducible VT during a 7.8-year follow-up period. Another study, which included various forms of repaired congenital heart disease, identified inducible VT as a risk factor for adverse outcome. In addition, the sensitivity of EP studies for detection of sustained VT has been significantly less than in patients with ischemic heart disease. Recently, noninvasive ECG abnormalities have been shown to have important prognostic implications. Several studies have found that patients with a QRS duration >180 ms are at increased risk for the development of sustained ventricular tachycardia.

These issues highlight the difficulties associated with determining the optimal management of ventricular arrhythmias in the adult tetralogy of Fallot population. While the general approach to treatment in these patients is similar to the management of patients with other forms of structural heart disease, specific differences evolve around the potential contribution of residual hemodynamic and ECG abnormalities. While sustained VT can be seen in the well-repaired patient, the patients at most risk would appear to be those with marked right ventricular dilatation, ventricular dysfunction, and prolonged QRS duration. Thus, some centers would advocate a more aggressive surgical approach in patients with both ventricular arrhythmias and significant residual right ventricular outflow tract obstruction or important pulmonary insufficiency with severe RV dilatation.

Although treatment of ventricular arrhythmias in the tetralogy of Fallot patient often requires arrhythmia expertise, the following guidelines can be suggested: Asymptomatic isolated PVCs should not be treated, although patients with more complex ventricular arrhythmias such as nonsustained VT may require more extensive investigation. In patients who have developed sustained VT, treatment options include antiarrhythmic drug therapy, map-guided ablation, surgery, and an implantable defibrillator. The patient who has survived a cardiac arrest is generally treated with an implantable defibrillator.

LONG-TERM FOLLOW-UP

Postoperative patients should have periodic physical examination, ECG, echocardiogram, and Holter monitoring. Periodic exercise testing also is employed in postoperative patients to assess for exercise-induced arrhythmias, to guide recommendations regarding exercise limitations, and to determine functional capacity.

Although most postoperative patients consider themselves to be asymptomatic, studies have shown a subnormal exercise response in many of these patients. This response may be due to long-standing pulmonary insufficiency and subclinical right ventricular dysfunction. It is suggested that postoperative tetralogy of Fallot patients avoid contact sports and extreme exercise under adverse conditions.

Pregnancy is generally well tolerated in women with stable hemodynamics after repair of tetralogy. The reported risk of congenital heart disease in offspring is approximately 3%.

PULMONARY ATRESIA WITH VENTRICULAR SEPTAL DEFECT (EXTREME TETRALOGY OF FALLOT)

The most important variant in the tetralogy group is the patient with pulmonary atresia. Such patients may have relatively normal-sized pulmonary arteries that can be repaired with a right ventricular outflow patch or with a right ventricle to pulmonary artery conduit, usually during infancy or childhood. However, others will have extremely small pulmonary arteries or no recognizable anatomic pulmonary arteries. Pulmonary blood flow is achieved by means of arterial collateral vessels, which may connect to normal pulmonary artery branches or supply a parallel circulation to one or both lungs (Fig. 10-6).

Management of these patients is variable. Surgical shunts can be placed into larger pulmonary artery branches in order to enlarge the caliber of the vessels, and at some centers, full repair may be carried out in neonates. Newer surgical techniques, including unifocalization of major arterial pulmonary collateral arteries (MAPCAs), have emerged, by which the right ventricle is connected to various segments of the pulmonary vascular bed via homograft or xenograft conduits. The procedure is usually performed in infancy or childhood. The VSD may be closed if pulmonary artery blood flow is adequate. Residual pulmonary artery hypertension is common in patients with predominant MAPCA circulations, and the result is never as satisfactory as that achieved for well-repaired, classic tetralogy patients. Reoperation for homograft replacement can be anticipated, (Figs. 10-7 and 10-8); such patients must be followed closely for progressive right ventricular outflow obstruction.

FIGURE 10-6

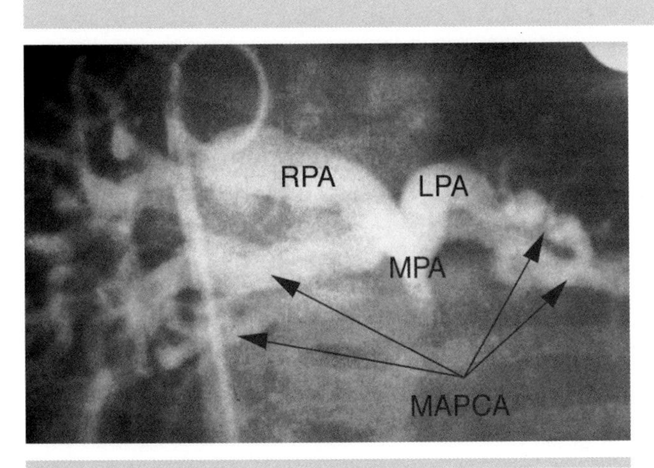

An aortogram in a patient with extreme tetralogy of Fallot with pulmonary atresia. The main pulmonary artery and branches are filled via an injection into the major arterial pulmonary collateral arteries. MPA, main pulmonary artery; RPA, right pulmonary artery; LPA, left pulmonary artery; MAPCA, major arterial pulmonary collateral arteries.

FIGURE 10-7

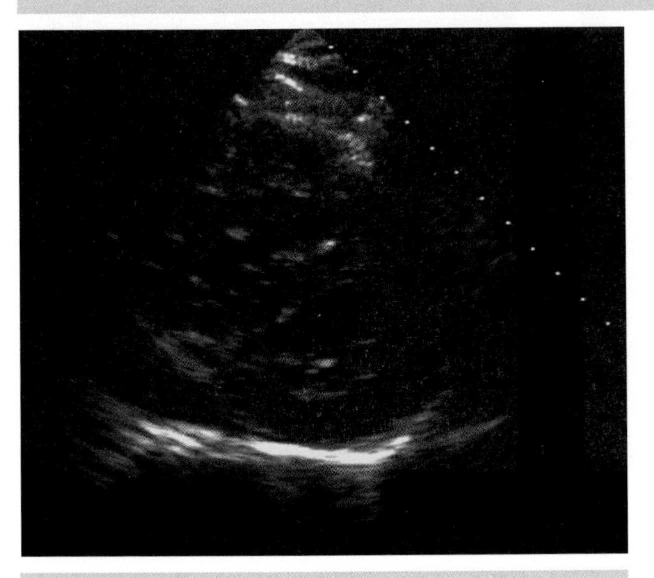

Parasternal short-axis view in a patient with a RV-PA obstruction. There is systolic flattening of the interventricular septum indicative of severe right ventricular hypertension.

FIGURE 10-8

High parasternal short-axis view of an adult with tetralogy of Fallot/pulmonary atresia, who has conduit obstruction in a right ventricle to pulmonary artery conduit. (*A*) The conduit is visualized anteriorly and extends posteriorly from the right ventricle to the pulmonary artery. (*B*) A color Doppler from the same patient shows turbulent flow during systole throughout the conduit. (*C*) A continuous wave Doppler within the conduit from the same patient shows a peak gradient of 72 mm Hg (arrow).

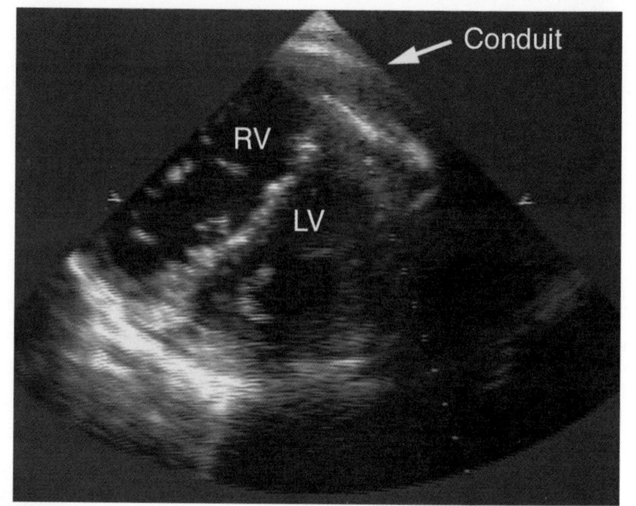

A

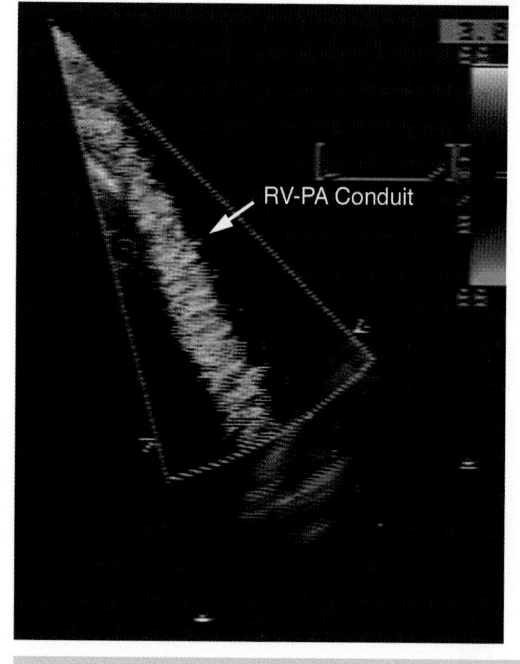

B

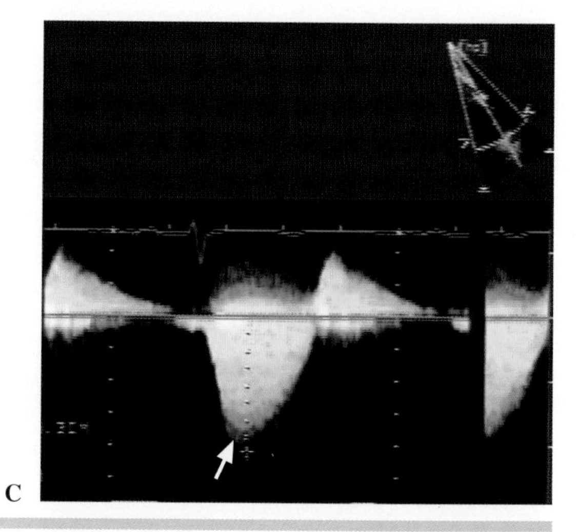

C

DOUBLE OUTLET RIGHT VENTRICLE

Double outlet right ventricle refers to a condition in which both great arteries arise from the right ventricle in conjunction with a large VSD. Conal tissue is present below the aortic valve, resulting in loss of mitral-aortic continuity. Oxygenated blood reaches the right ventricle and aorta through the VSD. Associated transposition of the great arteries and pulmonary stenosis are factors that influence the basic hemodynamics and management of such lesions. Discussion of this entity appears under various categories (e.g., VSD, see Chap. 3; D-TGA, see Chap. 11; L-TGA, see Chap. 8), depending on the associated anatomy and resultant physiology.

Double Outlet Right Ventricle with Normal Great Arteries and No Pulmonary Outflow Obstruction

Under these circumstances, left ventricular blood streams through the VSD directly into the aorta, with shunting also to the pulmonary artery. Because pulmonary resistance is lower than systemic resistance, a classic left-to-right shunt occurs with a presentation similar to that of the patient with a large VSD. The diagnosis is usually made in infancy, and early repair is carried out. A tunnel is constructed from the edges of the VSD, which directs blood from the left ventricle to the infundibular portion of the right ventricle, just below the aortic valve into the aorta. Once corrected, the prognosis is excellent, similar to that of a patient who has undergone standard VSD repair.

Double Outlet Right Ventricle with Normal Great Arteries and Subpulmonic Obstruction

This entity can be considered a variant of tetralogy of Fallot in which there is extreme overriding of the aorta, such that the aorta arises entirely from the right ventricular outflow tract. The VSD is closed as described earlier, and the right ventricular outflow tract obstruction is relieved as with any tetralogy patient. Late manifestations are similar to those described for tetralogy of Fallot.

Double Outlet Right Ventricle with Transposition of the Great Arteries

This is a complex congenital heart defect that requires complex surgical intervention (Fig. 10-9). Because the VSD is associated with the pulmonary artery, closure of the defect would create transposition of the great arteries, and therefore is not a solution to the abnormal hemodynamic status. Left ventricular blood must be tunneled through the VSD to the aorta, which is anterior to and a considerable distance from the left ventricle. In some cases this can be achieved, and a homograft from the right ventricle to the pulmonary artery completes the repair. When this approach is not possible, the VSD can be directed to the pulmonary artery, and an intra-atrial baffle procedure (Mustard or Senning operation) can correct the circulation. Double outlet right ventricle, almost invariably with malposi-

FIGURE 10-9

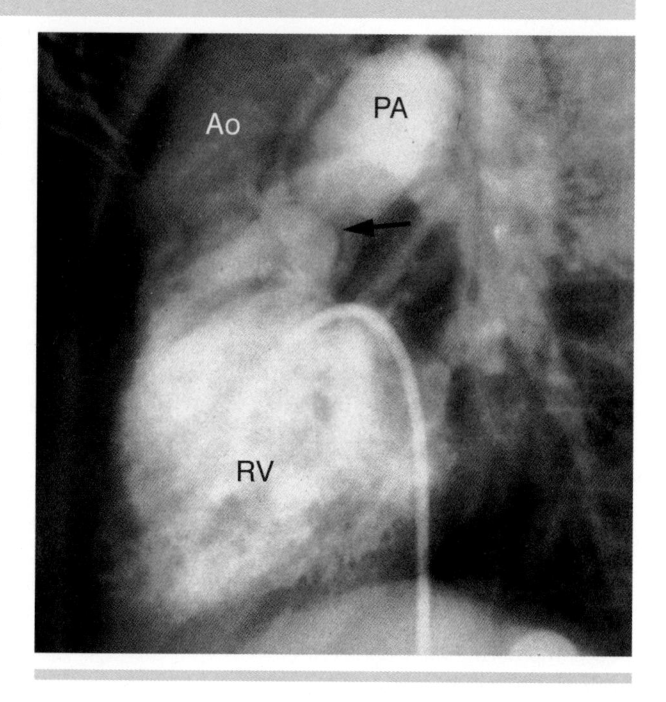

Right ventricular injection in a patient with double outlet right ventricle. There is both a subaortic and a subpulmonary infundibulum. Valvar pulmonary stenosis is present. Note the domed pulmonary valve cusps (arrow). RV = right ventricle, PA = pulmonary artery, Ao = aorta.

tion of the great arteries, often occurs in the presence of a single right ventricle. This entity is managed according to principles outlined for the care of patients with a single ventricle (see Chap. 12).

TETRALOGY OF FALLOT WITH ABSENT PULMONARY VALVE

A subgroup of tetralogy of Fallot includes patients with the four features of the disease, but with an absent pulmonary valve. The physiology is similar to that of other patients with tetralogy because the infundibular stenosis results in variable degrees of right-to-left shunt, depending on severity. However, the absent pulmonary valve results in a unique feature of the syndrome, which is that of markedly dilated pulmonary arteries. During infancy, this manifestation may result in impingement on airways, resulting in respiratory distress. In recent years, surgical techniques have been developed to diminish the size of the pulmonary arteries and relieve bronchial obstruction. When required, this surgery is usually carried out in early infancy.

Patients with this syndrome who are encountered in adult life most often have had corrective surgery for tetralogy of Fallot. The massive pulmonary artery dilation will be noted to persist. However, in a repaired tetralogy patient who does not have bronchial obstruction, the large pulmonary arteries are not of clinical significance. The angiographic pattern is extremely impressive (Fig. 10-10).

FIGURE 10-10

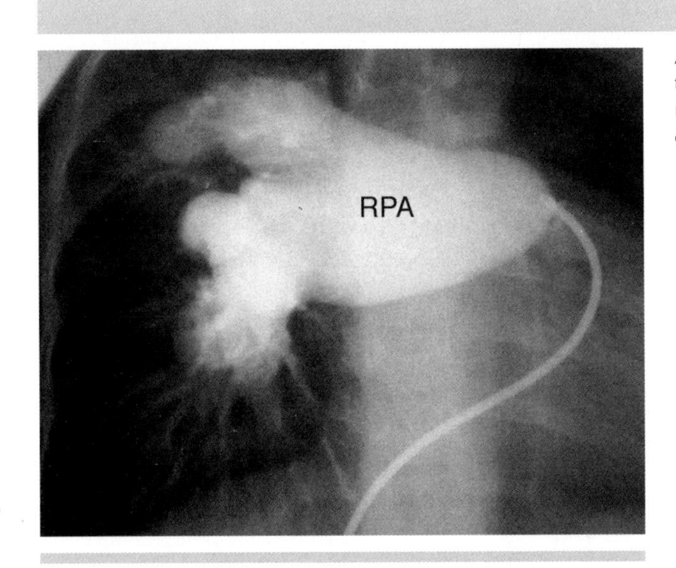

A right pulmonary artery angiogram in a patient with tetralogy of Fallot with absent pulmonary valve. The right pulmonary artery and its branches are massively dilated. RPA = right pulmonary artery.

Surgical repair of tetralogy of Fallot with an absent pulmonary valve may include a pulmonary valve replacement, although some centers do not include this component. Late reoperation because of pulmonary insufficiency may be required in some patients, similar to individuals who have had tetralogy repair with outflow patches, leaving essentially an absent pulmonary valve.

SUMMARY

The young adult with tetralogy of Fallot may present with a varied picture, depending on the original anatomy and subsequent surgical procedures.

Balanced Circulation: No Previous Operation

Such patients have moderate pulmonary stenosis with normal-sized pulmonary arteries. This syndrome is often referred to as a "pink tetralogy" or "balanced tetralogy." The pulmonary stenosis is not so severe that pulmonary blood flow is markedly limited; the patient is only mildly desaturated, and cyanosis is mild or difficult to detect. However, there is enough pulmonary stenosis to prevent increased pulmonary blood flow and pulmonary artery hypertension. Progressive right ventricular outflow obstruction will alter the hemodynamics and the patient may become increasingly cyanotic. Such patients may survive even into late adulthood without interventions, but they are at risk for stroke, endocarditis, and brain abscess. These patients are usually good candidates for surgical repair at any age. Successful surgery results in improvement in exercise capacity and improves life expectancy for the great majority of patients.

Previous Systemic-Pulmonary Arterial Shunt

These patients have had a previous shunt without intracardiac repair. If the shunt is large, pulmonary blood flow is high, producing a volume load on the left ventricle that may ultimately result in left ventricular dysfunction. In addition, late right ventricular dysfunction secondary to pulmonary artery hypertension may result from unrestricted flow at the site of shunt, most often from a Potts or Waterston side-by-side anastomosis, but occasionally from a modified Blalock or central shunt. If the shunt is sufficient to prevent severe cyanosis and polycythemia, but not large enough to result in pulmonary hypertension and undue left ventricular volume load (balanced), decades of stability are quite possible. However, in general, life expectancy is limited for uncorrected patients. Surgical repair markedly improves the outlook for such patients.

Post–Open-Heart Repair: Excellent Hemodynamic Result

The well-repaired patient with tetralogy of Fallot will most often be asymptomatic and acyanotic. There are no intracardiac shunts. The pulmonary outflow tract remains mildly obstructive and most often there is the murmur of pulmonary valve insufficiency. The mild valve abnormalities are well tolerated and the patient usually is active in all aspects of life, including recreational sports and other forms of physical exertion. Late hemodynamic abnormalities are rarely noted when the original repair has been excellent; however a few patients with chronic pulmonary insufficiency may develop late right ventricular dysfunction.

Post–Open-Heart Repair: Poor Result

A poor hemodynamic result occurs when there is a residual VSD or persistent severe obstruction to the right ventricular outflow tract, or both. If the former occurs in the context of total relief of the outflow tract, a persistent left-to-right shunt will occur. Such patients

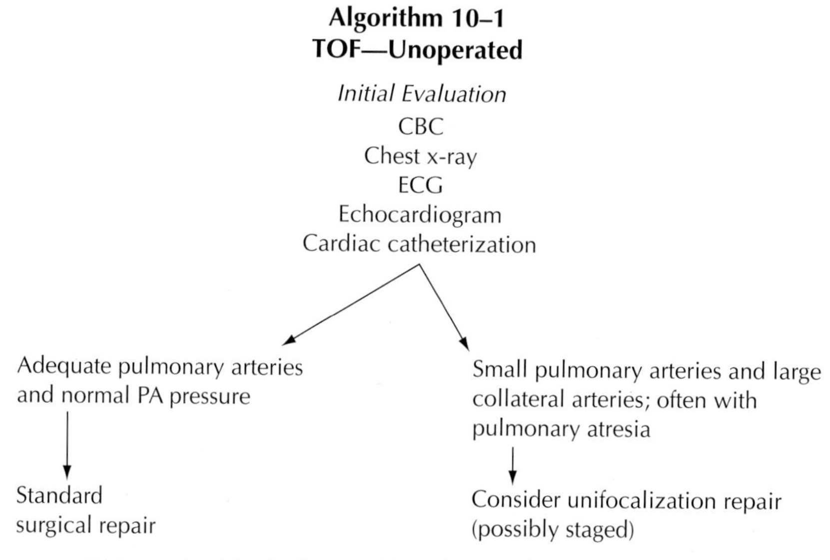

rarely present to the adult cardiologist late unless the VSD is small. In the presence of a large defect, reoperation is required almost immediately after the original surgery. When severe pulmonary stenosis persists with a closed ventricular defect, the clinical picture becomes that of isolated pulmonary stenosis, and, if uncorrected, right ventricular hypertrophy, dysfunction, and manifestation of right heart failure will ensue. Patients with severe pulmonary valve insufficiency and concomitant tricuspid insufficiency may develop right heart failure. Surgery should be performed before there is irreversible right ventricular dysfunction; in extreme cases, cardiac transplantation must be considered. Patients with ventricular arrhythmias and a poor hemodynamic result are more prone to ventricular tachyarrhythmias or sudden death than those patients in whom hemodynamics are excellent. Although rarely encountered in the modern era, patients with heart block require pacemaker implantation.

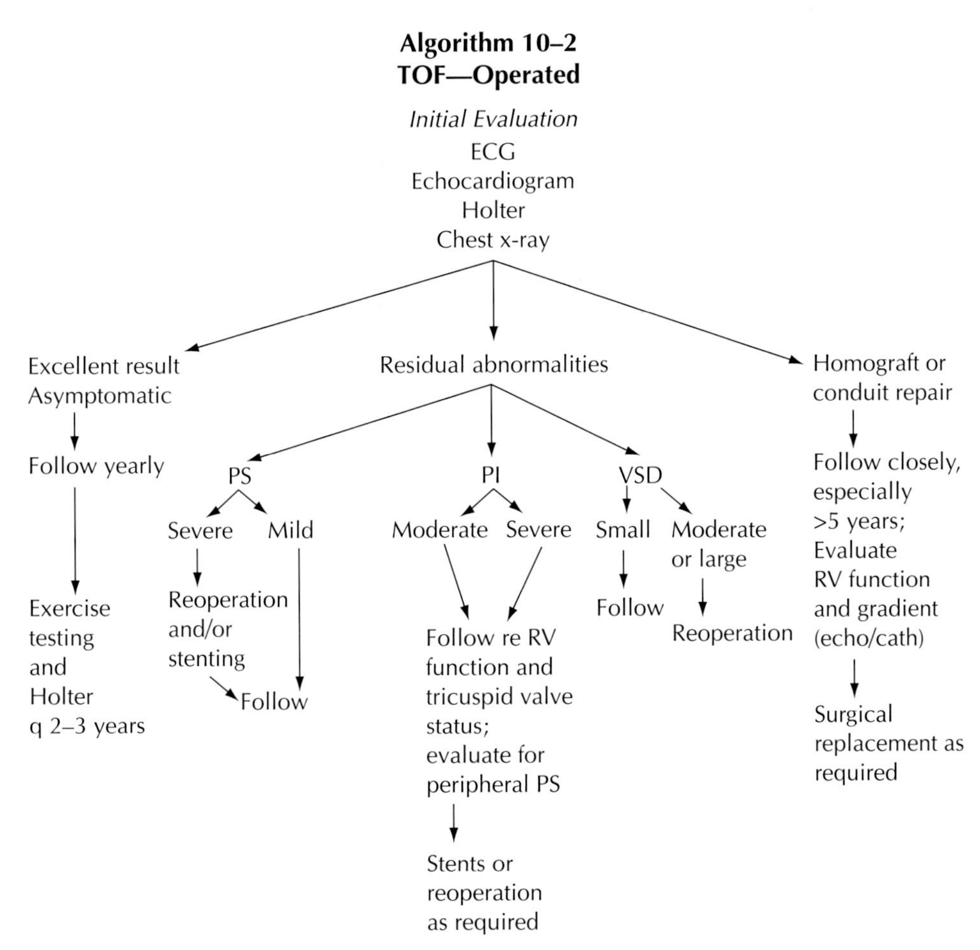

KEY: cath, catheterization; echo, echocardiogram; ECG, electrocardiogram; PI, pulmonary insufficiency; PS, pulmonary stenosis; RV, right ventricle; TOF, tetralogy of Fallot; VSD, ventricular septal defect.

BIBLIOGRAPHY

Ammash N, Warnes CA: Cerebrovascular events in adult patients with cyanotic congenital heart disease. *J Am Coll Cardiol* 28:768, 1996.

Bertranou EG, Blackstone EH, Hazelrig JB, et al: Life expectancy without surgery in tetralogy of Fallot. *Am J Cardiol* 42:458, 1978.

Blalock A, Taussig HB: Surgical treatment of malformations of the heart in which there is pulmonary stenosis or pulmonary atresia. *Am J Med* 128:189, 1945.

Castaneda AR, Sade RM, Lamberti J, Nicoloff DM: Reoperation for residual defects after repair of tetralogy of Fallot. *Surgery* 76:1010, 1974.

Deanfield JE, Ho S-Y, Anderson RH, et al: Late sudden death after repair of tetralogy of Fallot: A clinicopathologic study. *Circulation* 67:626, 1983.

Deanfield JE, McKenna WJ, Presbitero P, et al: Ventricular arrhythmia in unrepaired tetralogy of Fallot: Relation to age, timing of repair and haemodynamic status. *Br Heart J* 52:77, 1984.

Downar E, Harris L, Kimber S, et al: Ventricular tachycardia after surgical repair of tetralogy of Fallot: Results of intraoperative mapping studies. *J Am Coll Cardiol* 20:648, 1992.

Finck SJ, Puga FJ, Danielson GK: Pulmonary valve insertion during reoperation for tetralogy of Fallot. *Ann Thorac Surg* 45:610, 1988.

Grant GP, Garofano RP, Mansell AL, et al: Ventilatory response to exercise after intracardiac repair of tetralogy of Fallot. *Am Rev Respir Dis* 144:833, 1991.

Iyer KS, Mee RBB: Staged repair of pulmonary atresia with ventricular septal defect and major systemic to pulmonary artery collaterals. *Ann Thorac Surg* 51:65, 1991.

Kloevekorn WP, Meisner H, Paek SU, Sebering F: Long-term results after right ventricular outflow tract reconstruction with porcine bioprosthetic conduits. *J Cardiac Surg* 6:624, 1991.

Marelli AJ, Perloff JK, Child JS, Laks H: Pulmonary atresia with ventricular septal defect in adults. *Circulation* 89:243, 1994.

Murphy JG, Gersh BJ, Mair DD, et al: Long-term outcome in patients undergoing surgical repair of tetralogy of Fallot. *N Engl J Med* 329:593, 1993.

Park I-S, Leachman RD, Cooley DA: Total correction of tetralogy of Fallot in adults: Surgical results and long-term follow-up. *Tex Heart Inst J* 14:160, 1987.

Presbitero P, Prever SB, Contrafatto I, Morea M: As originally published in 1988: Results of total correction of tetralogy of Fallot performed in adults: Updated in 1996. *Ann Thorac Surg* 61: 1870, 1996.

Rosenthal A, Behrendt D, Sloan H, et al: Long-term prognosis (15 to 26 years) after repair of tetralogy of Fallot. I. Survival and symptomatic status. *Ann Thorac Surg* 38:151, 1984.

Sawatari K, Imai Y, Kurosawa H, et al: Staged operation for pulmonary atresia and ventricular septal defect with major aortopulmonary collateral arteries: New technique for complete unifocalization. *J Thorac Cardiovasc Surg* 98:738, 1989.

Schaff HV, DiDonato RM, Danielson GK, et al: Reoperation for obstructed pulmonary ventricle–pulmonary artery conduits. Early and late results. *J Thorac Cardiovasc Surg* 88:334, 1984.

Zhao HZ, Miller G, Reitz BA, Shumway NE: Surgical repair of tetralogy of Fallot: Long term follow-up with particular emphasis on late death and reoperation. *J Thorac Cardiovasc Surg* 89:204, 1985.

CHAPTER 11

D-TRANSPOSITION

D-transposition of the great arteries (TGA) is a relatively common cyanotic heart defect that when untreated almost invariably results in death in the neonatal period or infancy. In patients with this lesion, the great arteries arise from the opposite ventricles; thus, systemic venous return enters the right atrium, right ventricle, and aorta, whereas pulmonary venous return flows from the pulmonary veins to the left atrium, left ventricle (LV), and pulmonary artery (Fig. 11-1). When D-transposition (D-TGA) is present, the atria and ventricles are normally positioned and the great arteries are discordant, resulting in an anterior aorta arising from a right ventricular infundibulum (Fig. 11-2) and the pulmonary artery originating from the left ventricle. In this situation there is normal D-looping of the ventricles and fibrous continuity between the pulmonary and mitral valves. The majority of patients with D-TGA have an intact ventricular septum, but a significant number have a ventricular septal defect, patent ductus arteriosus, and/or other associated cardiac abnormalities.

To survive the neonatal period, a patient with D-TGA must have communications between the right and left sides of the heart to allow mixing of the two circulations. At the time of birth, patency of the foramen ovale allows sufficient mixing of the two circulations to permit survival, although with extremely low arterial oxygen saturation. These patients are severely cyanotic at birth and virtually never survive the neonatal period without intervention. Patients with large atrial septal defects, ventricular septal defects, and significant ductus arteriosus are less cyanotic and may live many months without surgical intervention if mixing is adequate. However, their ultimate prognosis remains grave without operative correction.

D-TGA should be contrasted with L-TGA (congenitally corrected transposition of the great vessels). In L-TGA, there is an L-ventricular loop that results in atrioventricular discordance and L-malposition of the aorta. This results in normal physiologic blood flow, although associated congenital anomalies are usually present (Chap. 8). Both D- and L-transposition of the great arteries also may be associated with many forms of single ventricle (Chap. 12).

CLINICAL FEATURES

Infancy and Childhood

Neonates with D-TGA and an intact ventricular septum present in the first day or two of life with severe cyanosis. If left untreated, these infants will die of severe hypoxemia,

FIGURE 11-1

D-transposition of the great arteries. The aorta (Ao) is anterior and arises from a normally positioned right ventricle (RV). The pulmonary artery (PA) is posterior and arises from a normally positioned left ventricle (LV).

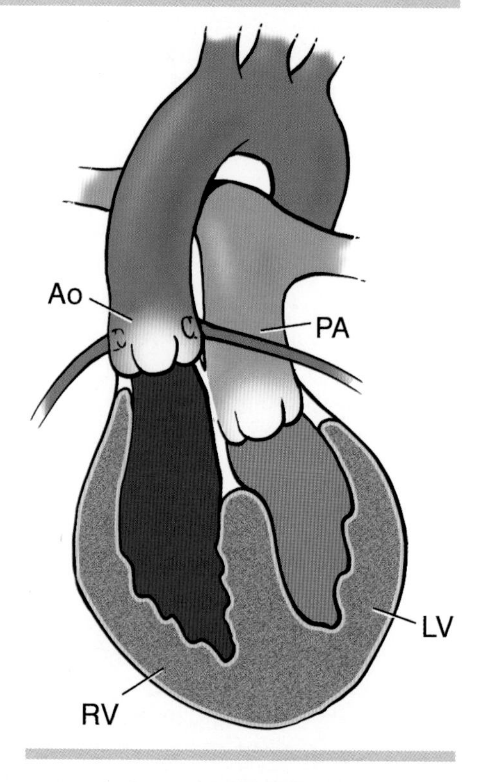

FIGURE 11-2

Parasternal long-axis view in a patient with D-transposition of the great arteries. The aorta is anterior and arises from the right ventricle. The posterior pulmonary artery arises from the left ventricle. The great vessels are parallel, consistent with transposition. LV, left ventricle; RV, right ventricle; PA, pulmonary artery; Ao, aorta.

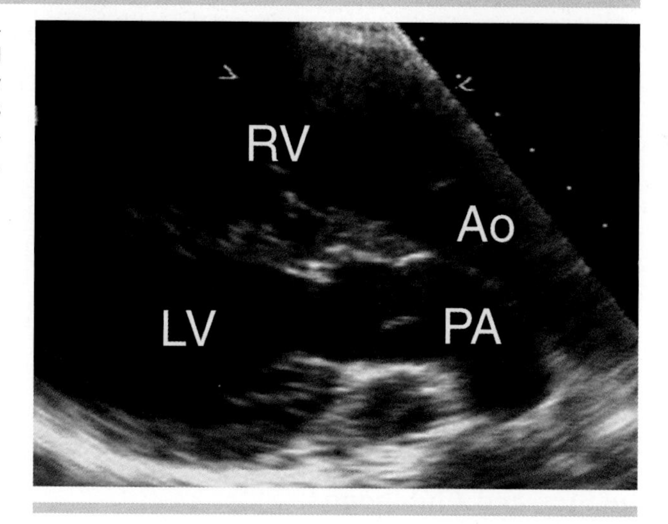

since there is insufficient mixing of the two circulations to allow adequate oxygenation of the peripheral tissues. Near the beginning of the surgical era, a number of innovative operations were devised to improve mixing of the parallel circulations at the atrial level. In 1950, the Blalock-Hanlon operation was developed, which created an ASD without the use of cardiopulmonary bypass. Three years later, the Baffes operation was performed, in which the IVC was diverted into the left atrium and the right upper pulmonary vein into the right atrium, improving oxygenation. In 1966, balloon atrial septostomy was introduced. In this procedure, a balloon-tipped catheter is passed across the foramen ovale into the left atrium. The balloon is inflated and pulled back into the right atrium, enlarging the atrial communication. This procedure, which is performed in the first days of life, increases mixing and allows adequate palliation until more specific surgical management could be carried out. In the past, a Senning or Mustard operation was performed within a few months of balloon septostomy. These procedures, although technically different, both route systemic venous return from the right atrium to the left ventricle and the pulmonary artery. Pulmonary venous return is baffled to the right ventricle, and oxygenated blood then enters the aorta (Fig. 11-3). The surgery results in physiologic correction of

FIGURE 11-3

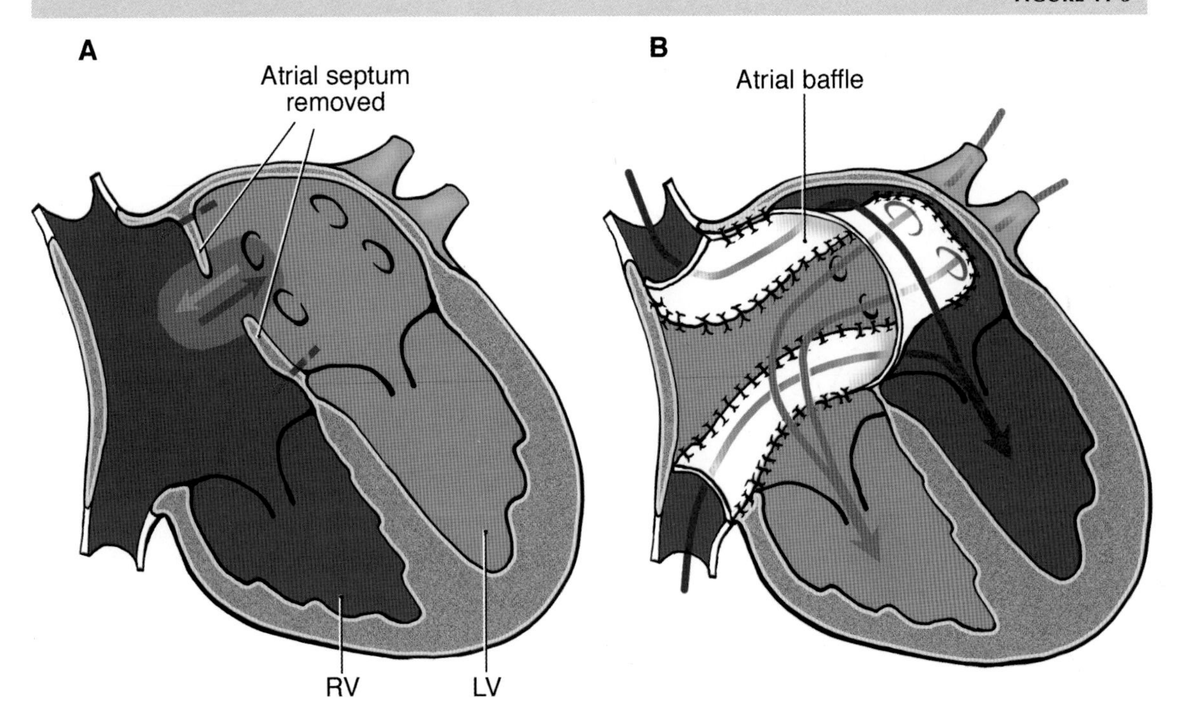

The Mustard operation for transposition of the great arteries. *A*. The atrial septum is removed. *B*. An atrial baffle is placed in such a manner that pulmonary venous blood flows over the baffle through the tricuspid valve into the systemic right ventricle and out the aorta. The superior and inferior vena caval blood flows inside the baffle through the mitral valve and into the left ventricle, which is connected to the pulmonary artery.

the circulation. A number of late problems are associated with these types of *atrial* switch operations. There remains a systemic right ventricle, which may result in abnormal right ventricular and tricuspid valve function. In addition, the extensive atrial surgery predisposes patients to sick sinus syndrome and atrial arrhythmias, particularly atrial flutter. Although the Mustard and Senning operations were lifesaving for many patients from the 1960s through the 1980s, over the past 10 to 15 years, these operations were replaced by the arterial switch operation (Jatene procedure). The *arterial* switch operation results in anatomic correction of patients with D-TGA. In this procedure, the ascending aorta and pulmonary artery are transected and reconnected to their anatomically correct ventricles. In addition, the coronary arteries, which arise from the anterior semilunar root, are transferred to the posterior semilunar root from which the aorta now arises. In patients with transposition and an intact ventricular septum, the operation must be performed shortly after birth before there is regression of the left ventricular mass as pulmonary vascular resistance falls (Figs. 11-4*A* through *D*; Figs. 11-5*A* and *B*). When the procedure is done in

FIGURE 11-4

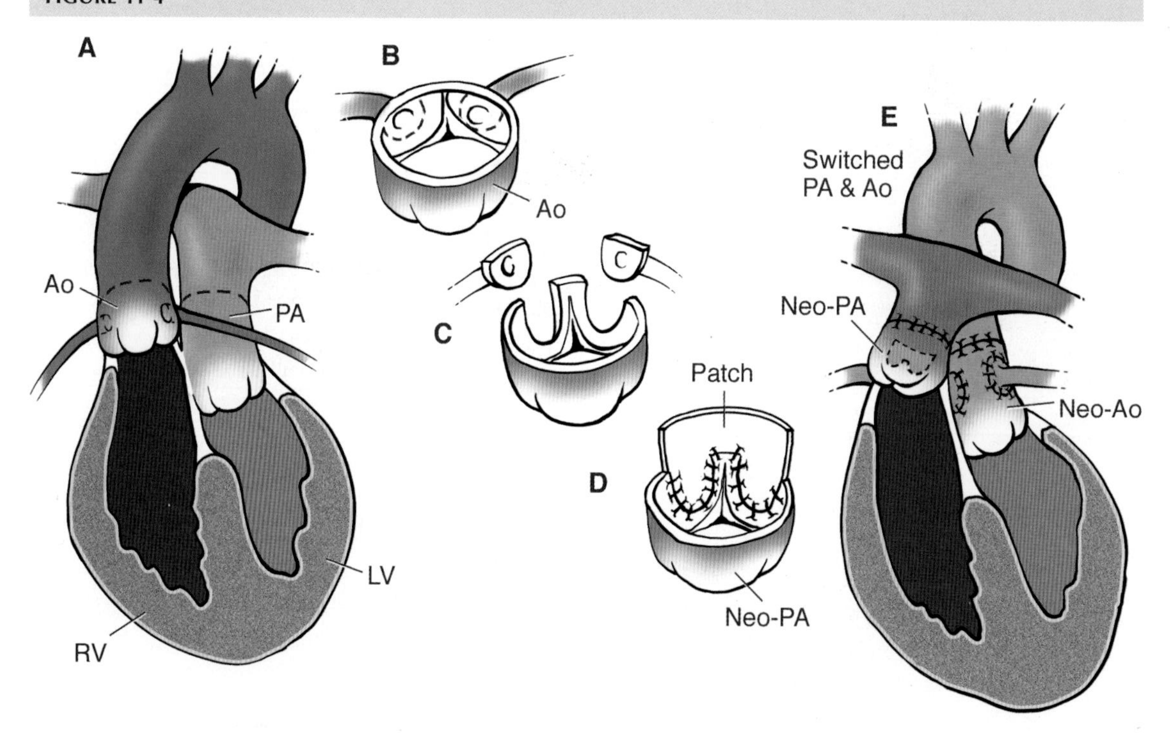

Arterial switch operation for D-transposition of the great arteries. *A*. The aorta is transected above the coronary ostia and the main pulmonary artery is transected in a parallel fashion. *B* and *C*. The coronary arteries are removed with a button of aortic tissue. *D*. The area of coronary resection is patched. *E*. The transected pulmonary artery is anastomosed to the semilunar root arising from the right ventricle, forming a neo-pulmonary artery (neo-PA). The ascending aorta is anatomosed to the new aortic root (neo-Ao) to which the coronary arteries have been transferred. This operation results in full anatomic correction of D-transposition of the great arteries.

FIGURE 11-5*A*

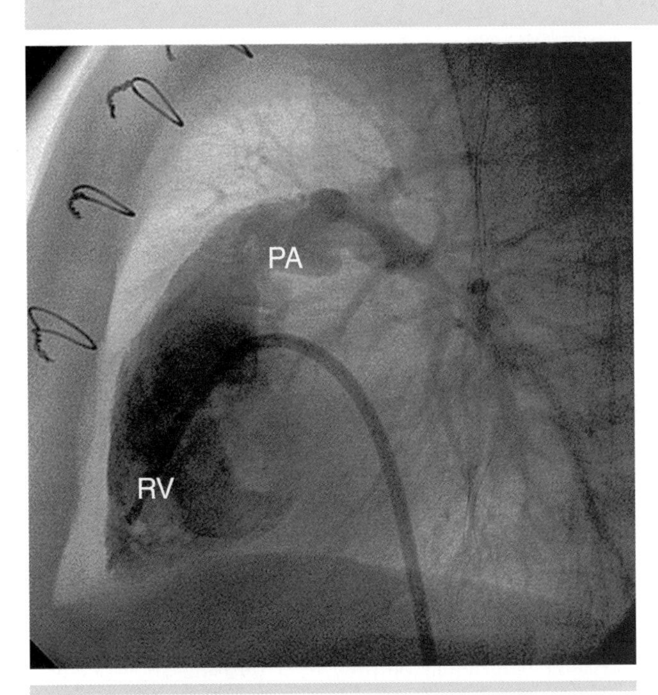

A right ventriculogram in the lateral projection in a patient who has undergone arterial switch repair. The pulmonary artery is now connected to the anatomic right ventricle. There is no evidence of right ventricular outflow obstruction. RV, right ventricle; PA, pulmonary artery.

FIGURE 11-5*B*

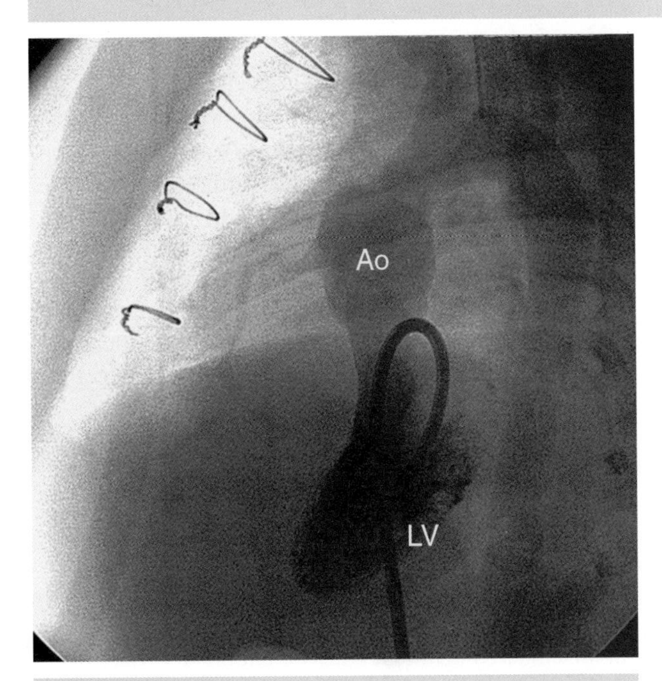

A left ventriculogram in the lateral projection in the same patient who has undergone arterial switch repair. The aorta is connected to the anatomic left ventricle. Note the enlargement of the neoaortic root. LV, left ventricle; Ao, aorta.

the first days of life, the operation can often be carried out without the necessity for a palliative balloon septostomy before surgery.

Infants with D-TGA and a ventricular septal defect (VSD) often present later in infancy. The VSD may allow adequate mixing of the two circulations, enabling some patients to survive for many months without surgery. However, in the presence of a large VSD, congestive heart failure may ensue, resulting in dyspnea, tachypnea, and failure to thrive. In the early years of cardiac surgery, patients with D-TGA and a large VSD underwent pulmonary artery banding to limit pulmonary artery blood flow, and at the same operation an atrial septal defect was created (Blalock-Hanlon procedure) to improve mixing and allow decompression of the left atrium. Modern management of this condition allows the initial surgical intervention to include the arterial switch and VSD repair in early infancy.

Some patients with D-TGA and a large VSD have naturally occurring pulmonary outflow obstruction; the clinical course and presentation of these patients depend on the degree of pulmonary stenosis. If pulmonary outflow tract obstruction is severe, a systemic artery to pulmonary artery shunt as well as a balloon atrial septostomy may be required. In balanced situations in which pulmonary stenosis is only moderate, the infants are essentially self-palliated and can survive for many years without intervention. Since abnormalities of the pulmonary valve would not allow an arterial switch operation to be carried out in these patients, eventual surgical treatment later in childhood would consist of a Rastelli operation. In this procedure, a patch is constructed that channels the LV blood flow through the VSD across the right ventricular outflow tract into the anterior aorta (Fig. 11-6). The isolated body of the right ventricle is then anastomosed to the pulmonary artery by a conduit or homograft. Blood flow from the LV to the main pulmonary artery is interrupted (Fig. 11-7*A* and *B*).

D-TGA in Adults

Patients with D-TGA virtually never reach adulthood without having had previous surgical interventions. The great majority of patients presenting to adult cardiologists have undergone a Senning or Mustard *atrial* switch operation or, less frequently, a Rastelli procedure. Since the *arterial* switch operation has been carried out in a large number of patients only in the last decade, few of these patients have reached adulthood. Medium-term follow-up indicates that the great majority will continue to do well in later years, although there have been some patients reported with coronary abnormalities after reimplantation.

The Adult Patient After the Mustard or Senning Operation

Late complications after both the Mustard and Senning atrial switch procedures are common in adult patients.

Residual atrial communications are not unusual and often consist of small, clinically unimportant left-to-right shunts. However, if there is some degree of baffle obstruction between the cavae and the left ventricle and the communication is proximal to the point of narrowing, a right-to-left shunt may occur.

Baffle obstruction will result in either systemic venous or pulmonary venous obstruction. Systemic venous obstruction can occur in either the inferior vena cava (IVC) or

FIGURE 11-6

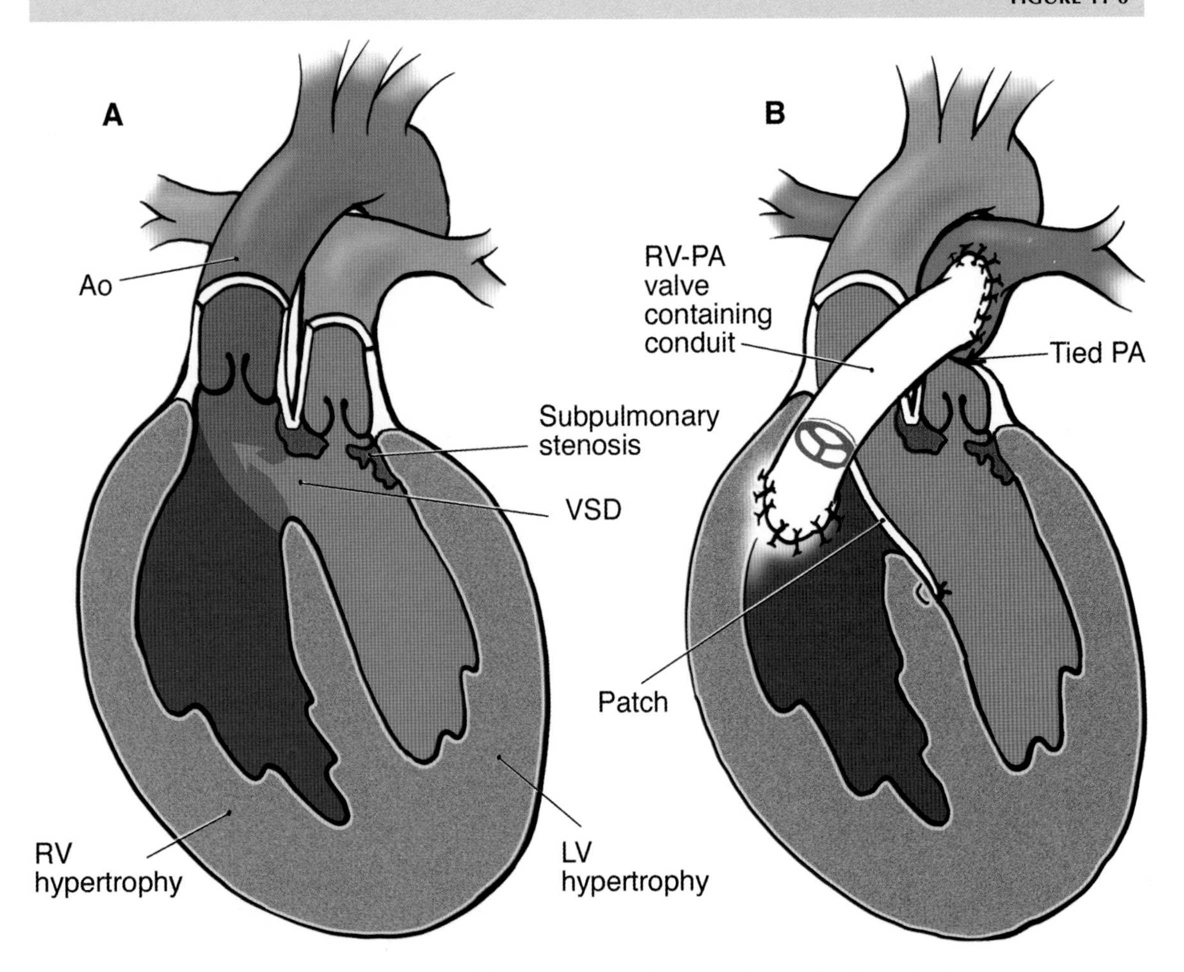

Rastelli operation for repair of (*A*) transposition of the great artery with ventricular septal defect and subpulmonary stenosis. The ventricular septal defect allows oxygenated blood to reach the aorta. *B*. The Rastelli repair includes tunneling of the left ventricle through the ventricular septal defect to the aorta. Right ventricular blood flow is via a homograft or valve-containing conduit. The proximal pulmonary artery is tied off (Tied PA).

the superior vena cava (SVC) limb of the baffle and results in various combinations of systemic venous obstructive symptoms (Fig. 11-8). Pulmonary venous obstruction produces elevated pulmonary venous and capillary pressure and, if severe enough, pulmonary hypertension. When significant, such obstructions present within months or a few years after the original operation and are not expected to be associated with severe symptoms beginning in adulthood. However, the possibility of mild to moderate obstruction must be considered in any patient with otherwise unexplained peripheral edema, hepatomegaly, ascites, low cardiac output, or pulmonary symptoms.

FIGURE 11-7*A*

Subcostal views in a patient who has undergone Rastelli repair for D-transposition of the great arteries with a ventricular septal defect and pulmonary stenosis. The aorta is anterior. There is an angled patch, which is echogenic and directs blood from the left ventricle into the aorta. Ao, aorta; LV, left ventricle; RV, right ventricle.

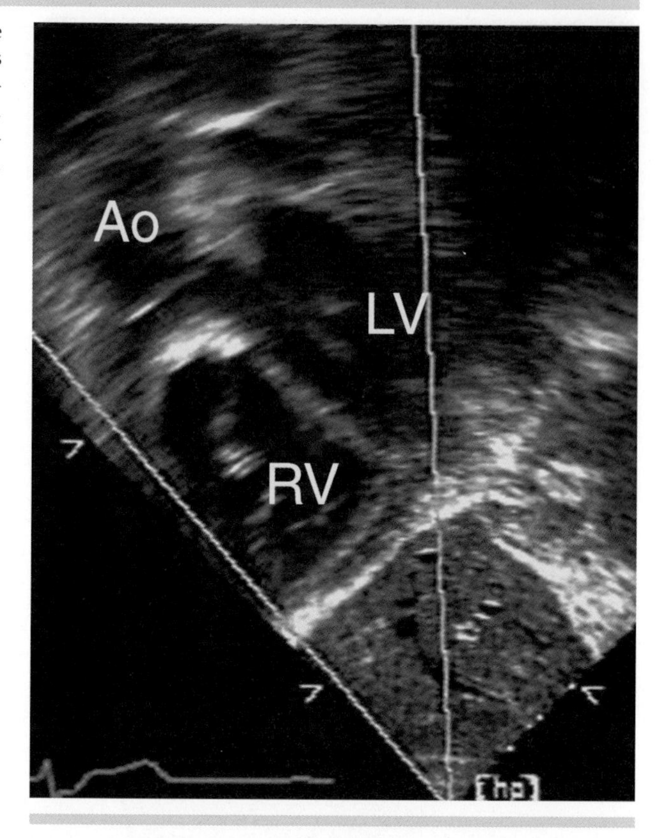

FIGURE 11-7*B*

Left ventriculogram in a patient who has had a Rastelli operation. Blood reaches the aorta through an outflow tunnel which utilizes the VSD. The metal ring (arrow) of a porcine valve conduit, which connects the right ventricle to the pulmonary artery, lies adjacent to the aorta. There is no contrast material in the right ventricle or pulmonary artery. LV, left ventricle; Ao, aorta.

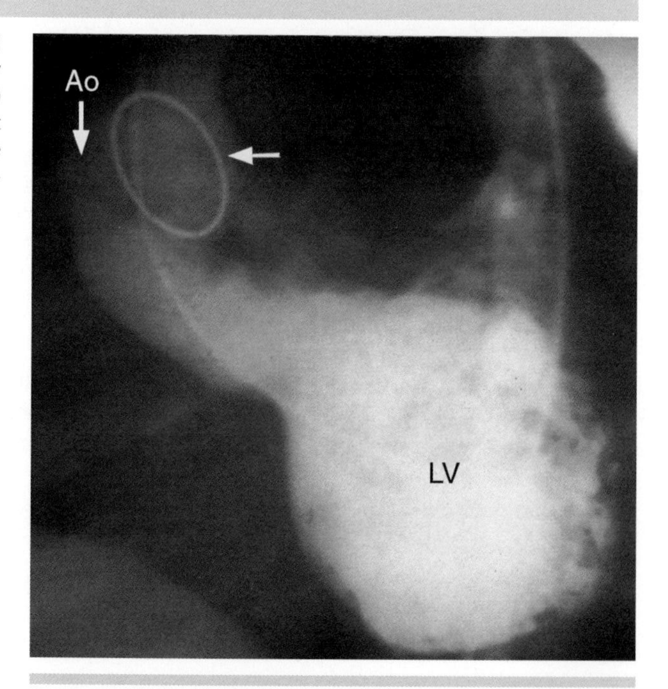

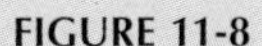

FIGURE 11-8

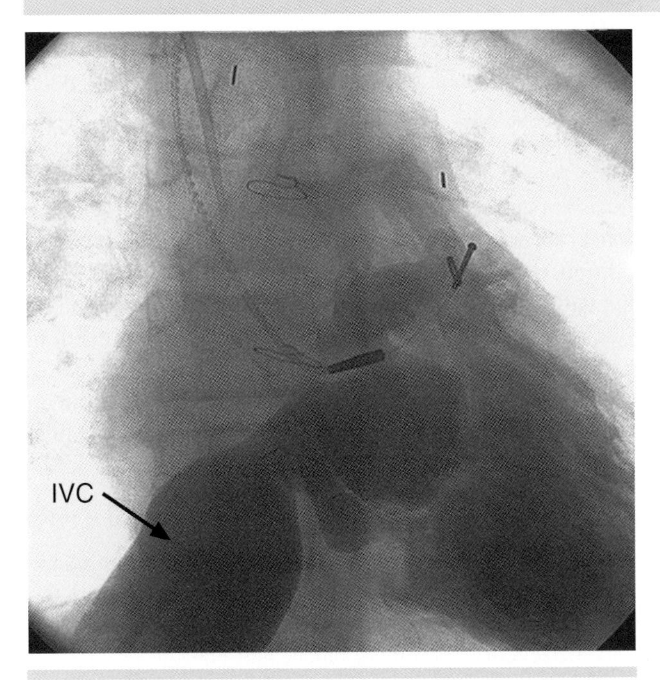

An IVC angiogram in an AP projection following Mustard repair. There is mild narrowing of the IVC limb. Blood flows from the IVC through the mitral valve and into the left ventricle, where it exits the pulmonary artery. An atrial pacemaker lead has been inserted from the SVC limb of the baffle into the left atrial appendage, which is part of the neo–right atrium. IVC, inferior vena cava; LV, left ventricle; PA, pulmonary artery.

Right ventricular (systemic) dysfunction may develop after *atrial* switch operations and this has important implications. Survival to age 20 in a large series of Mustard patients from Toronto was 76%; 40% of the late deaths were sudden. In general, a right ventricle that has not been subjected to abnormal afterload or preload or early cyanosis should function well into adulthood. This is also true for adults with L-TGA and no associated defects who occasionally are encountered in late adulthood without right ventricle dysfunction. However, in both of these lesions, right ventricular failure can occur in the absence of identifiable hemodynamic burdens. Thus, the ultimate fate of the systemic right ventricle after an *atrial* switch for D-tranposition also remains uncertain.

When right ventricular dysfunction does occur, it usually is found in conjunction with tricuspid insufficiency. Tricuspid insufficiency appears to be less well tolerated in a patient with a systemic right ventricle than in a patient with mitral regurgitation with a systemic left ventricle. Infundibular or aortic valve obstruction and insufficiency are extremely rare in patients with D-TGA.

Dynamic or anatomic left ventricular outflow tract obstruction that produces pulmonary stenosis is not unusual in patients after a Mustard or Senning operation. The ventricular septum is committed to the right ventricle, and the crescent-shaped low-pressure left ventricle occasionally is obstructed by a hypertrophied ventricular septum; in some cases, fibrous subvalvar subpulmonary intrusions also may be present. Most often, even moderately severe obstruction is well tolerated by the morphologic left ventricle.

Patients with D-TGA and VSD who are unoperated will develop *pulmonary vascular obstructive disease* within the first year of life in the great majority of cases. Even children who underwent septostomy for D-TGA with an intact ventricular septum can develop pulmonary vascular disease within a year or two. Pulmonary vascular disease is not an issue when switch procedures are done early in infancy.

Cardiac arrhythmias often are major findings in patients with D-TGA who have undergone an *atrial* switch operation. Twenty percent of neonates have abnormal sinus node function or junctional rhythm when discharged from the hospital after the *atrial* switch operation. It is well documented that increasing numbers of these patients gradually develop signs of sick sinus syndrome over the years. Late follow-up studies have shown sinus rhythm in only 40% of Mustard patients by age 20. Approximately 20% of *atrial* switch patients have had a pacemaker inserted because of severe bradyarrhythmias by the time they are young adults. In addition, these patients may develop atrial flutter with rapid AV conduction. Although patients with rapid atrial flutter can be markedly symptomatic, it is more likely that ventricular tachyarrhythmias are responsible for late sudden death in this population.

Identification of the high-risk patient is difficult because sudden death can occur in both symptomatic patients with RV dysfunction as well as in hemodynamically stable, asymptomatic patients.

Adult Patients After the Rastelli Repair

The Rastelli operation for patients with D-TGA, VSD, and pulmonary stenosis can be associated with late sequelae. Potential problems include obstruction of the tunnel from the left ventricle through the VSD into the aorta, resulting in subaortic stenosis; a residual left-to-right shunt from a defect at the level of the tunnel patch; and chronic pulmonary insufficiency or obstruction from the conduit or homograft connecting the right ventricle to the pulmonary artery. Cardiac arrhythmias also may occur in these patients.

Adult Patients After the Arterial Switch Operation

The major issue for patients who have had an *arterial* switch operation is the status of the coronary arteries. With the current state of the art in neonatal surgery, the coronaries can be transferred without kinking or obstruction by using a button technique (Fig. 11-4). In recent years, the incidence of clinically evident coronary insufficiency has been very low. Reports of late sudden death are rare. In a large series of the *arterial* switch patients, the incidence of unsuspected important coronary artery abnormalities was 3%. Whether these favorable findings will continue into adulthood remains to be seen, but currently there is no indication that a significant number of patients will develop late coronary manifestations as they grow older. Patients who have had a VSD closure with the *arterial* switch operation seem to have a similar outcome as those who originally had an intact ventricular septum. Rhythm disorders do not appear to be a problem after an *arterial* switch operation. Occasionally reoperation for supravalvar pulmonary stenosis has been necessary, but this complication has decreased in recent years. Dilatation of the neoaortic root with mild aortic regurgitation is a frequent finding and will require ongoing follow-up to determine whether these patients will develop late progressive aortic regurgitation.

PHYSICAL EXAMINATION

The features of the physical examination depend on the presence or absence of residual shunts or valvar abnormalities. The uncomplicated patient after an atrial switch operation has a loud single-second sound due to an anterior-positioned aortic valve. Since the right ventricle is the systemic pumping chamber, there is a right ventricular heave along the left sternal border. In the absence of associated defects, no significant murmurs are audible. The murmur of tricuspid insufficiency is similar in location to that of any patient with this abnormality, although after a Mustard or Senning operation, tricuspid insufficiency is functionally equivalent to mitral insufficiency in a normal heart. Patients with a residual VSD will have a harsh pansystolic murmur along the left sternal border. Valvar or subvalvar pulmonary stenosis results in a harsh systolic ejection murmur along the left midsternal border rather than at the left upper sternal border, because the pulmonary artery arises inferiorly, in the usual position of the aorta. The position of diastolic murmurs also relates to the reverse position of the great arteries with a systemic right ventricle. A tricuspid flow murmur is indicative of a large left-to-right shunt at the ventricular level or increased diastolic flow in the presence of tricuspid insufficiency. Patients with severe hemodynamic abnormalities will have the usual findings of cardiomegaly and a precordial heave. However, the precordial impulse tends to be more right ventricular or mixed than is noted in patients with severe heart failure and normally positioned ventricles.

Since the circulation has been "corrected" by the atrial switch operation, cyanosis will not be present unless there is a residual right-to-left shunt at the atrial level caused by obstruction or dysfunction of the atrial baffle. It is not unusual to note bradycardia or junctional rhythms, in keeping with the high incidence of sick sinus syndrome.

The typical cardiac exam after a Rastelli repair reveals a harsh systolic murmur along the left sternal border due to varying degrees of turbulence along the RV to PA conduit or homograft. Significant obstruction is usually associated with a louder and longer murmur. The systolic murmur of a residual VSD or subaortic obstruction within the interventricular tunnel can be obscured by the conduit murmur, or the reverse may be true. An early diastolic murmur along the left sternal border usually indicates pulmonary insufficiency. A right ventricular heave may accompany severe conduit obstruction.

The cardiac examination after an arterial switch is usually normal. A systolic ejection murmur at the left upper sternal border could suggest stenosis at the area of the anastomosis between the neopulmonary outflow tract and the pulmonary artery. Significant dysrhythmias have not been reported after the arterial switch operation.

NONINVASIVE EVALUATION

In patients who have had an atrial switch procedure, the *electrocardiogram* (ECG) shows right ventricular hypertrophy. Right axis deviation and large R waves in leads V_3R and V_1 are usual and often are associated with ST-T wave abnormalities. Sinus bradycardia and junctional rhythms of sick sinus syndrome are often present (Fig. 11-9). A normal ECG is expected in patients after successful arterial switch procedures.

The *chest x-ray* in a patient after an atrial switch operation indicates a right ventricular cardiac silhouette with a slight increase in the cardiothoracic ratio. The lung fields are usually normal. The chest x-ray may reflect associated defects; pulmonary congestion secondary to right ventricular dysfunction may be noted in symptomatic patients. The chest x-ray in patients after an arterial switch is usually normal.

The *echocardiogram* of a patient after an atrial switch procedure is characteristic. The ventricular septum is committed to the systemic right ventricle and bows posteriorly into

FIGURE 11-9

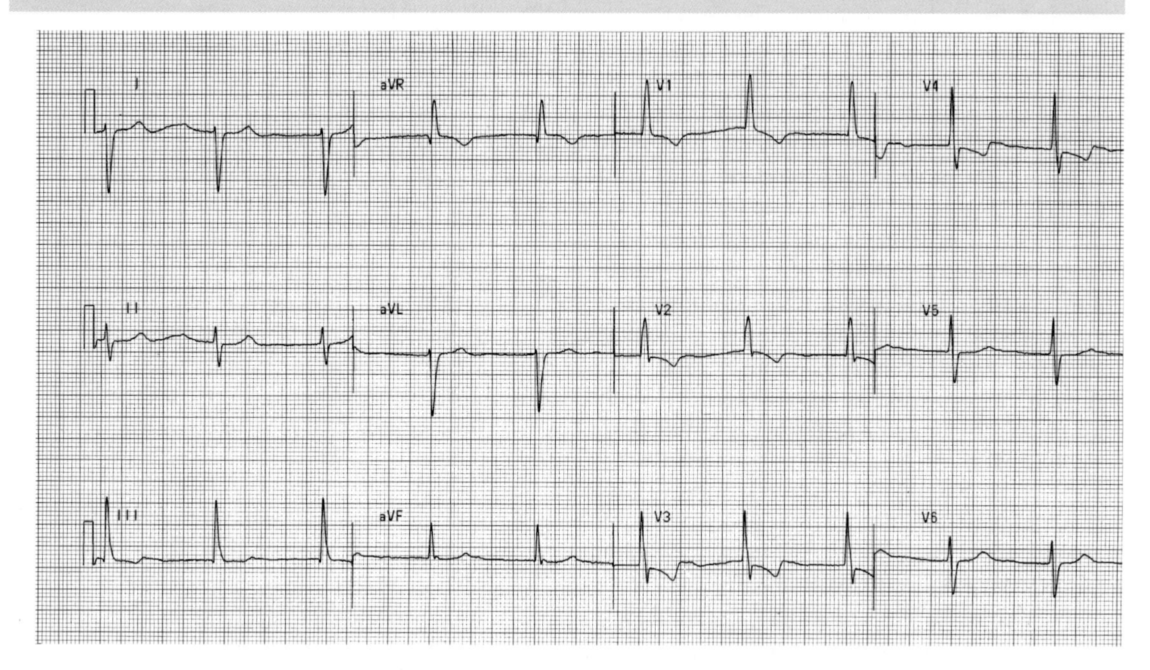

A 12-lead electrocardiogram in an adult following Mustard repair. The tracing shows a junctional rhythm with right ventricular hypertrophy.

the left ventricle (Fig. 11-10). A color Doppler study delineates the flow pattern across the systemic venous and pulmonary venous baffles to the left and right ventricles, respectively (Figs. 11-11*A* and *B*). Significant obstruction can usually be ruled out. Intra-atrial shunts may be difficult to assess by transthoracic imaging in adults. Right ventricular function, the status of the tricuspid valve, and the left ventricular outflow tract gradient can be assessed. Doppler-predicted gradients across abnormal valves or conduits are helpful in the clinical evaluation of postoperative patients with D-TGA. In adults, echocardiography may be limited for assessment of right ventricular function and cardiac magnetic resonance imaging (MRI) can be used for quantitative assessment of RV volume and ejection fraction. In addition, MRI shows excellent detail of the systemic and pulmonary venous pathways.

The evaluation of a Rastelli repair includes visualizing the intraventricular tunnel from the LV to the aorta and the status of the right ventricular–pulmonary artery (RV-PA) conduit or homograft. Right ventricular pressure can be assessed by TR jet if tricuspid regurgitation is present. Prediction of the conduit gradient is important but may not always be feasible in adult patients. Some adults may have a nonvalved right ventricular pulmonary artery (RV-PA) conduit that results in significant pulmonary insufficiency.

Patients who have had an arterial switch operation have a normal four-chambered heart. LV function and the presence of areas of ventricular dysfunction should be evalu-

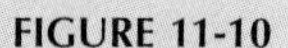

FIGURE 11-10

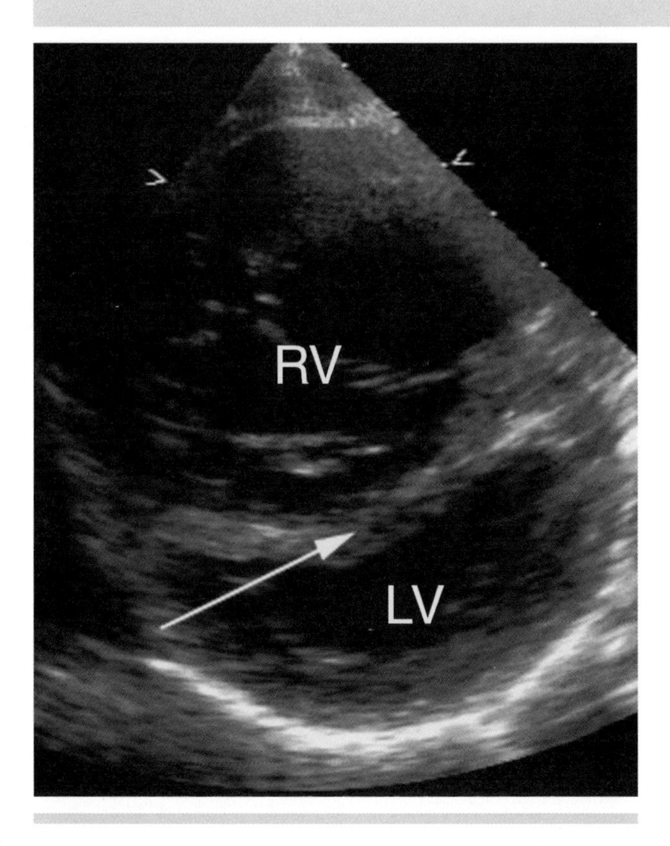

Parasternal short-axis view in a patient with a Mustard repair. There is posterior bowing of the interventricular septum (arrow) into the left ventricle due to compression of the left ventricle by the high-pressure systemic right ventricle. LV, left ventricle; RV, right ventricle.

ated. In addition, patients who had arterial switch procedures in the early years of such surgical treatment may display suprapulmonary stenosis in the area of the anastomosis. This obstruction can be delineated by echocardiography.

MANAGEMENT

Atrial Switch

All patients should have a complete history and physical examination, ECG, chest x-ray, echocardiogram, 24-h Holter monitor reading, and exercise test. On the basis of these studies and review of the early records, the patient's status can be determined. Small residual left-to-right atrial shunts or minimal right-to-left shunts are generally well tolerated, and no specific intervention is recommended in the absence of other significant hemodynamic abnormalities. Significant clinically important systemic venous or pulmonary venous obstruction is rare in adults; mild obstruction may be present and is well tolerated in an asymptomatic patient. However, in the presence of systemic or pulmonary congestion, intervention could be required. Relief of obstruction by surgical intervention or

FIGURE 11-11*A*

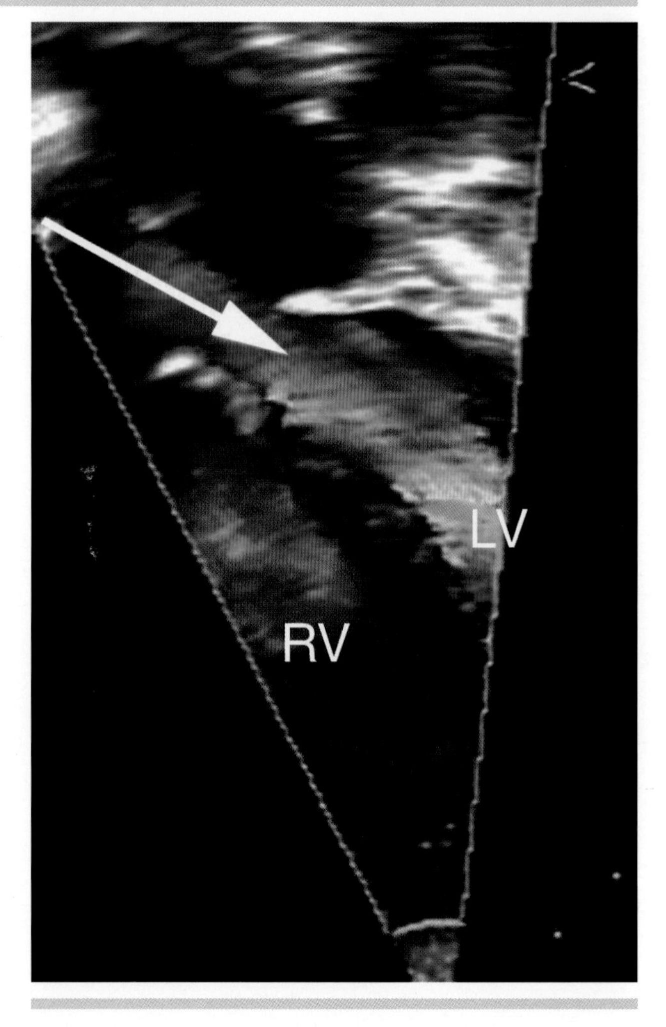

Color Doppler from an apical four-chamber view following a Mustard repair. The arrow points to unobstructed systemic venous inflow from the superior limb of the baffle, through the mitral valve, and into the left ventricle. RV, right ventricle; LV, left ventricle.

catheterization techniques using balloon dilation and/or stenting has been successful (Fig. 11-12*A* and *B*). Mild to moderate tricuspid insufficiency in the presence of good right ventricular function should be monitored closely, but valve repair or replacement should be reserved for patients with severe regurgitation and right ventricular dilatation. Tricuspid valve surgery may be only partially successful, thus suggesting conservative management for mild to moderate cases.

Left ventricular outflow tract obstruction to the pulmonary artery is generally well tolerated; surgical intervention may be difficult since the obstruction is most often dynamic or related to the geometry of the ventricular septum. Intervention should be reserved for severe obstruction, but patients with milder forms must be watched carefully for progression.

FIGURE 11-11*B*

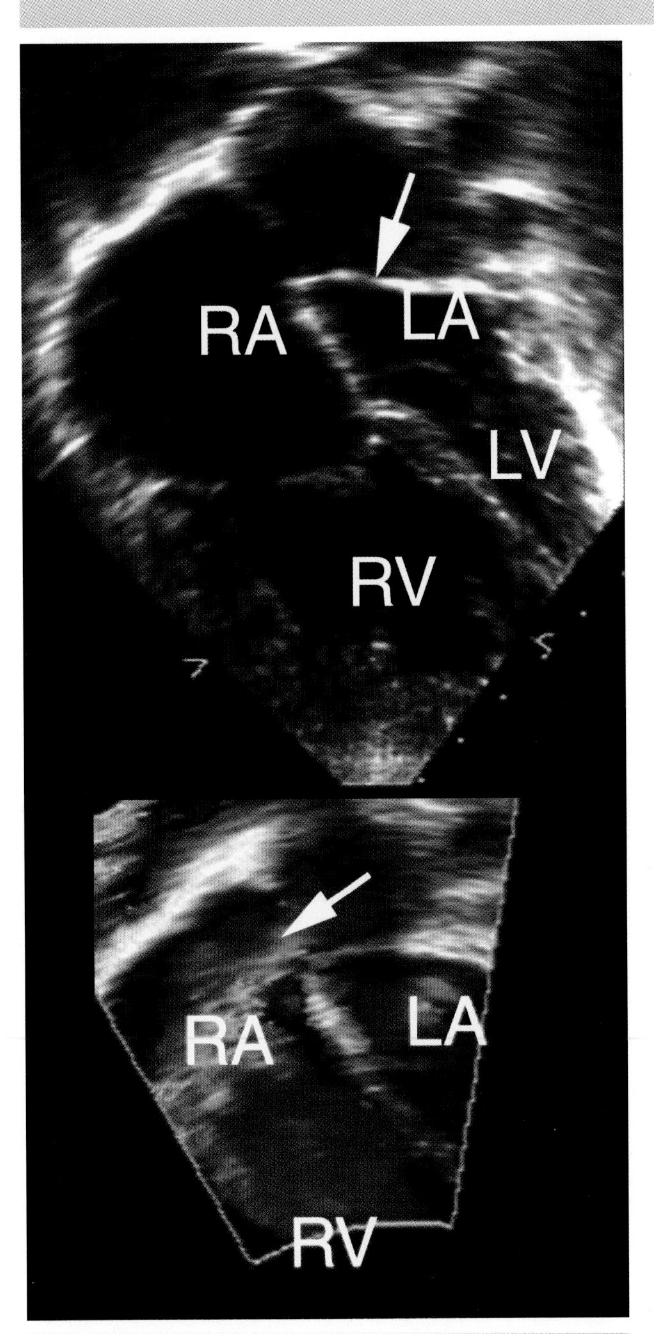

(Top) Apical four-chamber view following a Mustard repair. There is enlargement of the systemic right ventricle. The arrow points to a portion of the atrial baffle, which separates systemic venous and pulmonary venous blood. (Bottom) Color Doppler from the same patient showing unobstructed pulmonary venous inflow into the right atrial portion of the pulmonary venous atrium. RV, right ventricle; LV, left ventricle; RA, right atrium; LA, left atrium.

FIGURE 11-12*A*

An angiogram in the superior vena cava (SVC) in a patient with a Mustard repair. There is severe stenosis in the superior limb of the baffle. The proximal portion of the SVC is dilated and there is little antegrade flow through the obstructed baffle. A guide wire has been advanced through the baffle from the SVC into the left ventricle.

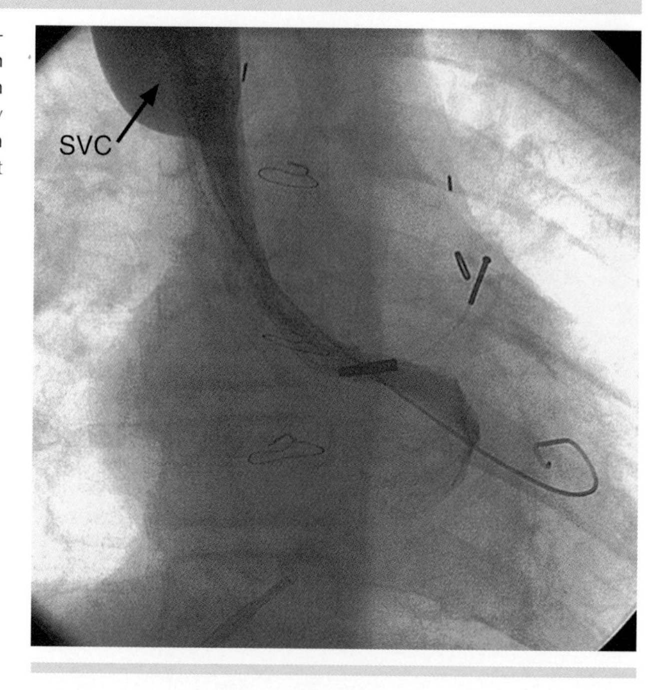

FIGURE 11-12*B*

An angiogram in the same patient showing successful dilatation of the SVC limb of the baffle with a stent.

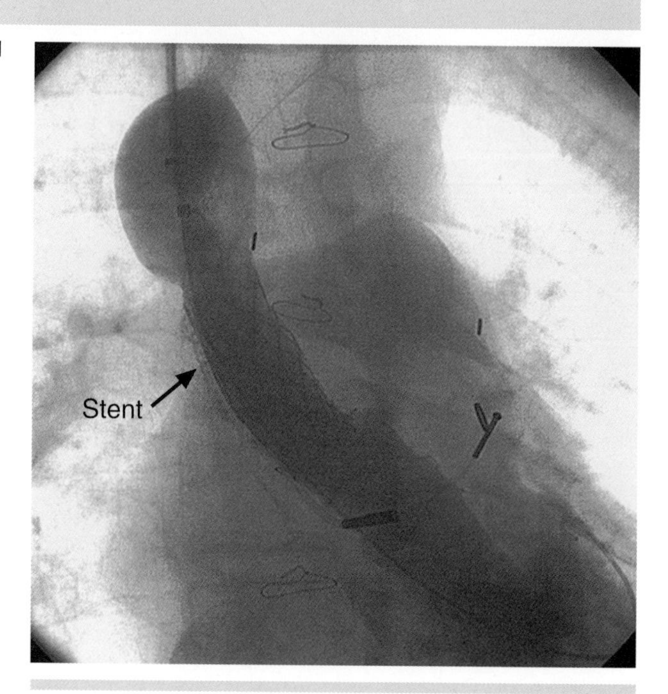

Yearly Holter recordings are suggested to assess cardiac rhythm. Management of sick sinus syndrome is similar to that of any patient with this rhythm disorder. Pacemaker insertion may be required in the presence of significant bradycardic symptoms or concomitant with the addition of certain antiarrhythmic drugs to control tachyarrhythmias. Atrial lead placement may be difficult in patients who have had an intraatrial baffle operation.

Right ventricular dysfunction should be treated with standard anticongestive measures, including digoxin, diuretics, and an angiotensin converting enzyme (ACE) inhibitor. Cardiac transplantation is a consideration in patients with intractable heart failure. A rare patient with severe right (systemic) ventricular dysfunction may be considered for conversion of an *atrial* switch to an *arterial* switch operation, but this requires pulmonary artery banding to increase left ventricular pressure and hypertrophy in order to function as a systemic ventricle. In contrast with PA banding in infancy to prepare the left ventricle of patients who did not have an early *arterial* switch as neonates, few successes have been reported in adults, and this approach is rarely recommended.

An occasional post–*atrial* switch patient will be encountered with chronic pulmonary vascular obstructive disease. During the 1960s and 1970s, a number of D-TGA patients had "palliative Mustard operations" in the presence of pulmonary vascular disease to improve arterial oxygen saturation by increasing mixing in the face of decreasing pulmonary blood flow. The procedure resulted in symptomatic improvement and greater longevity. Pulmonary vasodilator therapy is sometimes used in these patients, but heart-lung transplantation may be the only option for patients with intractable symptoms.

Patients who have had a Rastelli operation for D-TGA with VSD and PS must be observed carefully for a residual VSD (Fig. 11-13*A* and *B*), left ventricle to aorta tunnel obstruction, and/or RV-PA conduit obstruction. A TEE may be required to visualize a residual VSD or right ventricular outflow tract obstruction. Mild obstruction and insufficiency of the RV-PA conduit are well tolerated for many years but should be watched closely. The average longevity of the homograft or porcine xenograft is approximately 10 years, and as patients approach this limit, they should be evaluated with increased frequency. Atrial arrhythmias are less common after the Rastelli operation as compared with *atrial* switch patients, but regular follow-up for other rhythm disorders also is required.

Arterial Switch

Individuals who have reached adulthood after a successful *arterial* switch operation are likely to remain asymptomatic, but serial evaluation for myocardial ischemia during adulthood may be indicated. The presence of stenosis of the main pulmonary artery at the site of previous surgery must be assessed, but the absence of a significant left upper sternal border systolic murmur would indicate that obstruction is not present. Mild neoaortic valve regurgitation is common, and decision making in this context should be similar to that for any patient with aortic insufficiency. Cardiac MRI will be used more frequently to assess anatomic issues in older patients with limited echocardiographic windows.

The postoperative patient with D-TGA requires routine follow-up, and on the basis of specific indications, usually supravalvar pulmonary stenosis or coronary artery issues, cardiac catheterization and angiography may be required. The optimal noninvasive test for the assessment of myocardial ischemia has not yet been determined.

FIGURE 11-13*A*

A TEE in a patient with a Rastelli repair for D-transposition of the great arteries, showing partial separation of the interventricular tunnel producing a left to right shunt through the patch. The arrows delineate the location of the residual ventricular septal defect within the tunnel. RV, right ventricle; Ao, aorta.

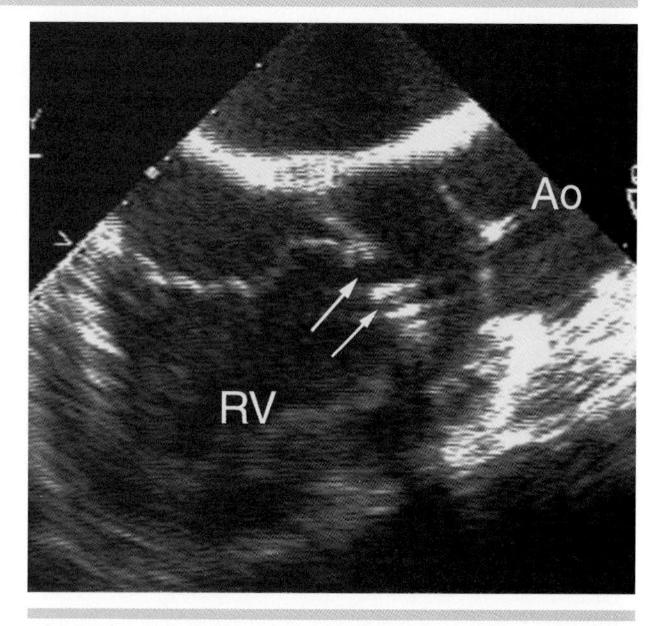

FIGURE 11-13*B*

Color Doppler from the same patient as in Fig. 11-13*A*. The arrows show abnormal color flow at the site of the residual left-to-right shunt within the interventricular tunnel, just below the aortic valve.

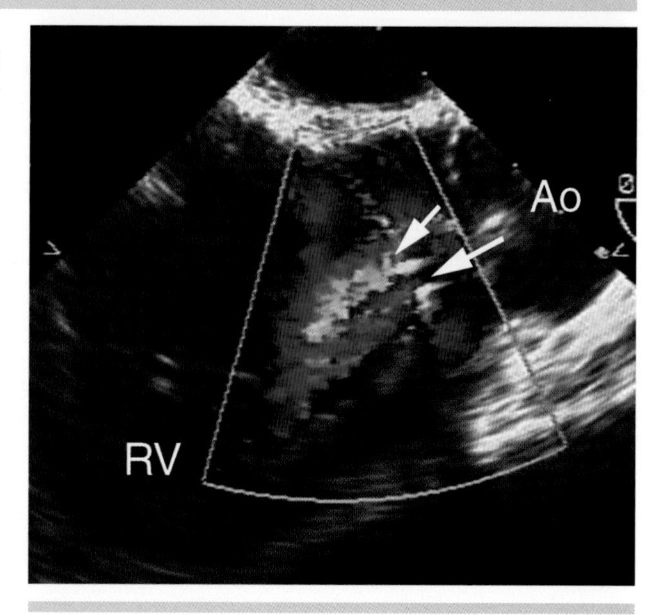

SUMMARY

Patients with D-TGA present to the adult cardiologist having had previous surgery. The modern management of this congenital lesion in the newborn period consists of the *arterial* switch procedure, but few of these patients are currently beyond adolescence. The great majority of the current population of adult patients with D-TGA has had an *atrial* switch operation (Mustard or Senning procedure) during infancy. A significant minority of patients with D-TGA, VSD, and pulmonary stenosis have had a Rastelli repair, which consists of a tunnel from the left ventricle to the aorta across the right ventricular outflow tract and placement of a homograft or porcine valve conduit from the right ventricular body to the main pulmonary artery.

D-TGA After Atrial Switch Procedure

Adult patients who have had an *atrial* switch procedure for D-TGA have a number of possible residual or late acquired problems, including the following:

1. Residual left-to-right or right-to-left atrial shunt. The latter occurs when there is also significant baffle obstruction downstream beyond the site of the atrial communication.
2. Significant systemic (tricuspid) AV valve regurgitation.
3. Right ventricular dysfunction.
4. Left ventricular outflow tract stenosis. This is usually dynamic, but can be discrete subvalvular.
5. Caval or pulmonary venous obstruction which is usually an early problem and rarely occurs in adulthood.
6. Sick sinus syndrome and atrial flutter. An increasing number of patients will emerge into adulthood requiring a pacemaker.
7. A rare young adult may present with pulmonary vascular obstructive disease which developed before an *atrial* switch, with or without VSD closure, could be performed. These patients should be managed in the same manner as any patient with pulmonary vascular obstruction disease.

D-TGA After Rastelli Repair for Associated Ventricular Septal Defect and Pulmonary Stenosis

Patients who have a systemic left ventricle entering the aorta through a tunnel across the VSD can have narrowing of the outflow region, creating subvalvar aortic stenosis. A residual VSD at the level of the patch from the VSD to the aorta can be present and may be associated with a significant left-to-right shunt. In addition, these patients must be observed for conduit obstruction at both proximal and distal sites as well as severe pulmonary insufficiency. Other associated lesions are rare.

Patients with D-TGA After Arterial Switch Operations

The major follow-up issues in these patients include coronary abnormalities secondary to the original operation and the potential for myocardial ischemia, although this has not been a prominent feature in patients followed into adolescence. Various degrees of obstruction at the supraneopulmonary valve level may be present, especially in patients operated on in the early years of arterial switch surgery, and an occasional patient eventually may require reintervention. Aortic root dilatation with mild aortic regurgitation is common, but has not been progressive. Long-term follow-up is required.

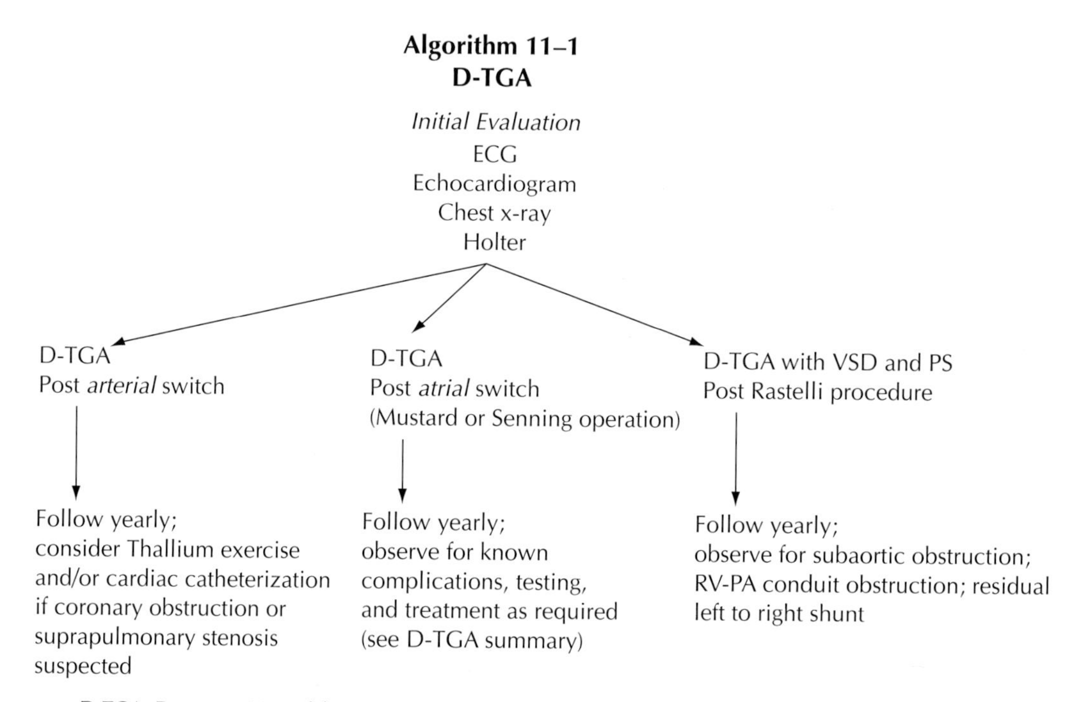

BIBLIOGRAPHY

Aziz KU, Paul MH, Idriss FS, et al: Clinical manifestations of dynamic left ventricular outflow tract stenosis in infants with D-transposition of the great arteries with intact ventricular septum. *Am J Cardiol* 44:290, 1979.

Bender HW Jr, Stewart JR, Merrill WH, et al: Ten years' experience with the Senning operation for transposition of the great arteries: Physiological results and late follow-up. *Ann Thorac Surg* 47:218, 1989.

Bical O, Hazan E, Lecompte Y, et al: Anatomic correction of transposition of the great arteries associated with ventricular septal defect: Midterm results in 50 patients. *Circulation* 70:891, 1984.

Ciaravella JM Jr, McGoon DC, Danielson GK, et al: Experience with the extracardiac conduit. *J Thorac Cardiovasc Surg* 78(6):920, 1979.

Cochrane AD, Karl TR, Mee RB: Staged conversion to arterial switch for late failure of the systemic right ventricle. *Ann Thorac Surg* 56:854, 1993.

Driscoll DJ, Nihill MR, Vargo TA, et al: Late development of pulmonary venous obstruction following Mustard's operation using a dacron baffle. *Circulation* 55(3):484, 1977.

Finn CJ, Wolff GS, Dick M, et al: Cardiac rhythm after the Mustard operation for complete transposition of the great arteries. *N Engl J Med* 310:1635, 1984.

Gelatt M, Hamilton RM, McCrindle BW, et al: Arrhythmia and mortality after the Mustard procedure: a 30-year single-center experience. *J Am Coll Cardiol* 29:194, 1997.

Gillette PC, Wampler DG, Shannon C, Ott D: Use of cardiac pacing after the Mustard operation for transposition of the great arteries. *J Am Coll Cardiol* 7:138, 1986.

Graham TP Jr: Hemodynamic residua and sequelae following intraatrial repair of transposition of the great arteries: A review. *Pediatr Cardiol* 2:203, 1982.

Hagler DJ, Ritter DG, Mair DD, et al: Clinical, angiographic, and hemodynamic assessment of late results after Mustard operation. *Circulation* 57:1214, 1978.

Hayes CJ, Gersony WM: Arrhythmias after the Mustard operation for transposition of the great arteries: A long term study. *J Am Coll Cardiol* 7:133, 1986.

Helbing WA, Hansen B, Ottenkamp J, et al: Long-term results of atrial correction for transposition of the great arteries: Comparison of Mustard and Senning operations. *J Thorac Cardiovasc Surg* 108:363, 1994.

Jenkins KJ, Hanley FL, Colan SD, et al: Function of the anatomic pulmonary valve in the systemic circulation. *Circulation* 84:III173, 1991.

Lecompte Y, Zannini L, Hazan E, et al: Anatomic correction of transposition of the great arteries: New technique without the use of a prosthetic conduit. *J Thorac Cardiovasc Surg* 82:629, 1981.

Lev M, Rimoldi HJA, Eckner FAO, et al: The Taussig-Bing heart: Qualitative and quantitative anatomy. *Arch Pathol Lab Med* 81:24, 1966.

Liebman J, Cullum L, Belloc NB: Natural history of transposition of the great arteries: Anatomy and birth and death characteristics. *Circulation* 40:237, 1969.

MacLellan-Tobert SG, Cetta P, Hagler DJ: Use of intravascular stents for superior vena caval obstruction after the Mustard operation. *Mayo Clin Proc* 71:1071, 1986.

Martin RP, Ettedgui JA, Qureshi SA, et al: A quantitative evaluation of aortic regurgitation after anatomic correction of transposition of the great arteries. *J Am Coll Cardiol* 12:1281, 1988.

Mustard WT, Keith JD, Trusler GA, et al: The surgical management of transposition of the great vessels. *J Thorac Cardiovasc Surg* 48:899, 1964.

Puley G, Siu S, Connelly M, et al: Arrhythmia and survival in patients >18 years of age after the Mustard procedure for complete transposition of the great arteries. *Am J Cardiol* 83:1080, 1999.

Rhodes LA, Wernovsky G, Keane JF, et al: Arrhythmias and intercardiac conduction after the arterial switch operation. *J Thorac Cardiovasc Surg* 109:303, 1985.

Senning A: Surgical correction of transposition of the great vessels. *Surgery* 50:773, 1959.

Seraf A, Lacour-Gayet F, Bruniaux J, et al: Anatomic correction of transposition of the great arteries in neonates. *J Am Coll Cardiol* 22:193, 1993.

Vetter VL, Tanner CS, Horowitz LN: Electrophysiologic consequences of the Mustard repair of D-transposition of the great arteries. *J Am Coll Cardiol* 10:1265, 1987.

Vouhe PR, Tamisier D, Leca F, et al: Transposition of the great arteries, ventricular septal defect and right ventricular outflow tract obstruction: Rastelli or Lecompte procedure? *J Thorac Cardiovasc Surg* 103:428, 1992.

Warnes CA, Somerville J: Transposition of the great arteries: Late results in adolescents and adults after the Mustard procedure. *Br Heart J* 58:148, 1987.

Williams WG, Trusler GA, Kirklin JW, et al: Early and late results of a protocol for simple transposition leading to an atrial switch (Mustard) repair. *J Thorac Cardiovasc Surg* 95:717, 1988.
Wilson NJ, Clarkson PM, Barratt-Boyes BG, et al: Long-term outcome after the Mustard repair for simple transposition of the great arteries: 28-year follow-up. *J Am Coll Cardiol* 32:758, 1998.
Wong KY, Venables AW, Kelly MJ, Kalff V: Longitudinal study of ventricular function after the Mustard operation for transposition of the great arteries: A long term follow up. *Br Heart J* 60:316, 1988.

CHAPTER 12

SINGLE VENTRICLE

Single ventricle is a term used to describe several different forms of congenital heart disease in which there is abnormal formation of the two ventricular chambers, resulting in a single functioning ventricular chamber. The nomenclature varies and includes the terms *single ventricle*, *common ventricle*, *double-inlet ventricle*, *univentricular heart*, and *univentricular atrial ventricular connection*. Tricuspid and mitral atresia also may be considered in this category, but mitral and/or aortic atresia with a tiny nonfunctional left ventricle (LV) generally is referred to as hypoplastic left heart syndrome. In addition, patients with other defects, for example, unbalanced atrioventricular (AV) canal and pulmonary atresia with an intact ventricular septum, may have single-ventricle physiology and require similar management.

A complete assessment of the anatomy of a patient with single ventricle includes an analysis of atrial situs, AV connection, ventricular morphology, great vessel relationships, and associated cardiac anomalies. Most patients with single ventricle have two ventricular chambers: a normal-size dominant chamber and a small rudimentary chamber that is connected through a bulboventricular foramen. If the dominant chamber is a morphologic LV, the rudimentary chamber will have features of a morphologic right ventricle (RV). Conversely, if the dominant chamber is a morphologic RV, the rudimentary chamber will have features of a morphologic LV. Some patients have a single ventricular chamber that may have an indeterminate trabecular pattern and no defined outflow ventricular chamber. With the exception of tricuspid atresia, almost all patients with single ventricle have transposed or malposed great arteries. A rare patient may have an absent ventricular septum without other anomalies (Holmes heart).

AV valve abnormalities are common in patients with single ventricle. Although most of these patients have two AV valves, other abnormalities may occur, such as overriding or straddling of one of the valves, AV valve atresia, and a common AV valve. A straddling AV valve refers to anatomy in which the papillary muscles of the valve apparatus arise from both the dominant and the smaller ventricular chambers.

DOUBLE-INLET LEFT VENTRICLE

Double-inlet LV is the most common form of single ventricle. In this lesion, two AV valves drain into a normal-size morphologic LV that is connected via the bulboventricular fora-

FIGURE 12-1

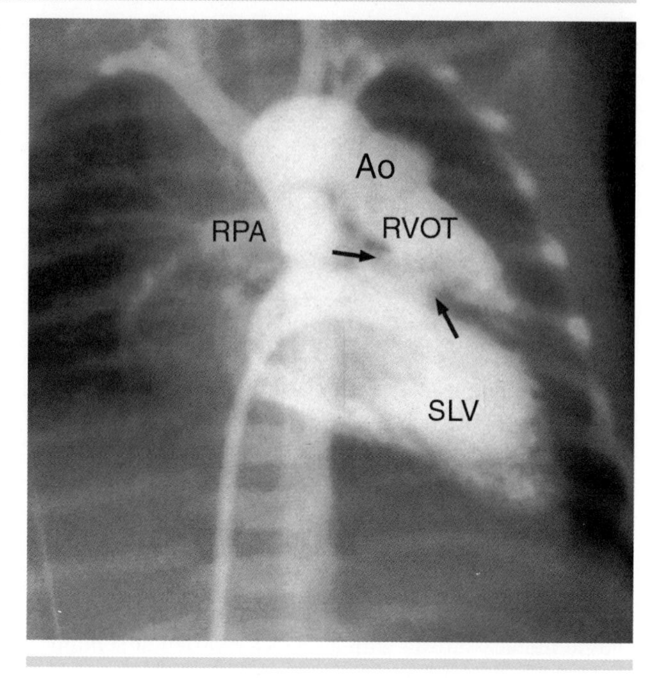

Single left ventricle. Angiogram demonstrates a single left ventricle connecting to a hypoplastic right ventricular outlet chamber and L-transposed aorta through a bulboventricular foramen (arrows). The origin of the pulmonary blood flow is not seen. SLV, single left ventricle; RVOT, right ventricular outlet chamber; RPA, right pulmonary artery; Ao, aorta.

men to a rudimentary RV chamber, most often leading to the malposed aorta (Fig. 12-1). The rudimentary chamber may be located anterosuperiorly on either the right or the left shoulder of the LV, depending on the atrial-ventricular relationship. Dextrocardia or mesocardia is not uncommon. Levocardia with abdominal situs inversus or heterotaxy and dextrocardia with situs solitus or heterotaxy are the most common forms; mirror image dextrocardia with situs inversus is rare. Many cases of single ventricle are a component of the asplenia or polysplenia syndrome; this often is referred to as right or left isomerism, respectively.

The vast majority of patients with double-inlet LV have L-looping of the ventricles and discordant ventriculoarterial connections in which the aorta arises from the infundibulum of the rudimentary RV chamber and the pulmonary artery arises from the dominant LV chamber with mitral valve–pulmonary valve continuity. The bulboventricular foramen, or ventricular septal defect (VSD), may be large and nonrestrictive; however, when the VSD is restrictive, subaortic stenosis results. Patients with a restrictive VSD are more likely to have coexisting coarctation of the aorta.

Subpulmonary stenosis may be present in patients with single ventricle as a result of posterior deviation of the infundibular septum, anomalous attachment of the AV valve across the outflow tract, or intrusion of fibrous tissue into the subpulmonary area. Valvar pulmonary stenosis may occur but is less common.

In 10% of cases of double-inlet LV, a D-loop ventricle and concordant ventricular–great artery connections are present. The dominant LV is posterior and to the left, while the rudimentary RV lies anterior and to the right. There may be two AV valves or a common AV valve. Pulmonary stenosis is common, and the VSD may be restrictive.

DOUBLE-INLET RIGHT VENTRICLE

In double-inlet RV, the AV connections are to a dominant RV that is connected to an inferoposterior rudimentary LV. Atrial situs inversus or situs ambiguous may be present. The ventriculoarterial connections are usually double-outlet from the dominant RV chamber or a single aortic outlet with pulmonary atresia. There may be two AV valves or a common valve.

DOUBLE-INLET INDETERMINATE VENTRICLE

This term is used when there is a single dominant ventricular chamber, usually an RV, without a recognizable rudimentary chamber. This lesion can be associated with atrial isomerism. Pulmonary stenosis is common, and the great vessels arise from the single ventricular chamber as a double-outlet connection or as a single outlet with pulmonary atresia.

TRICUSPID ATRESIA

Tricuspid atresia may be considered a unique form of single ventricle in which there is agenesis of the tricuspid valve. As a result, all the blood that enters the right atrium is diverted across an atrial septal defect or patent foramen ovale into the left atrium, mixes with pulmonary venous blood, and enters the LV (Fig. 12-2). A communication between the systemic circulation and the pulmonary circulation is required for survival, usually a VSD and occasionally a patent ductus arteriosus. The RV is typically small, consisting of a conus portion with little or no sinus component (Fig. 12-3).

The great arteries arise normally in 70% of cases, are D-transposed in 20%, and have more complicated great vessel relationships in the remainder of cases. When the great arteries are normally related, the pulmonary artery arises from the diminutive RV. When transposition of the great arteries is present, the pulmonary artery arises from the LV. Thus, a restrictive VSD can result in either subpulmonary or subaortic stenosis, depending on the position of the great arteries. When pulmonary atresia or an intact ventricular septum is present with normal great arteries, pulmonary blood flow is derived from a patent ductus arteriosus.

MITRAL ATRESIA AND OTHER FORMS OF HYPOPLASTIC LEFT HEART SYNDROME

In the presence of mitral atresia or other forms of hypoplastic left heart syndrome (HLHS), including combinations of severe mitral and aortic stenosis or atresia, pulmonary venous return reaches the right atrium and RV via a dilated foramen ovale or an atrial septal defect. Mitral atresia may be associated with various forms of single ventricle with variations in the position of the great arteries and in the presence and degree of pulmonary outflow obstruction. In HLHS, all cardiac output is provided by the single RV through the ductus arteriosus to the aorta. Blood flow is retrograde to the hypoplastic ascending aorta and coronary arteries and antegrade to the descending aorta and lower body.

FIGURE 12-2

A venous angiogram in a patient with tricuspid atresia demonstrates blood flow from the right atrium across the atrial septum into the left atrium and left ventricle. Large arrows delineate the large atrial septal defect. The small arrows indicate the site of tricuspid atresia. LV, left ventricle; LA, left atrium; CS, coronary sinus; IVC, inferior vena cava; RA, right atrium; SVC, superior vena cava; IV, innominate vein.

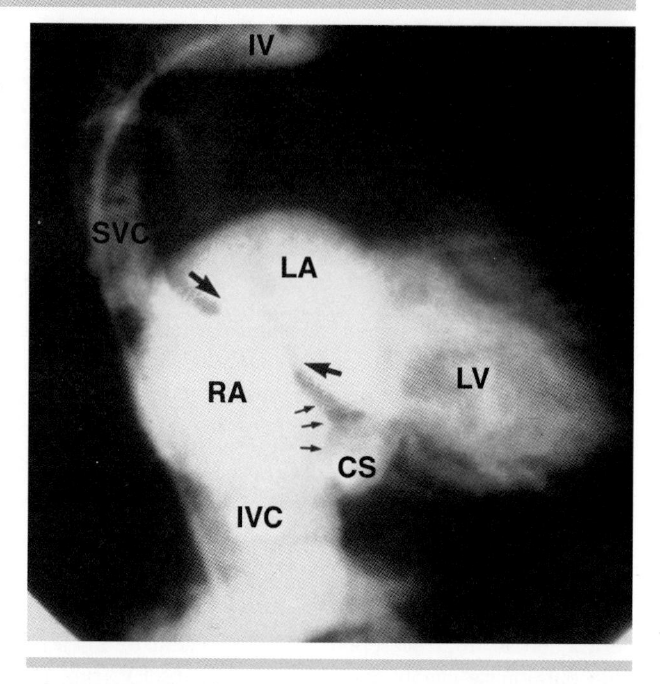

FIGURE 12-3

Left ventricular angiogram shows a large left ventricular chamber and a hypoplastic right ventricular infundibular component in a patient with tricuspid atresia. LV, left ventricle; RV, right ventricle; Ao, aorta.

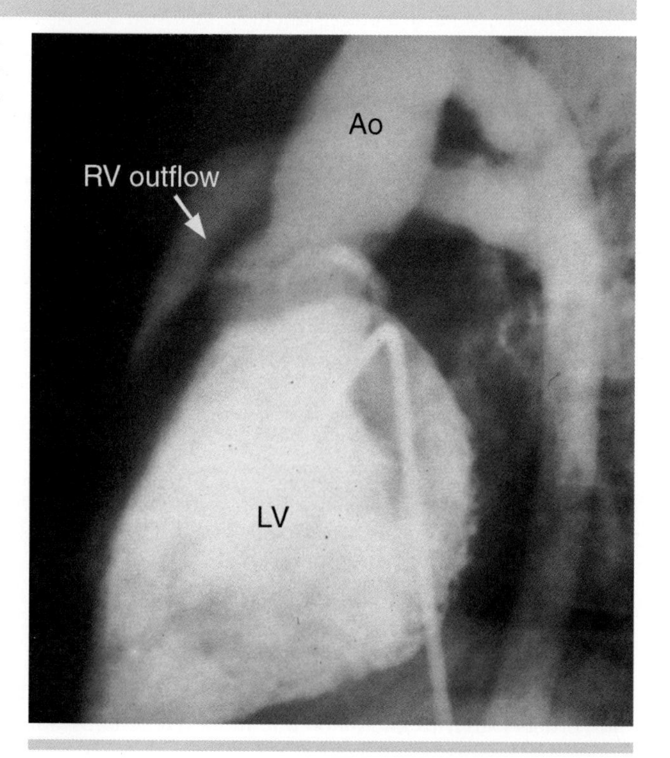

CLINICAL FEATURES

The clinical manifestations and prognosis for a patient with any form of single ventricle are related to pulmonary artery blood flow and pressure, which are determined by the presence and degree of pulmonary stenosis and the level of pulmonary vascular resistance. Two-thirds of patients with single ventricle have pulmonary stenosis or pulmonary atresia.

In the absence of pulmonary stenosis, pulmonary blood flow increases soon after birth in concert with the normal fall in pulmonary vascular resistance. A large left-to-right shunt subsequently ensues, resulting in increased pulmonary blood flow and volume overload of the single ventricle. Congestive heart failure is usually apparent within the first few weeks of life. The high ratio of pulmonary to systemic blood flow is reflected by high arterial oxygen saturation, which may exceed 90%. Unless pulmonary blood flow and pulmonary hypertension are controlled by the rapid development of a pulmonary outflow obstruction or by surgical intervention (pulmonary artery banding or an intracardiac repair), progressive heart failure and death are the result for most patients. A few infants survive long enough for significant pulmonary vascular obstructive disease to develop, and on a short-term basis, these patients improve and become relatively stable. Pulmonary blood flow falls, volume overload of the single ventricle declines, heart failure is alleviated, and cyanosis increases. However, as pulmonary vascular disease progresses, the opportunity for surgical repair disappears, and ultimately these patients are subjected to the late clinical course and complications of Eisenmenger's syndrome.

When pulmonary stenosis is present, pulmonary blood flow is determined by the degree of obstruction. Patients with severe pulmonary stenosis have diminished pulmonary blood flow and marked cyanosis and require early surgical intervention with a systemic–pulmonary artery shunt to increase pulmonary blood flow. Patients with lesser degrees of pulmonary stenosis may initially have adequate pulmonary blood flow and acceptable arterial saturation. Under these circumstances, surgery can be delayed until additional pulmonary blood flow is required, and a Glenn/Fontan type of repair can be carried out. An increase in cyanosis in a previously stable patient may be caused by an increase in the severity of pulmonary stenosis or may reflect inadequate blood flow relative to the growth of a patient with fixed pulmonary outflow obstruction.

In rare instances, an adolescent or adult with a single ventricle who has never had surgery will have adequate pulmonary blood flow and normal or slightly elevated pulmonary pressure as a result of a moderate degree of "natural" pulmonary stenosis. In this "balanced" situation in which arterial oxygen saturation is acceptable and pulmonary artery pressure remains low, the indications for late surgical intervention are less clear and require careful consideration of the long-term risks and benefits of a Fontan repair in a relatively asymptomatic adult.

Tricuspid Atresia

The clinical manifestations of tricuspid atresia depend on three factors: (1) the relationship of the great vessels, (2) the size of the VSD, and (3) the presence of pulmonary stenosis or atresia. These abnormalities determine whether pulmonary blood flow is normal, increased, or decreased. Most infants have diminished or normal pulmonary blood with varying degrees of cyanosis, but some initially have unrestricted pulmonary blood flow and develop heart failure from pulmonary overcirculation.

Tricuspid Atresia with Normally Related Great Arteries
If the VSD is initially small and/or there is obstruction of the RV outflow tract, diminished pulmonary blood flow will be present and cyanosis will be a prominent feature from the neonatal period. This is the usual presentation for patients with tricuspid atresia. If there is no connection between the pulmonary artery and the RV (pulmonary atresia), there is virtual absence of the RV outflow component. The magnitude of pulmonary blood flow is dependent on the size of the aortopulmonary communication, patent ductus arteriosus (PDA), and/or pulmonary collateral arteries.

When the VSD is large and pulmonary stenosis is absent, the result is a large left-to-right shunt through the VSD that produces high pulmonary blood flow and congestive heart failure during the first few months of life. This is the case at presentation in approximately 20% of infants with tricuspid atresia and normally related great arteries. If pulmonary blood flow is not reduced, the clinical picture is one of failure to thrive, pulmonary hypertension, and pulmonary congestion. Although early surgical intervention may be required, in most of these patients pulmonary blood flow decreases over the first few months of life because of diminution in the size of the VSD or development of RV outflow tract obstruction. As this occurs, the ratio of pulmonary to systemic blood flow falls, congestive heart failure improves, and aortic saturation declines. The shunts may remain balanced for a time, but as pulmonary blood flow is further restricted, cyanosis and polycythemia dominate the clinical picture.

Tricuspid Atresia with Transposition of the Great Arteries
The great vessels are D-transposed in approximately 20% of patients with tricuspid atresia. In this defect, the LV gives rise to the pulmonary artery and the aorta arises from the RV, which receives blood through the VSD. Valvar and/or subvalvar pulmonary stenosis or pulmonary atresia often is present, resulting in significant cyanosis. If there is no pulmonary stenosis, pulmonary overcirculation and early congestive failure ensues. If pulmonary blood flow is not controlled surgically, pulmonary vascular obstructive disease is to be expected among the survivors.

When significant pulmonary outflow obstruction is present, the VSD is usually large. If, however, there is no obstruction to pulmonary blood flow, the VSD size may be restrictive, causing subaortic obstruction.

Mitral Atresia and the Hypoplastic Left Heart Syndrome

Patients with mitral atresia and HLHS do not survive infancy without early balloon atrial septostomy and/or surgical intervention. Systemic blood flow is dependent on an adequate atrial communication as well as a patent ductus arteriosus. Severe congestive heart failure and death within the first few weeks occur as these fetal connections become restrictive. Surviving patients with forms of single ventricle associated with mitral atresia with an intact ventricular septum and a hypoplastic left side of the heart have been treated with the three-stage Norwood operation. Initially, in the neonate this involves widely opening the atrial septum, anastomosing the main pulmonary artery to the ascending aorta, and controlling pulmonary blood flow by means of a Blalock-Taussig shunt. In the second operation later in the first year of life, the arterial shunt is eliminated, and a bidirectional Glenn procedure (superior vena cava [SVC] to pulmonary artery) is carried out. In the third stage, the Fontan procedure is completed by directing the inferior vena cava (IVC) to the pulmonary artery, resulting in a total cavo-pulmonary connection with a single systemic RV. Some patients with mitral atresia have two functioning ventricles with a VSD and may or may not have pulmonary stenosis. Thus, either pulmonary artery banding or a Blalock-Taussig shunt is done early in life as well as a balloon atrial septostomy to allow unimpeded blood flow from the left atrium to the right atrium and ventricle. Those patients will need a surgical atrial septectomy within a few months after the original balloon septostomy palliation.

Physical Examination

Physical examination varies among unoperated patients with single ventricle, depending on anatomy, hemodynamic status, and associated cardiac abnormalities. Infants with normal pulmonary vascular resistance and high pulmonary blood flow have findings of a large left-to-right shunt with signs of ventricular volume overload on examination. As long as pulmonary vascular resistance is normal, patients manifest little or no cyanosis, with an O_2 saturation approaching 90%. An active and heaving precordium is typically present, reflecting the large volume load on the single ventricle. A diastolic rumble may be audible as a result of increased blood flow across an AV valve. For unoperated patients who survive childhood because pulmonary vascular obstructive disease develops, pulmonary blood flow falls and signs of ventricular volume overload gradually disappear. Arterial O_2 saturation decreases, and secondary polycythemia develops.

The great majority of adult patients have pulmonary stenosis, and their status can be recognized clinically by the presence of a harsh systolic ejection murmur along the left sternal border. The second heart sound is single. The murmur of pulmonary stenosis may be confused with the murmur of bulboventricular foramen obstruction. The latter murmur refers to a restrictive connection between the dominant chamber and the rudimentary chamber. In tricuspid atresia, it is a VSD that is restrictive, resulting in subpulmonary stenosis when the great arteries are normally related and subaortic stenosis when the great arteries are transposed.

AV valve regurgitation is not uncommon in patients with a single ventricle. The murmur is typically holosystolic and is audible at the lower sternal border and apex. Since the AV valves are associated with the right atrium, a jugular venous V wave and/or a pulsatile liver may be present.

Noninvasive Evaluation

There is considerable variability in the *electrocardiogram* (ECG) of patients with a single ventricle. Varying degrees of ventricular hypertrophy or intraventricular conduction defects and ST abnormalities are typically present in older patients. In patients with tricuspid atresia, ECG may be useful in predicting certain anatomic features of this lesion.

When the great arteries are normally related, ECG typically shows a left superior QRS axis (0 to −90 degrees), right atrial hypertrophy, and LV hypertrophy. When the great vessels are transposed, the axis is usually between 0 and +90 degrees.

The *chest x-ray* findings vary with pulmonary blood flow. When pulmonary blood flow is decreased, the cardiac silhouette may be normal or mildly enlarged with diminished pulmonary vascularity. Cardiomegaly and increased pulmonary vascularity are prominent in patients in whom pulmonary blood flow is increased because of an arterial–pulmonary artery shunt, and the classic large main pulmonary arteries and tapering peripheral vessels are noted in the presence of pulmonary vascular obstructive disease.

Echocardiography provides critical information in patients with single ventricle, including anatomy (Fig. 12-4), ventricular function, presence of AV valve regurgitation, pulmonary obstruction, bulboventricular foramen obstruction, and pulmonary and systemic venous anomalies. While most of this information usually can be obtained in children, the imaging of adults is usually more limited, and additional studies, such as transesophageal echocardiography (TEE), cardiac magnetic resonance imaging (MRI) (Fig. 12-5), and cardiac catheterization, are required to delineate all the pertinent anatomy.

FIGURE 12-4

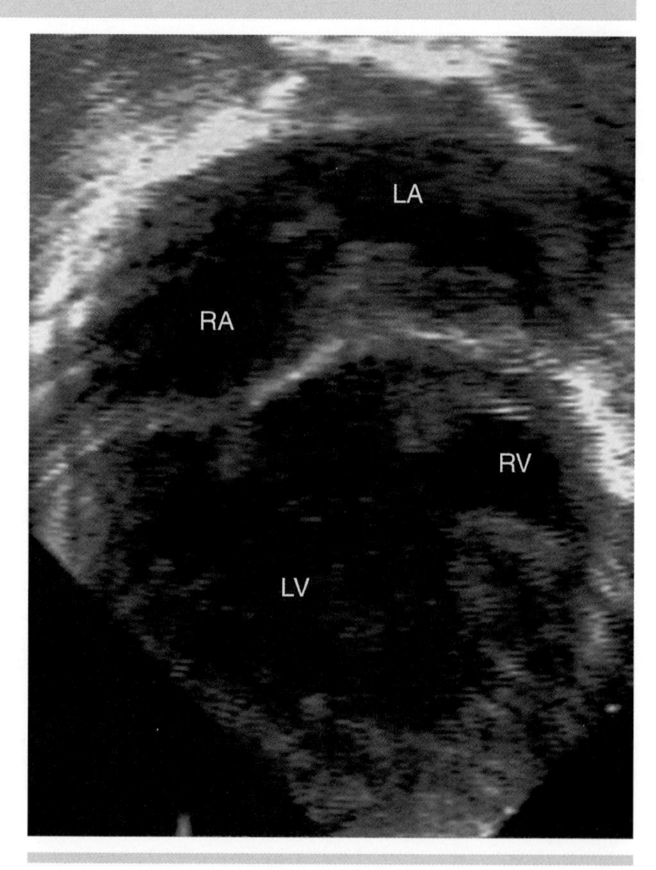

Apical four-chamber view of a patient with univentricular heart of the left ventricular (LV) type. There is atrioventricular discordance. A rudimentary right ventricle (RV) arises from the left basal section of the heart from which the aorta (not shown) arises. The outlet from the LV to the small RV is known as the bulboventricular foramen. RA, right atrium; LV, left ventricle; RV, right ventricle; LA, left atrium.

FIGURE 12-5

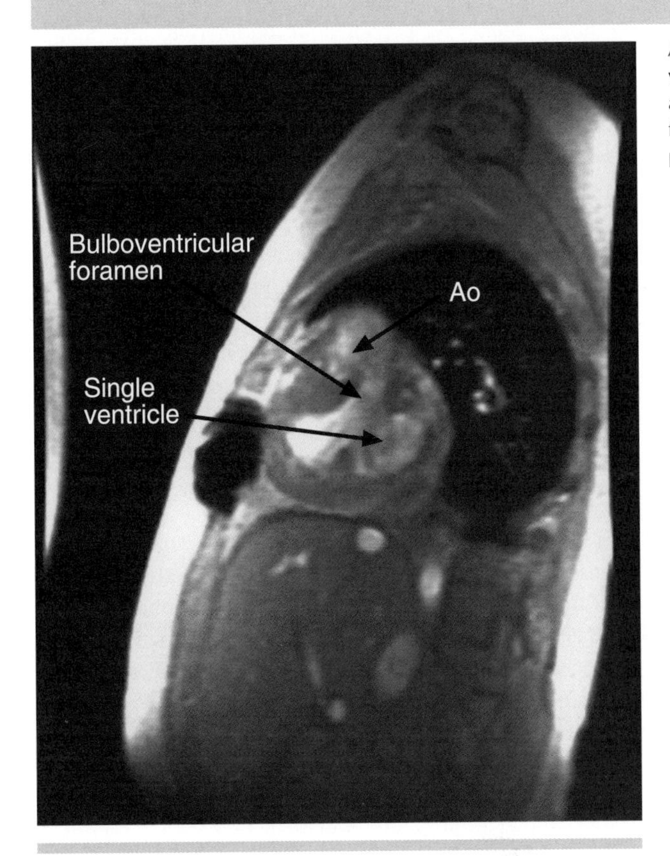

A cardiac MRI in a patient with a single ventricle. The ventricle is hypertrophied. The aorta (Ao) arises from a small outlet chamber above the bulboventricular foramen. The pulmonary arteries are not seen in this plane.

Echocardiography of tricuspid atresia specifically reveals the absence of a tricuspid valve orifice, a large atrial communication, the relationships of the great vessels, the size of the right ventricle, the presence and size of a VSD, and proximal pulmonary artery anatomy. Color Doppler and MRI are useful to assess for the presence of a PDA or aortopulmonary collaterals as well as the presence of left AV valve regurgitation.

Cardiac Catheterization

The role of cardiac catheterization in patients with single ventricle has evolved in recent years as a result of improvements in noninvasive imaging modalities. Since the diagnosis of single ventricle and tricuspid atresia can be readily established with echocardiography and cardiac MRI, the need for diagnostic cardiac catheterization has diminished over the years.

The indications for cardiac catheterization vary with the patient's age and clinical status. Invasive studies during the neonatal period often are required to determine the pulmonary artery anatomy before the placement of a shunt in patients with pulmonary stenosis or atresia. A complete intracardiac study often can be deferred until more definitive surgery is contemplated, at which time the ventricular function, AV valve abnormalities, systemic venous and pulmonary artery anatomy, presence of collaterals, and hemodynamics become critical in determining the surgical options. Since some of these questions will have been answered by echocardiography, the extent to which these findings need to be confirmed during the study will vary.

In patients with tricuspid atresia, the catheterization technique is straightforward. A venous catheter is advanced into the right atrium and across the atrial septal defect into the left atrium and left ventricle. Since all the right atrial blood empties into the left atrium, there is complete mixing of pulmonary venous and systemic venous blood in the left atrium. As a result, oxygen saturations will be similar in the left and right ventricles, pulmonary artery, and aorta.

The right atrial pressure may be slightly higher than the left atrial pressure but will be significantly higher if the atrial communication is restrictive, which is uncommon. If the VSD is large, the left and right ventricular pressures will be equal. If the VSD is restrictive, there will be a gradient between the left and right ventricles. In an adult who has not had a Fontan repair, the atrial communication is almost always nonrestrictive and the VSD and/or right ventricular outflow tract is obstructive.

The pulmonary artery pressure may be measured by advancing the catheter into the RV through the VSD or by retrograde catheterization from the aorta when a shunt or ductus arteriosus is present. The size of the pulmonary arteries should be determined as well as the site of any branch stenoses that would require repair as part of a reparative operation. In addition, before a Glenn procedure is planned, the presence or absence of a left SVC must be determined by angiography.

Virtually all adult patients with tricuspid atresia and normally related great arteries have restriction of pulmonary blood flow and low pulmonary artery pressure unless an overly large systemic–pulmonary artery shunt is in place. If tricuspid atresia and D-transposition of the great arteries are present in an adult, subvalvar or valvar pulmonary stenosis almost always coexists. Since after a Fontan operation the LV blood flow must continue to reach the aorta through the VSD, the size of the VSD must be determined and the gradients must be measured.

In the era before echocardiography, the diagnosis of tricuspid atresia typically was made angiographically with a right atrial angiogram. The studies showed antegrade flow of contrast into the left atrium and reflux into the IVC without direct opacification of the RV. The anatomy and size of the RV can be visualized angiographically, but since the ventricle almost never is incorporated in a surgical repair today, this information is rarely useful.

MANAGEMENT

Treatment of patients with a single ventricle varies according to anatomy. Palliative procedures for infants to increase or limit pulmonary blood flow and direct systemic venous blood to the lungs include a systemic–pulmonary artery shunt to increase pulmonary blood flow and pulmonary artery banding to limit pulmonary blood flow. The classic Glenn anastomosis, a bidirectional Glenn, and the more definitive Fontan operation usually are performed during early childhood, but on occasion an unoperated adult with balanced hemodynamics is encountered who is a candidate for a Fontan operation.

When additional pulmonary blood flow is required during early infancy, a systemic–pulmonary artery shunt is performed. Although the modified Blalock shunt (Gortex tube from subclavian artery to pulmonary artery) is currently the procedure of choice, adults who were treated two or more decades ago during childhood may have received other types of shunts, such as a classic Blalock (subclavian artery to upsilateral pulmonary arteries), Potts (descending aorta to left pulmonary artery), or Waterston shunt [ascending aorta to right pulmonary artery (RPA)]. The Potts and Waterston shunts are not performed today because of their propensity to cause distortion of the pulmonary arteries and result in hyperkinetic pulmonary hypertension, which in turn leads to pulmonary vascular obstructive disease.

Blalock-Taussig Shunt

The classic Blalock shunt, in which the subclavian artery is directly anastomosed to the pulmonary artery, has been replaced by the modified Blalock, in which a Gortex graft is used to connect the subclavian artery with the ipsilateral pulmonary artery. Unlike the Potts and Waterston shunts, the smaller caliber of the Blalock shunt usually prevents excessive pulmonary blood flow and pulmonary hypertension. The modified Blalock-Taussig shunt produces adequate pulmonary blood flow for growth and development during infancy. Although a shunt is effective in increasing pulmonary blood flow and raising arterial saturation, it does produce an excess volume load on the single ventricle, can distort pulmonary arteries, and usually becomes inadequate with growth of the patient or the development of an obstruction at the anastomosis. This is manifested clinically by increasing cyanosis and polycythemia as well as diminished exercise capacity. At any age, if it is established that additional pulmonary blood flow is required, further surgery is indicated. Before the era of the Fontan repair, patients were managed with another shunt or a Glenn anastomosis.

Glenn Operation

The Glenn anastomosis was developed in the mid-1950s as a method of partially bypassing the right heart. In this operation, the SVC is transected just above its entrance into the right atrium and anastomosed end to end to the distal portion of the RPA. The previously divided proximal RPA and distal SVC are oversewn. If a left SVC is present, it is ligated. This results in unidirectional low-pressure flow of SVC blood into the RPA (Fig. 12-6). The classic Glenn shunt had the advantage of allowing a direct connection of systemic venous blood to the right lung at low pressure, eliminating the possibility of pulmonary hypertension from an overly large systemic-pulmonary shunt, and preventing marked ventricular volume loading. The Glenn operation was used as an alternative to the classic Blalock-Taussig shunt in patients with tricuspid atresia, and was considered long-term palliation before the advent of the Fontan operation.

In the present era, the classic end-to-end SVC–right pulmonary artery (RPA) Glenn operation is almost never done, having been replaced by the bidirectional Glenn. This procedure, which directs SVC blood flow to the right and left pulmonary arteries, usually precedes the full Fontan procedure. Nevertheless, a significant number of adult patients still have the original SVC-RPA anastomosis. Thus, it is important to understand the clinical manifestations and potential complications associated with this operation.

FIGURE 12-6

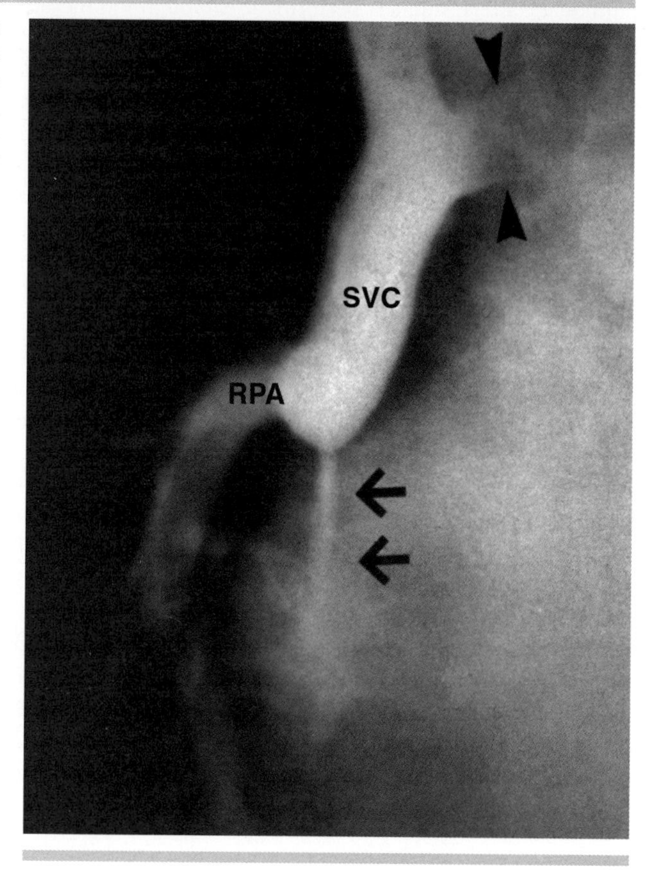

Angiogram showing classic Glenn anastomosis. The superior vena cava has been anastomosed to the right pulmonary artery. There is a leak through the previously ligated connection between the superior vena cava and the right atrium (small arrows). The large arrows point to the innominate vein. SVC = superior vena cava, RPA = right pulmonary artery.

The Glenn shunt improves oxygen saturation more efficiently than does an arterial shunt without increasing pulmonary artery pressure or ventricular overload. The risk of the procedure is extremely low. Potential complications include transient SVC obstruction, pleural effusion, chylothorax, and pericardial effusion. Despite the excellent results with the Glenn anastomosis, the operation is palliative, having no effect on the desaturated blood that enters the heart from the IVC.

The status of blood flow to the LPA must be considered after a Glenn operation is performed. If a contralateral arterial shunt to the LPA is also present, the additional blood flow into that artery should not be excessive enough to cause pulmonary hypertension. Conversely, too little flow into the LPA may cause underdevelopment of the pulmonary artery and compromise the success of a Fontan repair.

Patients who have had a classic Glenn operation for a decade or more are at risk for the development of pulmonary arteriovenous fistulas. Intrapulmonary right to left shunting through a pulmonary AV fistula increases over time. This process may be suspected clinically because of a gradual increase in cyanosis that is not due to intracardiac shunting. The diagnosis may be established by an echo "bubble" study from the right arm that shows the rapid appearance of bubbles into the left atrium or a lung scan that shows increased uptake in the brain, kidneys, and contralateral lung. Pulmonary angiography can delineate the fistula and shows rapid emptying of contrast into the pulmonary veins. Coil embolization of important pulmonary AV fistulas can be performed in some patients, with improvement in oxygen saturation.

The Glenn anastomosis typically provides excellent palliation for 6 to 8 years before increasing cyanosis or exercise intolerance develops. If a Blalock shunt to the contralateral lung is also patent, the patient is frequently asymptomatic with an oxygen saturation in the middle to upper 80s and only a mildly increased hemoglobin. When clinical deterioration occurs in a patient with a Glenn shunt, it may be related to (1) the development of venous collaterals from the SVC to the IVC, resulting in diminished blood flow through the Glenn, possibly as a result in part of failure of growth of the SVC-RPA anastomosis, (2) pulmonary AV fistula, and (3) diminished blood flow to the LPA because of stenosis or occlusion of a contralateral shunt. In patients with tricuspid atresia there may also be restriction of the VSD size or progressive RV outflow tract obstruction, which limits blood flow to the LPA.

Once the patient develops symptoms related to inadequate pulmonary blood flow, such as fatigue, exercise intolerance, and increasing polycythemia, cardiac catheterization is indicated to determine the hemodynamic status. In the modern era, an adult with a Glenn shunt could still be a candidate for a more definitive Fontan operation if the LPA was normal and other important criteria were meant. Since the classic Glenn anastomosis is an end-to-end anastomosis from the SVC to the RPA and isolates the RPA from the rest of the pulmonary trunk, the next stage of surgery in a modified Fontan operation is to direct IVC blood to the LPA. In the past, this was accomplished with an atriopulmonary connection, in which the right atrium is anastomosed to the main or LPA. An alternative approach in the current era would be to restore continuity between the right and left pulmonary artery and channel the IVC through the right atrium into the underside of the pulmonary arteries, establishing a total cavopulmonary anastomosis. In rare instances, a patient who is not a candidate for additional surgery may benefit from the construction of a right axillary arteriovenous fistula to increase blood flow through the Glenn shunt.

Bidirectional Glenn Operation

In recent years, the classic Glenn operation has been replaced by the bidirectional Glenn shunt, in which the SVC is anastomosed to the RPA, which remains in continuity with the LPA (Fig. 12-7). The SVC-RA connection is ligated as it is in the classic Glenn anastomosis. In addition, the azygous vein and left SVC, if present, are ligated to prevent a "steal" away from the bidirectional Glenn shunt (Fig. 12-8). In cases where the left SVC is isolated from the right SVC, the left SVC is directly anastomosed to the pulmonary artery.

The bidirectional Glenn allows SVC blood to be distributed to both the right and left pulmonary arteries. To complete the modern Fontan repair, blood from the IVC is baffled through or external to the atrium into the underside of the RPA. As a result, all the vena caval blood flows into the pulmonary arteries, which are in continuity. Other sources of competitive flow into the pulmonary arteries, such as a patent arterial shunt and significant aortopulmonary collaterals, usually are eliminated perioperatively, although some

FIGURE 12-7

A venous angiogram in a patient with cavopulmonary anastomosis. The catheter is advanced from the inferior vena cava (IVC) through the right atrium into the superior vena cava (SVC). An angiogram in the SVC shows a bidirectional Glenn anastomosis, which fills both the right and left pulmonary arteries. SVC, superior vena cava; RPA, right pulmonary artery; LPA, left pulmonary artery.

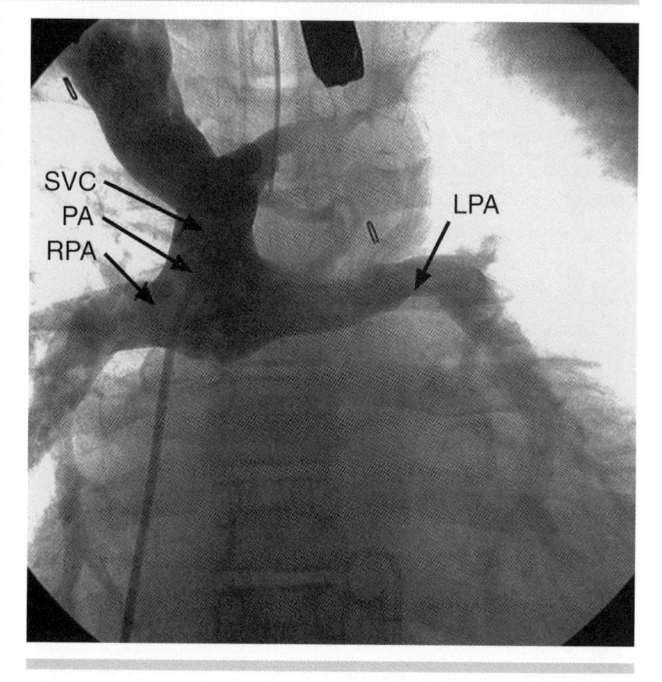

FIGURE 12-8

An innominate vein angiogram performed in a patient with a cavopulmonary anastomosis. This angiogram shows patency of a left superior vena cava (LSVC), which drains directly into the left atrium (LA), resulting in an obligatory right-to-left shunt and arterial desaturation. The catheter was passed from the inferior vena cava through the lateral tunnel and into the superior vena cava (SVC) and innominate vein. The arrow points to the LSVC off the innominate vein.

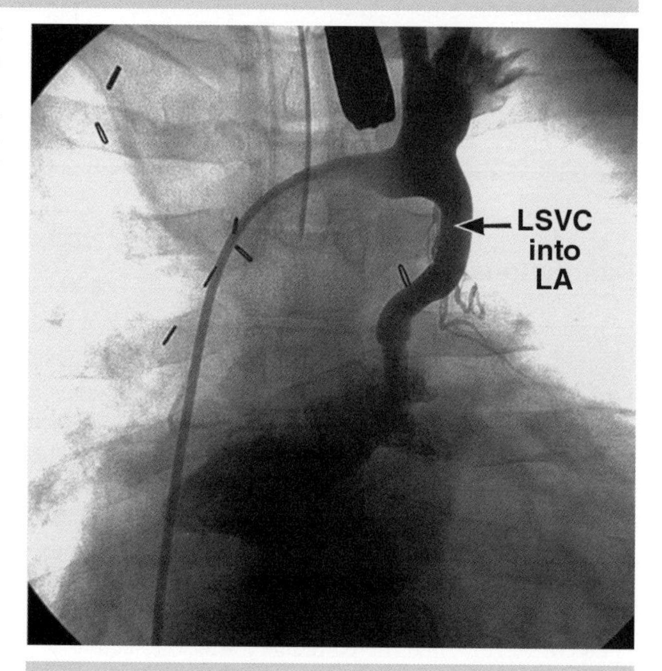

antegrade blood flow through a stenotic pulmonary valve may be left by some surgeons. Since the bidirectional Glenn usually is carried out in anticipation of completion with the Fontan procedure, there are less often specific late complications since it rarely remains as a freestanding operation.

Fontan Operation

In the modern era, the Fontan operation is the most definitive procedure for patients with the various forms of a univentricular heart. The Fontan operation was first performed in 1968 for patients with tricuspid atresia. The operation has undergone multiple modifications over the years to improve hemodynamics and decrease the incidence of supraventricular arrhythmias.

Pulmonary blood flow is achieved by an anastomosis between the right atrium or venae cavae and the pulmonary arteries. Blood flow through the pulmonary arteries is passive and is dependent on unimpeded flow through the pulmonary arteries and low filling pressures of the single ventricle. The preoperative hemodynamic assessment is therefore critical in determining whether a patient is a Fontan candidate. The ideal patient has unobstructed pulmonary arteries with low pulmonary vascular resistance, normal systolic function of the ventricle, a normal end-diastolic pressure ($<$12 mm Hg), and no AV valve regurgitation.

Originally, the criteria for candidacy for the Fontan operation were strict, and most patients who underwent the operation had tricuspid atresia with excellent anatomy and hemodynamics. It was felt that very young or older patients would not benefit from the procedure. However, over the last decade, the criteria for the Fontan operation have been broadened considerably. The operation can be performed at any age in patients with pulmonary arteries that are normal or can be repaired by surgical angioplasty or stenting at the time of the operation. Patients with single right, left, or primitive ventricles are also candidates as long as ventricular function is adequate. In some cases, a severely insufficient AV valve can be repaired or replaced prior to or at the time of the Fontan procedure. Patients with pulmonary hypertension secondary to pulmonary vascular obstructive disease are not candidates for surgery. However, a mild degree of pulmonary hypertension caused by high pulmonary blood flow from a systemic–pulmonary artery shunt may not be a contraindication for Fontan surgery if the pulmonary vascular resistance is normal.

RA-PA Anastomosis

The original procedure as described by Fontan for tricuspid atresia consisted of a Glenn shunt, closure of the atrial septal defect, insertion of valves at the IVC–right atrial junction, and at the anastomosis of the right atrial appendage to the LPA, and ligation of the main pulmonary artery. Preexisting shunts or aortopulmonary communications were ligated to prevent competing sources of blood flow into the pulmonary artery. It was subsequently appreciated that the placement of valves within the Fontan circulation not only was unnecessary for forward flow but created gradients within the venous system that obstructed venous outflow to the pulmonary artery. Subsequently, the insertion of venous valves was eliminated from the procedure (Figs. 12-9*A* and 12-10).

FIGURE 12-9*A*,*B*, AND *C*

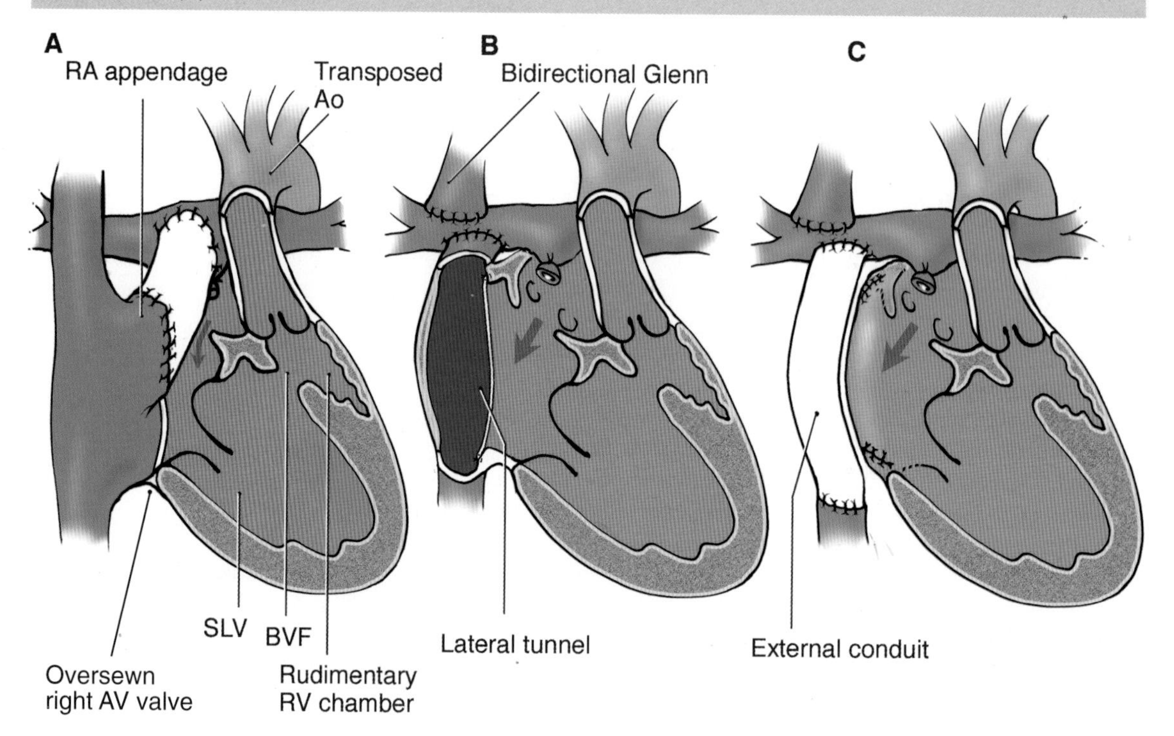

A. The classic Fontan operation is illustrated for a patient with a single left ventricle (D-TEA) and a rudimentary right ventricular outflow chamber. The right atrial appendage is broadly anastomosed to the pulmonary artery. The right AV valve and atrial communication are closed surgically. Oxygenated blood from the left atrium reaches the single ventricle and the aorta via the tricuspid valve and bulboventricular foramen. Thus, the single ventricle serves as a left ventricle. In tricuspid atresia (not shown), the atrial communication is closed and oxygenated blood enters the left ventricle through the mitral valve. *B*. The lateral tunnel operation is illustrated in a patient who had had an earlier bidirectional Glenn shunt. A tunnel from the inferior vena cava to the proximal superior vena cava and pulmonary artery is constructed within the atrium. *C*. In the external conduit procedure the inferior vena cava blood reaches the pulmonary artery directly through an interposed external tunnel. SLV, single left ventricle; BVF, bulboventricular foramen; AV, atrioventricular.

Lateral Tunnel

The direct right atrial–pulmonary artery anastomosis functioned well for many years, but turbulent flow within the large dilated right atrium resulted in energy loss, stasis, and diminished right-sided blood flow. Moreover, it was recognized that atrial contraction does not create pulsatile flow to the pulmonary arteries. Blood flow through the Fontan is passive and critically dependent on single ventricle function, normal pulmonary vascular resistance, and preserved AV conduction. The dilated right atrium also predisposes to clot formation and supraventricular arrhythmias.

To improve the efficiency of venous flow into the pulmonary arteries, the Fontan operation was modified to a direct systemic venous–pulmonary artery connection. The

FIGURE 12-10

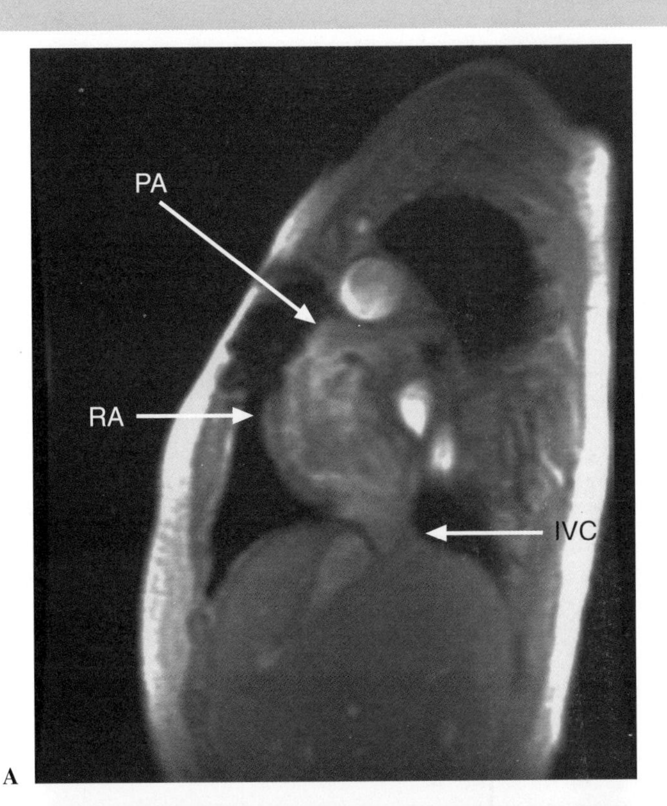

A

A. A cardiac MRI in a patient with an atriopulmonary anastomosis. Note the massive dilatation of the right atrium and its connection to the pulmonary artery.

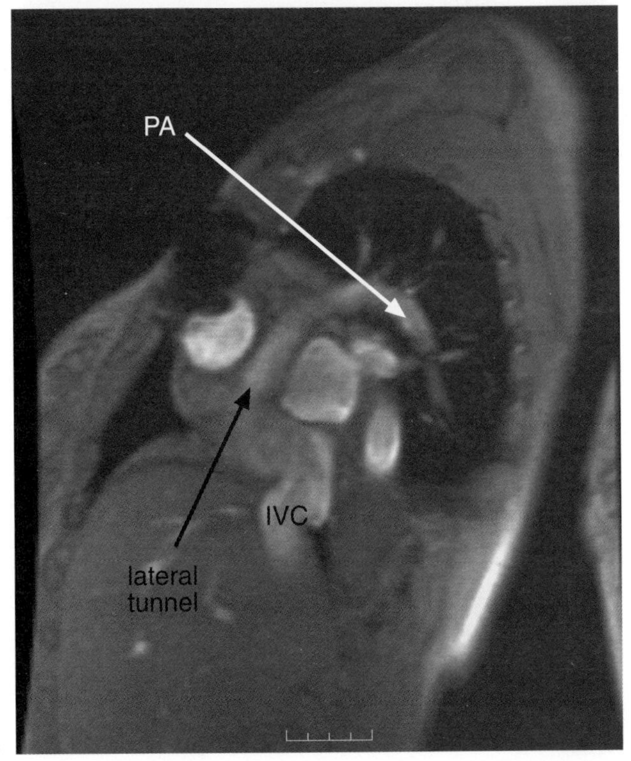

B

B. A cardiac MRI in a patient with a modified Fontan procedure consisting of a lateral tunnel. The study delineates the anastomosis from a portion of the right atrium into the pulmonary artery. PA, pulmonary artery; RA, right atrium; IVC, inferior vena cava.

lateral tunnel procedure, along with the bidirectional Glenn anastomosis, completes a total cavopulmonary anastomosis. In this operation, a tunnel is constructed by pericardium or Dacron along the lateral portion of the right atrium, connecting the IVC with the underside of the RPA (Fig. 19-9*B*). The SVC is transected at the level of the RPA, and both portions of the SVC are anastomosed to the RPA (Fig. 12-11). Although follow-up for this operation is shorter than for the atriopulmonary anastomosis, it is generally thought that circulatory dynamics are improved and the complications related to the interposed dilated right atrium are less as blood is directed through a tunnel rather than through a dilated right atrium. As a component of both the right atrial–pulmonary artery connection and lateral tunnel Fontan, many centers advocate creating a fenestration between the right atrium and the left atrium. This allows runoff of blood from the higher-pressure right atrium to the left atrium and systemic circulation, which is thought to result in a less complicated postoperative course with better cardiac output and fewer and less prolonged pleural effusions. The spectrum of use of the fenestration is broad; some centers fenestrate virtually every patient and others reserve the procedure for high-risk individuals in whom low pulmonary blood flow through the Fontan may be expected. Right-to-left shunting across the fenestration can preserve cardiac output. As a result, these patients are more cyanotic in the postoperative period and beyond. Some fenestrations close spontaneously over time, and others may require device closure.

Extracardiac Connection

In recent years, some surgeons have modified the Fontan operation further by connecting the IVC to the pulmonary arteries with an extracardiac tube (Fig. 12-9*C*). Proponents of

FIGURE 12-11

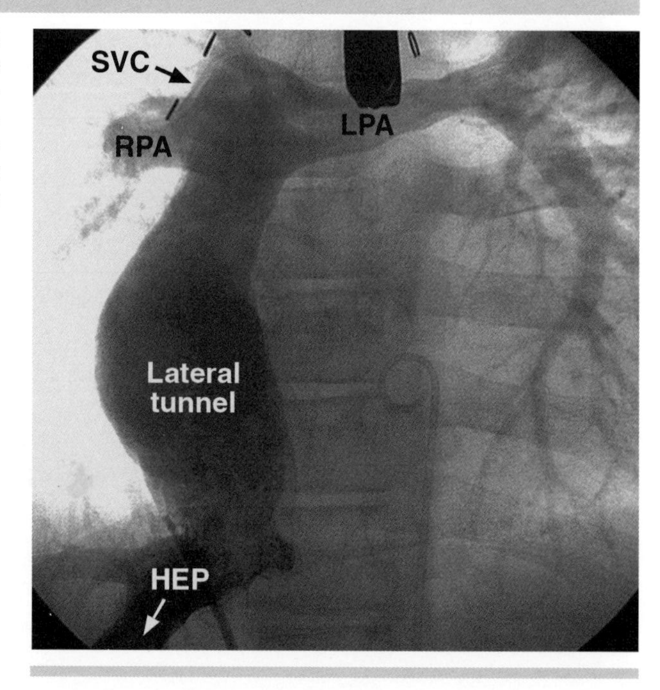

An angiogram is performed within the lateral tunnel in a patient with a modified Fontan operation. The cavopulmonary anastomosis is visualized with no evidence of obstruction. There is back filling of the hepatic veins. The proximal pulmonary arteries are unremarkable. SVC, superior vena cava; Hep V, hepatic vein. RPA, right pulmonary artery; LPA, left pulmonary artery.

this operation argue that this approach may prevent the late atrial tachyarrhythmias that are responsible for significant late morbidity in older Fontan patients. The extracardiac Fontan eliminates most of the atrial suture lines and the high venous pressures within the right atrium, which are the likely cause of atrial arrhythmias. A potential disadvantage of this approach is the use of prosthetic materials that may be subject to clot formation and obstruction. Fenestration of an extracardiac Fontan connection is more difficult to place and requires that the conduit be sutured directly to the right atrial wall. Since the follow-up of patients with an extracardiac Fontan is short and the late outcome is uncertain, some surgeons reserve the procedure for situations in which the intracardiac anatomy is more suitable than a lateral tunnel.

RA-RV Fontan

In a small number of patients with tricuspid atresia, the RV can be large enough to incorporate into the repair, often in conjunction with a Glenn anastomosis. In these patients, blood flow from the right atrium to the RV is achieved by using a porcine valved conduit, a homograft, or a nonvalved anastomosis. The atrial and ventricular septal defects are closed to prevent intracardiac shunting.

Although the right atrium–right ventricle (RA-RV) modified Fontan has the potential advantage of a right-sided pumping chamber, the operation is rarely performed today. Whereas RV repair might result in RV growth, a small and poorly compliant RV most often results in nonpulsatile pulmonary blood flow, as in the standard Fontan operation. Since obstruction within the RA-RV conduit or homograft is inevitable and generally occurs within 10 years after surgery, this approach incurs the necessity for reoperation to replace the conduit and relieve obstruction, with little or no apparent benefit over the cavopulmonary anastomosis. Nevertheless, some patients have reached adult life and have had stable hemodynamics with the "four-chamber" Fontan.

Surgical Issues and Controversies

It is essential that early palliative procedures not cause anatomic or hemodynamic abnormalities that will jeopardize the success of a future Fontan repair in a patient with single ventricle. Potential contraindications include obstruction or occlusion of a pulmonary artery, elevation of pulmonary vascular resistance from persistent pulmonary hypertension, and LV dilatation from volume overload induced by a large shunt.

Infants with Decreased Pulmonary Blood Flow

In most forms of single ventricle, pulmonary blood flow usually is restricted during infancy, and often a shunt is required to improve oxygenation and relieve polycythemia. In the current era, a modified Blalock-Taussig shunt is the procedure of choice for neonates with obstructive pulmonary blood flow in the context of single ventricle. Later in the first year of life, a bidirectional Glenn operation generally is performed in preparation for a total cavopulmonary anastomosis, often because additional pulmonary blood flow is required. Many institutions perform the bidirectional Glenn operation as a staged procedure in preparation for the Fontan operation. However, some patients may be stable for a longer period of time with adequate pulmonary blood flow and can undergo the full Fontan operation without the intermediate bidirectional Glenn operation.

Infants with Increased Pulmonary Blood Flow

If a single ventricle has no obstruction to pulmonary outflow, with no gradient between the LV and the pulmonary artery, early surgical intervention is necessary to restrict pulmonary blood flow. If blood flow is not controlled, severe congestive heart failure and, among survivors, pulmonary vascular obstructive disease will ensue. Excessive pulmonary blood flow causes progressive ventricular dilatation and volume overload, elevated end-diastolic pressure, and ventricular dysfunction. If this process is not interrupted during infancy, the probability of a successful Fontan repair lessens until the operation is no longer feasible.

Pulmonary artery banding has been the procedure performed to restrict pulmonary blood flow and prevent LV volume overload and pulmonary hypertension. The clinical course after pulmonary artery banding is one of gradually progressive pulmonary stenosis that results in diminished pulmonary blood flow and increased cyanosis. Once additional pulmonary blood flow is required, a bidirectional Glenn shunt or complete Fontan repair is carried out. The classic Glenn procedure is no longer used. A well-recognized complication seen after pulmonary artery banding is the development of bulboventricular foramen obstruction. Significant obstruction, which produces subaortic stenosis, must be remedied surgically to prevent progressive ventricular hypertrophy and obstruction.

Obstruction of the VSD or Bulboventricular Foramen

An important issue both pre-Fontan and later is the size of the VSD or bulboventricular foramen (BVF). If the communication is restrictive, a pressure gradient will be present between the left and right ventricles. This is the functional equivalent of subaortic stenosis in patients with a transposed aorta arising from a small RV outflow ventricle or pulmonary stenosis in the presence of tricuspid atresia and normal great artery position. Significant obstruction at the VSD or BVF level complicates a Fontan repair by causing ventricular hypertrophy, decreased LV compliance, and increased LV end-diastolic pressure. This problem is encountered most frequently in patients who have undergone pulmonary artery banding or repair of anomalies of the aortic arch. Whether the development of obstruction at the VSD-BVF level is related to pulmonary artery banding or the natural history of this lesion is not clear, but regardless of the cause, if significant subaortic obstruction develops before or after a Fontan repair, surgery may be required to enlarge or bypass the VSD or BVF. Direct enlargement of the VSD or BVF is the most obvious approach, but early attempts were not effective. Often the enlargement was insufficient, and obstruction recurred; complete heart block or injury to other intracardiac structures was not unusual. However, in recent years, by means of resection of muscular septum inferior to the VSD or BVF, larger communications can be made with fewer complications, and more complex surgical approaches can be avoided. This has again become the procedure of choice at some centers.

If obstruction at the level of the VSD is present during infancy or seems likely to develop, another surgical approach is to perform a Damus-Kaye-Stansel procedure. In this operation, the pulmonary artery is ligated and the proximal portion is anastomosed to the ascending aorta. This arrangement permits unobstructed blood flow into the aorta from the LV and proximal pulmonary artery, avoiding the restrictive VSD. There remain two systemic semilunar valves, either of which could become insufficient at a later time. Pulmonary blood flow into the distal pulmonary arteries is achieved by a modified Blalock shunt. A third approach to a restrictive VSD or BVF in selected patients is to perform an arterial switch that restores continuity between the LV and the aorta. The resultant subpulmonary obstruction may be sufficient to control pulmonary blood flow without pulmonary artery banding.

A Fontan repair can proceed at a later stage regardless of the operative approach to relieve VSD or BVF obstruction. In some patients, relief of obstruction can be done at the time of the Fontan procedure. Among both children and adults, VSD or BVF obstruction may develop or progress years after an earlier Fontan procedure, resulting in the need for reoperation.

One-Stage, Two-Stage, or No Fontan

In the present era, infants after the neonatal Norwood operation for HLHS are treated with an early bidirectional Glenn procedure, with a Fontan operation done later. This limits the length of time the ventricle is exposed to increased LV volume from the systemic to pulmonary artery shunt as well as allowing the final procedure to be done in a somewhat older patient. The Fontan operation carried out in the first year of life carries an increased risk of mortality and morbidity compared to older infants and children. It is somewhat controversial whether the two-stage procedure should be done for every Fontan candidate. In the presence of controlled pulmonary blood flow with only a mild increased ventricular preload, some patients can have the more definitive Fontan operation done later. There are many patients with reasonable pulmonary blood flow, normal pulmonary artery pressure, and only minimal increased ventricular volume who have successful Fontan operations done even in adulthood, without an earlier bidirectional Glenn operation.

Because of late complications after the Fontan operation, a few centers have advocated only a bidirectional Glenn operation and an associated arterial shunt instead of completing the Fontan procedure. It may be argued that the arterial shunt needed to keep arterial saturations at an acceptable level in adult life will be too large, resulting in unacceptable long-term ventricular volume loads. Thus, this approach generally has not been utilized.

Fenestration or No Fenestration

The fenestration procedure at the time of the Fontan operation allows improved systemic cardiac output at the cost of increased cyanosis. Many of these patients are apt to have a less complicated postoperative course with fewer pleural effusions and shorter hospital stays. Later, the fenestration closes spontaneously, is closed by a device at cardiac catheterization, or is left open indefinitely. On a long-term basis, it is not advisable to leave an atrial communication in a patient with higher than normal right atrial pressure with the potential for paradoxical embolization. Anticoagulation is generally recommended for adults under these circumstances. Whether all patients require a fenestration as part of the Fontan operation is controversial; many centers carry out very few fenestrations, whereas others fenestrate on a routine basis.

Lateral Tunnel versus External Conduit

IVC–pulmonary artery anastomosis is a basic component of Fontan repair. The lateral tunnel operation creates a channel from the IVC to the pulmonary artery within the right atrium and has the advantage of avoiding an artificial external tube that might be prone to obstruction. In addition, if a fenestration is used, later catheterization device closure can be achieved without difficulty. The external conduit is somewhat easier to place surgically, and long suture lines within the right atrium are avoided. A "sutureless" atrium may not be as prone to late arrhythmias as it is with the extensive intraatrial surgery required for the lateral tunnel. How the theoretical advantages and disadvantages of each approach will eventually be translated into outcome data will determine whether one or the other becomes the standard for the Fontan procedure.

EVALUATION OF A PATIENT WITH SINGLE VENTRICLE WHO HAS NOT HAD A FONTAN PROCEDURE

Adult patients with single ventricle typically fall into one of three groups: (1) patients who were palliated with a systemic to pulmonary artery shunt and/or a Glenn procedure who have remained relatively stable, (2) patients who have pulmonary vascular obstructive disease or pulmonary artery abnormalities that preclude a Fontan repair, and (3) patients who have undergone a Fontan repair.

Most adults seen today have had a Fontan repair during childhood or adolescence or were considered for the procedure but were not found to fit the criteria for surgery. It is distinctly unusual for an adult to remain asymptomatic after only palliative shunt surgery during childhood.

The history and physical examination provide important clues about the clinical situation in a patient with single ventricle who has not had the Fontan operation. When exercise intolerance, fatigue, and cyanosis are the major symptoms, the problem is usually inadequate pulmonary blood flow. This can occur when there is significant pulmonary stenosis and low pulmonary artery pressure or, at the other extreme, when pulmonary hypertension and high pulmonary vascular resistance are present. If a continuous murmur is audible, it usually implies that the shunt is patent and no more than mild elevation of pulmonary artery pressure is present. These patients still may be candidates for a Fontan repair if the hemodynamics, ventricular function, and pulmonary artery anatomy are acceptable. Patients deemed inoperable for a Fontan procedure in the past nevertheless may be candidates today, because the operative criteria are less stringent.

If a continuous murmur is not audible but was present previously, it is indicative of pulmonary hypertension or occlusion of a previous shunt. If the shunt is occluded, the pulmonary artery pressure is likely to be low and the patient may be suitable for a Fontan operation. A prominent systolic murmur representing significant pulmonary stenosis is almost always present in adults with single ventricle who have not had a Fontan procedure. The absence of the murmur with progressive cyanosis is apt to indicate pulmonary hypertension with elevated pulmonary vascular resistance.

The chest x-ray and echocardiography provide information about LV function, the presence of AV valve regurgitation, and/or whether there is obstruction at the VSD or BVF level. However, essential information about pulmonary artery pressure, pulmonary vascular resistance, and pulmonary artery anatomy must be obtained by cardiac catheterization.

If the cardiac catheterization demonstrates normal pulmonary vascular resistance with adequate-size pulmonary arteries and preserved ventricular function with a normal ventricular end-diastolic pressure, the patient is a candidate for a Fontan operation. If the pulmonary vascular resistance is elevated, the operation is not possible. If the pulmonary arteries are not in continuity or have been isolated by a previous shunt or Glenn anastomosis, a careful assessment of the resistance in each pulmonary artery will determine whether there are surgical options that include pulmonary arterioplasty and/or reconnection. If a Glenn shunt is present, an angiogram in the SVC will assess blood flow into the RPA, narrowing at the anastomosis, the presence of pulmonary arteriovenous fistulas, and venous collateral flow from the SVC to the IVC.

When an adult with single ventricle or tricuspid atresia is evaluated initially, the pertinent issues are: (1) pulmonary artery anatomy and resistance, (2) ventricular function, (3) arrhythmias, and (4) the status of the AV valve. The presence of AV valve regurgitation does not necessarily preclude a Fontan repair if AV valve repair or replacement can be performed. If the LV end-diastolic pressure is elevated, it must be established whether that is due to LV volume overload from high pulmonary blood flow or is the result of irreversible myocardial disease, which would preclude an operation. Patients in the high-pulmonary-flow group who have good ventricular function still may be candidates for a Fontan repair. These individuals will have an aortic saturation in the upper 80s, normal pulmonary vascular resistance, and normal or only mildly elevated pulmonary artery and LV end-diastolic pressure.

Examination of a patient with a Glenn anastomosis reveals elevated jugular venous pressure that reflects mean pulmonary artery pressure in the absence of any gradient between the SVC and the RPA. The increased venous pressure represents the transpulmonary gradient of 6 to 7 mm Hg that is necessary for blood to flow through the pulmonary vascular bed into the left side of the heart. Blood flow within the Glenn shunt does not produce a cardiac murmur.

EVALUATION OF A PATIENT AFTER THE FONTAN OPERATION

Although the Fontan operation must be viewed as a palliative operation, the long-term outlook is better than for patients with only systemic to pulmonary artery shunts. Outcomes are expected to continue to improve as a result of better myocardial protection during surgery, a lower incidence of reoperation, and modifications of the procedure.

Five- and 10-year survivals of 88 and 78%, respectively, have been reported. Late deaths have resulted from myocardial failure and arrhythmias. Risk factors for an adverse outcome after a Fontan operation include AV valve regurgitation, LV dysfunction, postoperative right atrial pressure $>$20 mm Hg, obstructive pulmonary arteries, and the presence of New York Heart Association (NYHA) class III and IV clinical status.

Patients who are stable after a Fontan operation have preserved ventricular systolic function and normal ventricular end-diastolic pressure with little or no AV valve regurgitation and sinus rhythm. With a ventricular end-disatolic pressure $<$12 mm Hg and a transpulmonary gradient of 6 to 7 mm Hg, a systemic venous pressure between 12 and 19 mm Hg is required to drive blood through the pulmonary circuit. If the preoperative LV end-diastolic pressure is $>$12 mm Hg and is not due to a remediable problem such as excessive pulmonary blood flow, subaortic obstruction, or AV valve regurgitation, systemic venous pressure after surgery may exceed 20 mm Hg, which leads to persistent pleural effusions, ascites, and peripheral edema. Such patients benefit from ACE inhibitors and an atrial fenestration, which increases cardiac output at the cost of cyanosis. Other findings suggesting persistent abnormalities after the Fontan operation include a continuous murmur from aortopulmonary collaterals or a patent systemic to pulmonary artery shunt; a systolic murmur resulting from pulmonary or subaortic stenosis or AV valve insufficiency; and diastolic murmurs indicating AV valve stenosis or aortic regurgitation. Right-to-left shunting across an atrial communication, cardiac arrhythmias, and protein-losing enteropathy also are potential late complications.

An adult with a Fontan repair requires ongoing medical follow-up. Particular attention should be directed to ventricular function, the development of left AV valve regurgitation and atrial arrhythmias, and the potential for obstruction within the Fontan.

Physical Examination

The physical examination of a patient after a Fontan repair can provide important information about the status of the repair. Most patients in whom there are no significant residual hemodynamic problems will have an unremarkable examination. There are often no audible cardiac murmurs; S_2 is single, and the only other demonstrable abnormality may be an elevated jugular venous pressure, which reflects the pressure within the Fontan circuit. However, in patients with residual problems, physical examination may reveal evidence of right-sided congestion with ascites, hepatomegaly, and peripheral edema. The liver may be enlarged secondary to elevated venous pressure. A pulsatile liver occurring with the A wave of atrial systole may be noted.

A nearly normal oxygen saturation is expected in a patient with an uncomplicated Fontan. However, varying degrees of arterial desaturation may be present in some patients, and it is important that the etiology be established. Cyanosis can be caused by an intracardiac or an intrapulmonary right-to-left shunt. Intracardiac shunting may be due to (1) a leak across the intraatrial baffle that separates systemic venous blood from pulmonary venous blood, (2) a previously unrecognized left SVC, which usually drains into the coronary sinus but occasionally drains directly into the left atrium, (3) a communication from the right atrium through a leak in a previously oversewn right-sided AV valve into the single ventricle, or (4) a right-to-left atrial shunt that was placed intentionally to decompress the Fontan circulation into a lower-pressure left atrium (fenestration).

In addition to intracardiac causes of cyanosis, intrapulmonary shunting from a pulmonary AV fistula can produce late cyanosis in patients who have had a classic Glenn anastomosis. This complication also can occur in patients who have a bidirectional Glenn anastomosis but is seldom encountered.

MANAGEMENT ISSUES AFTER A FONTAN OPERATION

Obstruction within the Fontan Circulation

Obstruction within the Fontan anastomosis is uncommon when a direct atriopulmonary or cavopulmonary anastomosis is performed. When obstruction is present, it usually occurs early after surgery and is at the site of the surgical anastomosis or uncorrected pulmonary artery stenosis. Late obstruction occasionally may be recognized and managed by surgical modification or stent placement (Fig. 12-12*A* and *B*). In addition, patients with

FIGURE 12-12*A*

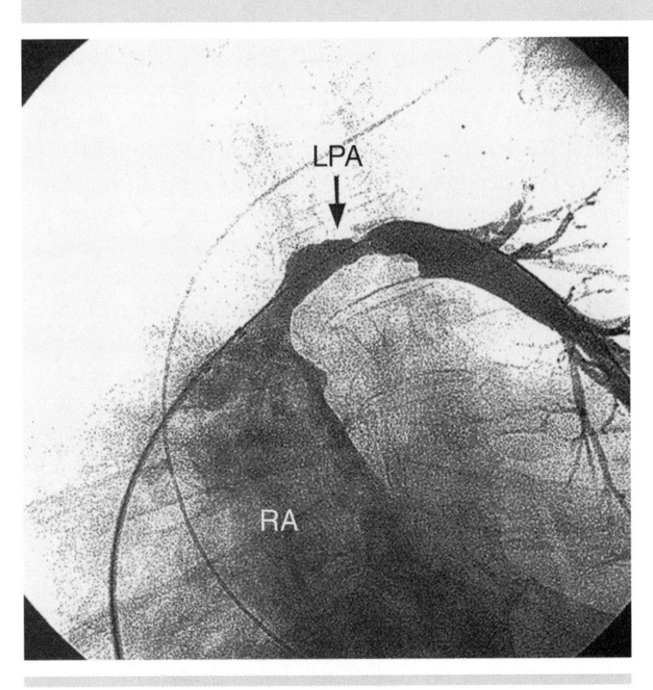

Severe obstruction is demonstrated in the anastomosis between the right atrium and the left pulmonary artery in a patient with a modified Fontan repair. LPA, left pulmonary artery; RA, right atrium.

FIGURE 12-12*B*

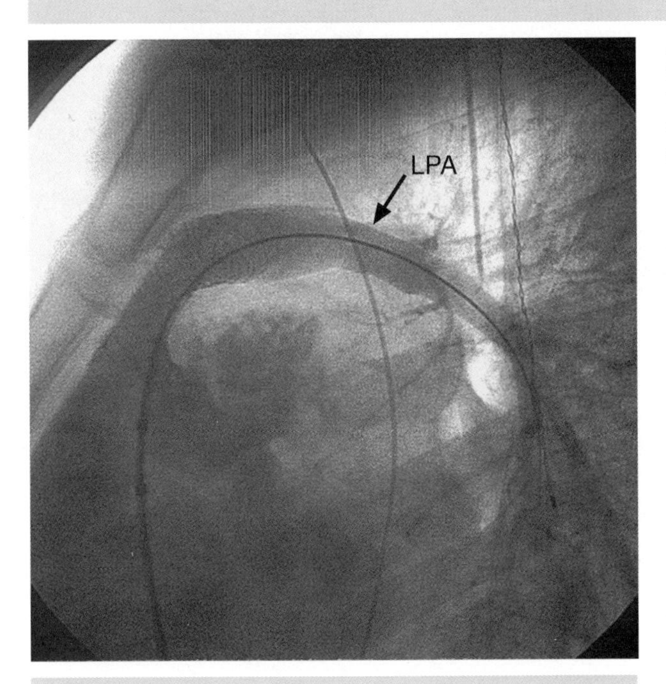

An angiogram performed in the same patient following placement of a stent within the graft between the right atrium and the left pulmonary artery. There is no evidence of residual obstruction. LPA, left pulmonary artery.

persistent pulmonary arterial collaterals may have elevated pulmonary artery and systemic venous pressures because of higher resistance to venous flow in the distal pulmonary arteries. Finally, right pulmonary venous obstruction by a dilated right atrium has been observed in patients who have had a right atrial–pulmonary artery anastomosis (Fig. 12-13).

In the rare patient with an RA-RV connection for tricuspid atresia, the late development of porcine conduit or homograft obstruction should be anticipated. The majority of porcine-valved conduits have required reoperation after 10 years. The symptoms of conduit obstruction are variable. Some patients may experience a decline in exercise capacity or manifest evidence of right-sided congestion. If a Glenn anastomosis is also present, conduit obstruction may be less obvious because a significant portion of pulmonary blood flow is maintained through the SVC-RPA anastomosis. Once significant conduit obstruction develops, reoperation is indicated. The site of obstruction varies among patients and includes valvar obstruction, diffuse narrowing of the conduit secondary to the development of an intimal peel, or sternal compression and narrowing at the proximal or distal anastomosis.

AV Valve Insufficiency

AV valve insufficiency is poorly tolerated in the Fontan circulation. Elevation of left atrial pressure raises pulmonary artery and systemic venous pressure within the Fontan circuit and results in "right heart" failure and low cardiac output. Unless there is concomitant repair or replacement of a severely insufficient AV valve, the Fontan operation is contraindicated on this basis. The same problem arises for a patient who develops progressive AV valve insufficiency after having undergone a Fontan operation earlier in life. Late worsening of tricuspid insufficiency in patients with a single right ventricle may occur, and the resultant ventricular dysfunction is poorly tolerated in the context of Fontan physiology. Although AV valve regurgitation must be considered in a different context for Fontan patients than in patients with a normal heart, nonetheless, it is often a difficult decision to proceed with reoperation for AV valve repair or replacement in these patients. When it is determined that surgery is necessary, a decision must be made whether AV valvu-

FIGURE 12-13

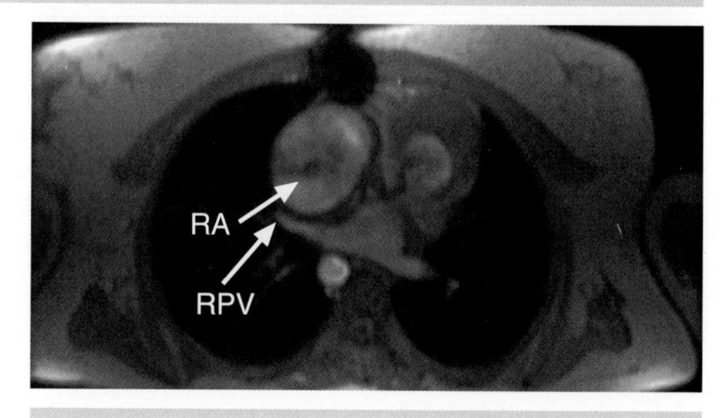

Cardiac MRI of an adult 13 years after a modified Fontan operation using an atriopulmonary anastomosis. The right atrium (RA) is severely enlarged and is producing compression of the right pulmonary vein (RPV).

loplasty would be effective or whether an AV valve replacement is required. Replacement of a tricuspid valve in a patient with a systemic right ventricle may be difficult.

Thromboembolic Complications

There is a small but significant incidence of thromboembolic complications following a Fontan procedure. Potential etiologies include: (1) the large patulous right atrium seen with atriopulmonary connections, (2) a persistent right-to-left shunt through a residual right atrium–left atrium communication, either inadvertent or from a persistent fenestration, (3) the development of atrial tachyarrhythmias, and (4) chronic low cardiac output.

Most centers advocate daily antiplatelet doses of aspirin on a routine basis, and for high-risk patients, anticoagulation is recommended. Treatment practices vary concerning the use of prophylactic anticoagulants in these patients; many advocate the use of warfarin once intracardiac thrombus is suspected or after the development of atrial fibrillation or atrial flutter. Transesophageal echocardiography (TEE) plays an important role in assessing the possibility of a thrombus in the Fontan circulation.

Arrhythmias

Atrial tachyarrhythmias have been the most difficult problem facing older patients with a Fontan repair. The most common arrhythmias are intraatrial reentrant tachycardia and atrial fibrillation (Fig. 12-14). Treatment of recurrent atrial tachyarrhythmias in Fontan patients continues to be difficult and must be individualized. Patients who develop atrial fibrillation typically experience marked fatigue and fluid retention and are at risk for intraatrial thrombus formation. The loss of AV synchrony is poorly tolerated in most Fontan patients, presumably related to the rise in left atrial pressure and its effect on flow through the Fontan. Whether patients who were repaired with a lateral tunnel or extracardiac conduits will have a reduced incidence of arrhythmias during late follow-up compared with those with the direct RA-PA Fontan is not yet known, since these operations have not been in use as long as the classic atriopulmonary anastomoses have. Similarly, a decrease in the incidence of rhythm disorders with the external conduit compared to the lateral tunnel has been suggested but as yet is unproven.

Restoration of sinus rhythm in patients with atrial fibrillation or atrial flutter is the goal of treatment, and careful management is required. If the duration of the atrial arrhythmia cannot be determined accurately but is not felt to be recent in onset, a 4-week course of anticoagulation is usually recommended before cardioversion is attempted in a stable patient. Echocardiographic studies of Fontan patients with atrial fibrillation and atrial flutter frequently show "smoke" in the right atrium, consistent with sluggish blood flow.

Recurrences of atrial tachyarrhythmias are common and generally require chronic antiarrhythmic drug therapy in an attempt to maintain sinus rhythm. However, antiarrhythmic drug therapy can be complicated in this population because of limited drug efficacy and underlying abnormalities of the sinus node and AV conduction system. In addition, ventricular dysfunction may limit antiarrhythmic drug options. Amiodarone is often used in patients with refractory arrhythmias. Permanent pacing may also be problematic. Epi-

FIGURE 12-14

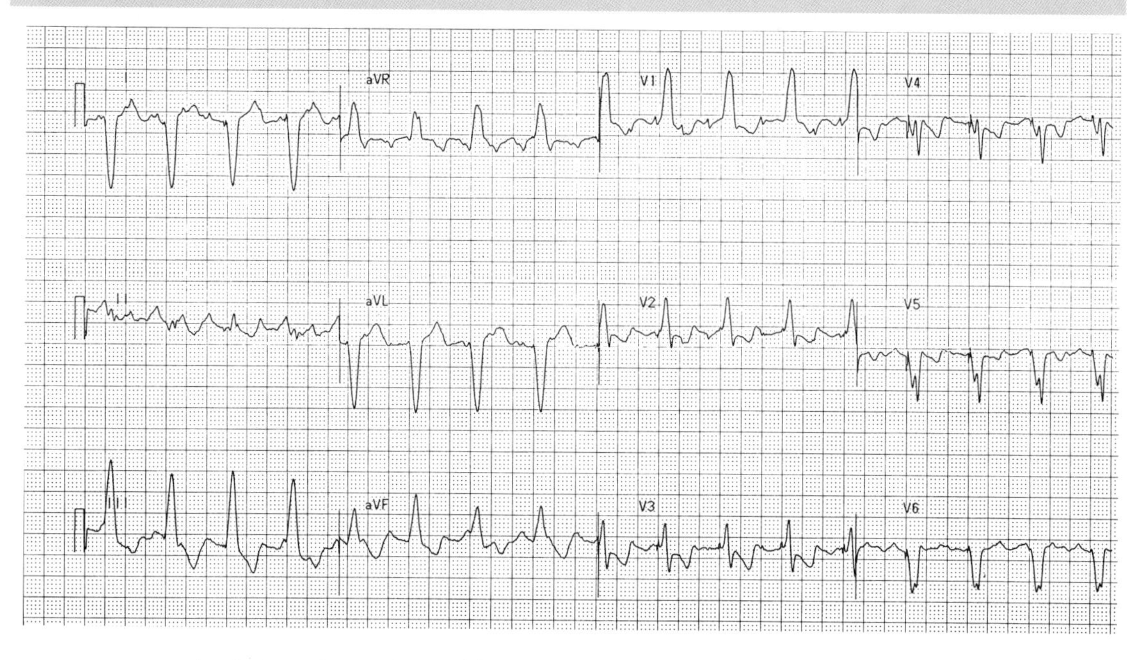

An electrocardiogram in an adult patient with an atriopulmonary anastomosis showing atrial tachycardia with 2:1 AV block.

cardial leads are preferred over the transvenous route to avoid the potential for thrombus formation and to permit dual-chamber pacing.

Radio frequency ablation has been somewhat effective in Fontan patients with recurrent atrial flutter or atrial tachycardia. However, these procedures require considerable expertise and specialized equipment for precise mapping of the tachycardia circuit.

Surgical revision of the Fontan has been used with some preliminary success in Fontan patients with refractory atrial tachyarrhythmias, but experience is limited. The operation is formidable, consisting of conversion from an atriopulmonary anastomosis to a lateral tunnel or extracardiac cavopulmonary connection in conjunction with intraoperative ablation and a MAZE procedure. The goal is to prevent recurrent atrial fibrillation and reentrant atrial tachycardia and to improve the hemodynamic status. Many of the patients referred for Fontan revision have had additional abnormalities prompting reoperation, abnormalities such as right pulmonary vein compression or right atrial thrombus.

Protein-Losing Enteropathy

The development of protein-losing enteropathy (PLE) is a serious complication of the Fontan operation. This entity generally occurs late after the operation and has been reported in 10 to 15% of late Fontan survivors. The development of PLE may be more likely in patients with significant hemodynamic abnormalities, but PLE also can occur as an isolated problem in a Fontan patient who has done well otherwise. Chronic low cardiac output may be an important predisposing factor.

Treatment of PLE is very difficult. Diuretics are standard; high-dose spironolactone may be helpful for fluid management. Modification of diet does not seem to confer a significant benefit, and the use of steroids and heparin has resulted in only anecdotal improvement. Treatable causes of abnormal hemodynamic abnormalities should be sought and corrected, if feasible. A cardiac catheterization often is advised to assess hemodynamics and pulmonary artery anatomy. More recently, cardiac MRI has been an excellent imaging tool to delineate the Fontan circuit and can provide anatomic details about regions that are more difficult to observe on angiography, most notably pulmonary vein compression by an enlarged right atrium.

In extreme cases, fenestration of the Fontan has been performed in the hope that reducing venous pressure will improve the PLE. Surgical revision of the Fontan from an atriopulmonary connection to a cavopulmonary anastomosis also has been used for this purpose. Some success has been reported with these modalities, but cardiac transplantation may be necessary in refractory cases; PLE most often disappears after a successful heart replacement.

Hepatic Dysfunction

Late hepatic dysfunction can occur after a Fontan repair. Patients can present with signs of hypersplenism such as thrombocytopenia or with hepatic congestion and ascites. Although some of these older patients are found to have transfusion-related hepatitis, in others, hypersplenism appears to be related solely to the chronic elevation of venous pressure.

Acquired Cardiac Disease

Since few Fontan patients have reached the age in which ischemic heart disease becomes manifest, we do not yet know what impact acquired heart disease will have on their clinical course. It is reasonable to assume that certain acquired problems such as coronary artery disease and cardiomyopathy will have an especially adverse effect on patients with the Fontan circulation.

Pregnancy creates unique problems for the Fontan patient. The hemodynamic changes during pregnancy, which include an expansion in blood volume and compression of the IVC during the third trimester, cause significant changes in preload (Chap. 17). The situation is also complicated by the need for cardiotonic and antiarrhythmic medications in some patients, which could pose an additional risk to the developing fetus.

Failed Fontan

Patients who have had a Fontan operation early in life may be encountered who have had numerous complications and in whom over time, medical and surgical therapy are no longer effective in preventing progressive symptoms and allowing an acceptable quality of life. Signs and symptoms include right-sided heart failure, low cardiac output, arrhythmias, cyanosis, and extremely poor exercise tolerance. Conversion of RA-PA Fontan to a lateral tunnel or external conduit has been tried in some cases, when a large patulous right atrium with resultant energy loss is considered the key causative factor. However, most patients with refractory symptoms ultimately become candidates for cardiac replacement. Although the risks are increased in these patients due to multiple operations, the need for extensive reconstruction, or nutritional issues, including the presence of PLE, heart transplantation offers these patients an alternative when the clinical situation has deteriorated. The experience with heart transplantation in some patients with a failed Fontan has been positive. It has been reported that these individuals have amelioration of symptoms and are similar to other heart transplantation patients in terms of their day-to-day life and prognosis. Of course, they are also subject to the sometimes difficult management strategies and frequent reevaluations that are necessary for the care of any patient after heart transplantation.

SUMMARY

Single ventricle refers to a cardiac defect or combination of defects that results in a single functioning ventricular chamber. The basic entities classified as single ventricle include (1) double-inlet LV with a small-outlet RV chamber, usually leading to a transposed aorta, (2) double-inlet RV with a small LV chamber often associated with mitral obstruction, (3) indeterminate ventricle, (4) tricuspid atresia, and (5) absent ventricular septum with otherwise normal atrial–ventricular–great artery connections (Holmes heart), a rare variation. In addition, an unbalanced AV canal, pulmonary atresia with an intact ventricular septum, and HLHS with mitral/aortic atresia all result in single-ventricle physiology and may have similar management considerations. However, the latter defects often are not formally classified under the heading of single ventricle.

Patients with single ventricle who have survived to adult life under all these classifications usually have had one or more cardiac operations. During infancy, management depends on the state of the pulmonary outflow tract. Patients with unobstructed pulmonary blood flow require an early operation (pulmonary artery banding, an arterial switch procedure, or another palliative operation). Infants with obstructed pulmonary blood flow require an arterial-to-pulmonary shunt procedure.

Most of these patients who reach adult life have undergone one or more operative procedures. The majority of patients who have had a Fontan operation originally had an arterial shunt that was replaced in one or two stages by an atriopulmonary or a total cavopulmonary anastomosis; some have had the Fontan operation as the primary procedure in late childhood or as an adult. An occasional unoperated patient may be encountered who has reached adulthood with balanced pulmonary blood flow, absence of other severe cardiac abnormalities, and good ventricular function. Although such a patient may have reached adolescence and beyond without a previous operation, he or she still may be eligible for a Fontan operation upon indication.

The physical examination of a patient with single ventricle varies with the anatomy and physiology. Patients who have undergone a Fontan operation with no residual AV valve insufficiency, bulboventricular obstruction, or LV outflow tract obstruction will have no significant cardiac murmurs. Fontan patients with a loud murmur will have an associated abnormality, usually obstruction at the VSD level, BVF obstruction, AV valve insufficiency, or other associated abnormalities. The presence of cyanosis most often indicates a residual intracardiac right-to-left shunt.

Most unoperated patients with single ventricle who survive childhood and adolescence will have enough pulmonary outflow obstruction to prevent pulmonary hypertension but still have sufficient pulmonary blood flow to avoid severe cyanosis and allow growth and development. Late survivors with single ventricle who have unobstructed pulmonary outflow obstruction will have pulmonary vascular obstruction with limited pulmonary blood flow, and these patients have the usual late course of increasing cyanosis associated with Eisenmenger's syndrome.

Laboratory studies vary, depending on the operative history and present physiology. "Ideal" Fontan patients have unencumbered blood flow from the cavae to the pulmonary artery either directly or through the right atrium, depending on the type of Fontan procedure. Those with good ventricular function with no AV valve regurgitation or ventricular outflow obstruction have a central venous pressure, which reflects pulmonary artery pressure, in the range of 12 to 15 mm Hg.

In most cases, echocardiography, either transthoracic or TEE, will delineate the anatomy of patients with single ventricle. Cardiac MRI can be used for pulmonary and systemic venous drainage when needed. Cardiac catheterization and angiography are necessary to determine operability in candidates for the Fontan operation or to document late pathophysiology in symptomatic patients who have had a Fontan operation earlier in life.

The modern Fontan operation consists of directly anastomosing the superior and inferior vena cavae into the pulmonary artery. The IVC is tunneled within the right atrium or externally. However, many adults, perhaps the majority with a Fontan operation, have a direct right atrial–pulmonary artery anastomosis type of connection, which for the most part is not utilized today. The direct caval anastomosis results in laminar blood flow, and energy loss from turbulent blood currents is avoided. The incidence of late arrhythmias may be decreased compared with the direct RA-PA connection, in which the capacious right atrium may be more prone to rhythm disturbances. Long-term data are not available.

There are many unresolved questions and issues related to the Fontan operation, ranging from management of infants to that of adults. (1) Should all infants have a two-stage repair: a bidirectional Glenn shunt followed by the complete Fontan operation? (2) Is an external conduit preferable to a lateral tunnel procedure to connect the IVC to the pulmonary artery? (3) Should every patient be fenestrated at the time of a Fontan operation and later have device closure, or should this technique be utilized only for high-risk patients? (4) If there is an intracardiac obstruction from a VSD (in tricuspid atresia) or BVF, should the communication be made larger directly within the ventricle, or should a bypass procedure be utilized (Damus-Kaye-Stansel operation)? (5) Which patients with an atrial–pulmonary artery connection and low cardiac output/frequent rhythm abnormalities should be converted to a lateral tunnel or extracardiac Fontan repair? (6) How can PLE be prevented or treated more effectively? (7) Does a single LV Fontan have a better prognosis than a single RV Fontan? As data accumulate in the adult population, many of these questions will be answered, but at present, many decisions regarding single ventricle and the Fontan operation must be made on an empirical basis.

Algorithm 12–1
Single Ventricle
(Unoperated or Systemic-Pulmonary Arterial Shunt Only)

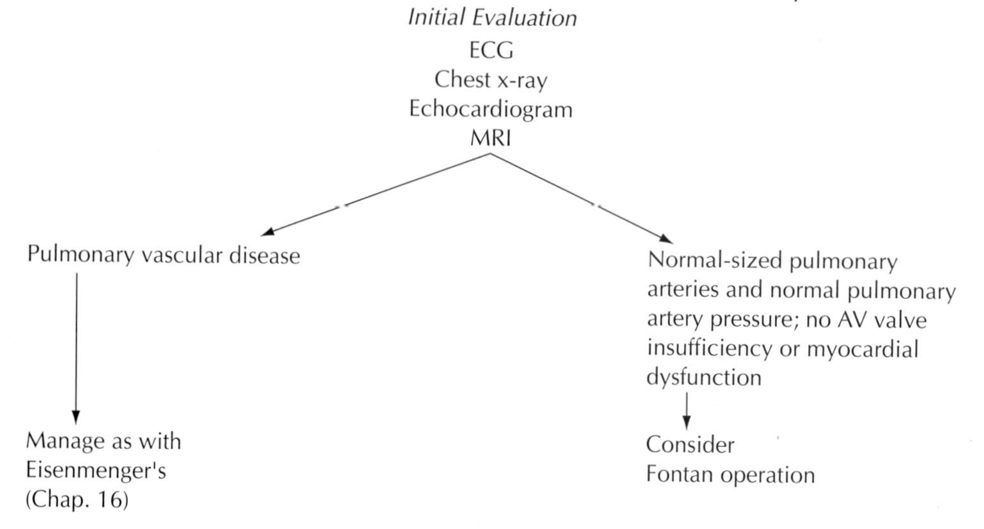

KEY: AV, atrioventricular; ECG, electrocardiogram; MRI, magnetic resonance imaging.

Algorithm 12–2
Single Ventricle (Post Fontan Operation)

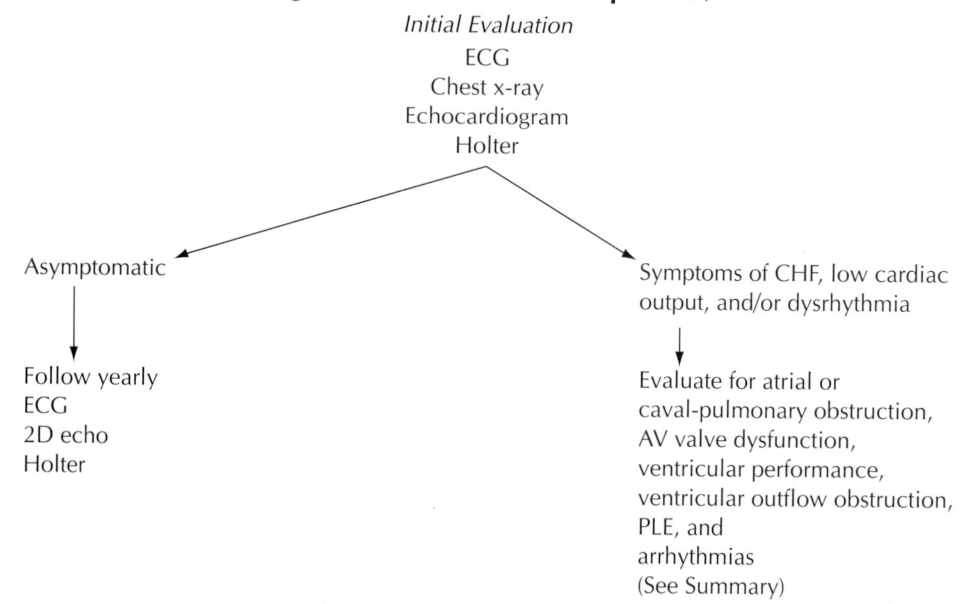

KEY: CHF, congestive heart failure; ECG, electrocardiogram; PLE, protein-losing enteropathy.

An unoperated patient with a single ventricle will be a candidate for a Fontan procedure at any age if: (1) the pulmonary artery anatomy is normal or can be repaired by surgical angioplasty, (2) pulmonary artery pressure and vascular resistance are normal, (3) AV valve function is normal, (4) there is no ventricular outflow obstruction across a BVF or restrictive VSD, (5) ventricular function is preserved, and (6) atrial arrhythmias are controlled. Intracardiac repair of AV valve abnormalities or VSD/BVF obstruction sometimes can be carried out during Fontan surgery if other criteria are met. The Fontan operation is a palliative procedure, but the prognosis is better than it is for patients who in the pre-Fontan era had systemic arterial–pulmonary artery shunts only and were subject to long-term volume load on the single ventricle.

A patient who becomes symptomatic late after a Fontan operation must be evaluated for a number of potential late complications, including subtle obstruction of the right atrium or vena cava to pulmonary artery connection, AV valve and/or ventricular dysfunction, ventricular outflow obstruction, PLE, cardiac arrhythmias, and superimposed acquired heart disease. In most cases, these problems can be approached medically and/or surgically, with improvement to be expected, but among patients who continue to deteriorate despite vigorous management modalities, cardiac transplantation has been a successful final alternative.

BIBLIOGRAPHY

Bjork VO, Olin CL, Bjarke BB, Thoren CA: Right atrial-right ventricular anastomosis for correction of tricuspid atresia. *J Thorac Cardiovasc Surg* 77:452, 1979.

Brestcker M, Myers J, Cyran SE: Conversion of modified Fontan-Kreutzer connection to total cavopulmonary connection: Results in improved exercise tolerance and quality of life. *Circulation* 92(Suppl I):I-55, 1995.

Bridges ND, Lock JE, Castaneda AR: Baffle fenestration with subsequent transcatheter closure. *Circulation* 82:1681, 1990.

Conte S, Gewillig M, Eyskens B, et al: Management of late complications after classic Fontan procedure by conversion to total cavopulmonary connection. *Cardiovasc Surg* 7(6):651, 1999.

Deal BJ, Mavroudis C, Backer CL, et al: Impact of arrhythmia circuit cryoablation during Fontan conversion for refractory atrial tachycardia. *Am J Cardiol* 83(4):563, 1999.

De Leval MR, Liner P, Gewilling M, Bull C: Total cavopulmonary connection: A logical alternative to atriopulmonary connection for complex Fontan operations: Experimental studies and early clinical experience. *J Thorac Cardiovasc Surg* 96:682, 1988.

Driscoll DJ, Offord KP, Feldt RH, et al: Five to fifteen year follow-up after Fontan operation. *Circulation* 85:469, 1992.

Feldt RH, Driscoll DJ, Offord KP, et al: Protein-losing enteropathy after the Fontan operation. *J Thorac Cardiovasc Surg* 112(3):672, 1996.

Fernandez G, Costa F, Fontan F, et al: Prevalence of reoperation for pathway obstruction after Fontan operation. *Ann Thorac Surg* 48:654, 1989.

Fontan F, Kirklin JW, Fernandez G, et al: Outcome after a "perfect" Fontan operation. *Circulation* 81:1520, 1990.

Gates RN, Laks H, Drinkwater DC Jr, et al: The Fontan procedure in adults. *Ann Thorac Surg* 63(4):1085, 1997.

Gewillig MH, Lundstrom UR, Bull C, et al: Exercise responses in patients with congenital heart disease after Fontan repair: Patterns and determinants of performance. *J Am Coll Cardiol* 15: 1424, 1990.

Girod DA, Fontan F, Deville C, et al: Long-term results after the Fontan operation for tricuspid atresia. *Circulation* 75(3):605, 1987.

Glenn WWL: Circulatory bypass of the right heart: II. Shunt between superior vena cava and distal right pulmonary artery: Report of a clinical application. *N Engl J Med* 259:117, 1958.

Grant G, Mansell A, Garfano R, et al: Cardiorespiratory response to exercise after the Fontan procedure for tricuspid atresia. *Pediatr Res* 24:1, 1988.

Gross G, Jonas R, Castaneda AR, et al: Maturational and hemodynamic factors predictive of increased cyanosis after bidirectional cavopulmonary anastomosis. *Am J Cardiol* 74:705, 1994.

Gundry SR, Razzouk AJ, del Rio MS, et al: The optimal Fontan connection: A growing extracardiac lateral tunnel with pedicled pericardium. *J Thorac Cardiovsc Surg* 114:552, 1997.

Kao JM, Alejos JC, Grant PW, et al: Conversion of atriopulmonary to cavopulmonary anastomosis in management of later arrhythmias and atrial thrombosis. *Ann Thorac Surg* 58:1510, 1994.

Koff GH, Laks H, Stansel H, et al: Thirty year follow-up of superior vena cava pulmonary artery (Glenn) shunt. *J Thorac Cardiovasc Surg* 100:662, 1990.

Knott-Craig CJ, Danielson GK, Schaff HV, et al: The modified Fontan operation: An analysis of risk factors for early postoperative death or takedown in 702 consecutive patients from one institution. *J Thorac Cardiovasc Surg* 109:1237, 1995.

Kreutzer J, Keane JF, Lock JE, et al: Conversion of modified Fontan procedure to lateral atrial tunnel cavopulmonary anastomosis. *J Thorac Cardiovasc Surg* 111(6):1169, 1996.

Kreutzer J, Lock JE, Jonas RA, Keane JF: Transcatheter fenestration dilation and/or creation in postoperative Fontan patients. *Am J Cardiol* 79:228, 1997.

Kreutzer C, Schlichter AJ, Kreutzer GO: Cavoatriopulmonary anastomosis via a nonprosthetic medial tunnel. *J Card Surg* 12:37, 1997.

Mair DD, Hagler DJ, Julsrud PR, et al: Early and late results of the modified Fontan procedure for double-inlet left ventricle: The Mayo Clinic experience. *J Am Coll Cardiol* 18:1727, 1991.

Mair DD, Puga FJ, Danielson GK: Late functional status of survivors of the Fontan procedure performed during the 1970s. *Circulation* 86(Suppl 5):II–106, 1992.

Marcelletti C, Corno A, Giannico S, Marino B: Inferior vena cava pulmonary artery extracardiac conduit: A new form of right heart bypass. *J Thorac Cardiovasc Surg* 100:228, 1990.

Marcelletti CF, Hanley FL, Mavroudis C, et al: Revision of previous Fontan connections to total extracardiac cavopulmonary anastomosis: A multicenter experience. *J Thorac Cardiovasc Surg* 119(2):340, 2000.

Mertens L, Hagler DJ, Sauer U, et al: Protein-losing enteropathy after the Fontan operation: An international multicenter study: PLE study group. *J Thorac Cardiovasc Surg* 115(5):1063, 1998.

Milo S, Ho SY, Macartney FJ, et al: Straddling and overriding atrioventricular valves, morphology and classification. *Am J Cardiol* 44:1122, 1979.

Moodie DS, Ritter DG, Tajik AJ, et al: Long-term follow-up in the non-operated univentricular heart. *Am J Cardiol* 53:1124, 1984.

Peters NS, Somerville J: Arrhythmias after the Fontan procedure. *Br Heart J* 68:199, 1992.

Rhodes J, Garofano RP, Bowman FO Jr, et al: Effect of right ventricular anatomy on the cardiopulmonary response to exercise: Implications for the Fontan procedure. *Circulation* 81(6):1811, 1990.

Rosenthal D, Friedman A, Kleinman CH, et al: Thromboembolic complications after Fontan operations. *Circulation* 92(Suppl II):II-287, 1995.

Shiraishih Silverman NH: Echocardiographic spectrum of double inlet ventricle: Evaluation of the intraventricular communication *J Am Coll Cardiol* 15:1401, 1990.

Sluysmans T, Sanders S, Van der Velde M, et al: Natural history and patterns of recovery of contarctile function in single left ventricle after Fontan operation. *Circulation* 86:1753, 1992.

Thompson LD, Petrossian E, McElhinney DB, et al: Is it necessary to routinely fenestrate an extracardiac Fontan? *J Am Coll Cardiol* 34(2):539, 1999.

Van Pragh R, Ongley P, Swan H: Anatomic types of single or common ventricle in man: Morphologic and geometric aspects of 60 necropsied cases. *Am J Cardiol* 13:367, 1964.

Van Son JA, Mohr FW, Hambsch J, et al: Conversion of atriopulmonary or lateral atrial tunnel cavopulmonary anastomosis to extracardiac conduit Fontan modification. *Eur J Cardiothorac Surg* 15(2):150, 1999.

Vargas FJ, Mayer JE Jr, Jonas RA, Castaneda AR: Atrioventricular valve repair or replacement in atriopulmonary anastomosis: Surgical considerations. *Ann Thorac Surg* 43:403, 1987.

Vitullo DA, DeLeon SY, Berry TE, et al: Clinical improvement after revision in Fontan patients. *Ann Thorac Surg* 61:1797, 1996.

CHAPTER 13

TRUNCUS ARTERIOSUS

Truncus arteriosus is a relatively rare congenital cardiac abnormality that results from failure of the development of the conus arteriosus. This structure divides the primitive truncal valve into two semilunar valves, pulmonary and aortic, and merges with the developing ventricular septum inferiorly. During normal cardiac development, the great arteries are delineated superiorly by the spiral septum in which the proximal pulmonary arteries rise from the ascending aorta just above the aortic valve. In the absence of a conus arteriosus and spiral septum, there is a nonrestricted outflow ventricular septal defect, and blood from both ventricles is ejected across a single truncal valve into the truncus arteriosus. The valve often has four cusps. The pulmonary arteries emerge from the ascending aorta as a common trunk (type 1) (Fig. 13-1*A* and *B*) or, less often, arise separately from the lateral portion of the ascending truncus (type 2). When there appear to be no pulmonary arteries from a large aorta, pulmonary blood flow is provided by collateral vessels. In the past, this condition was also considered to be a form of truncus arteriosus, then referred to as type IV under a different system of nomenclature. However, a tiny, perhaps microscopic, right ventricular outflow tract is present; therefore, this anatomy is no longer classified as truncus arteriosus, but belongs in the category of extreme tetralogy of Fallot with pulmonary atresia. A significant percentage of patients with truncus arteriosus have DiGeorge syndrome and a chromosomal abnormality known as 22q11 deletion (see Chap. 18).

CLINICAL FEATURES

Infancy and Childhood

Truncus arteriosus results in complete mixing of systemic and pulmonary venous blood in the ascending aorta and almost always unrestricted pulmonary blood flow. At birth, pulmonary blood flow is limited by elevated pulmonary resistance. However, as pulmonary vascular resistance falls in the first days or weeks of life, a large left-to-right shunt develops and congestive heart failure ensues. The increase in pulmonary blood flow creates a large volume load on the left ventricle. Some degree of truncal valve insufficiency is not unusual, and may be severe, thus contributing to ventricular preload. Affected infants characteristically present with the findings of severe cardiac decompensation; bounding pulses are common because of diastolic runoff into the pulmonary arteries or truncal valve

FIGURE 13-1*A*

Anterior–posterior projection. An aortogram in an AP projection showing a patient with type 1 truncus arteriosus. The pulmonary artery emerges from the ascending aorta. Ao, aorta; PA, pulmonary artery.

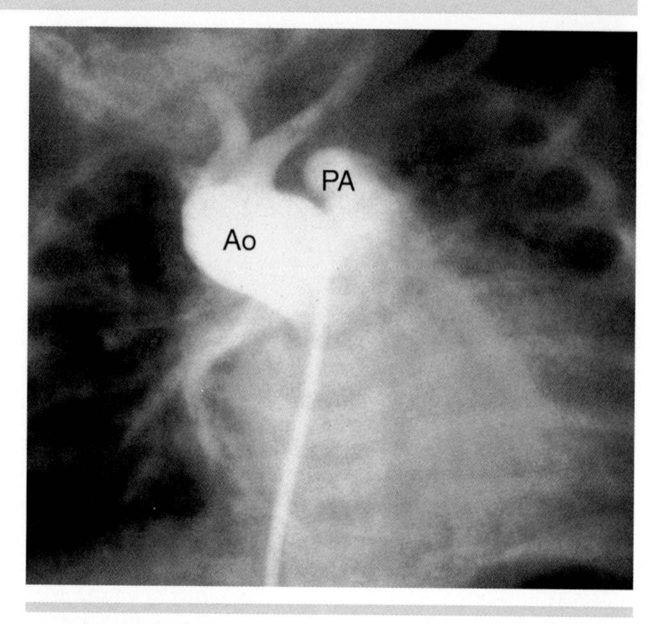

FIGURE 13-1*B*

Aortogram in a patient with type I truncus arteriosus (lateral view). The pulmonary artery emerges posteriorly from the aorta as a single branch and bifurcates to the left and right pulmonary arteries. Ao, aorta; MPA, main pulmonary artery; RPA, right pulmonary artery; LPA, left pulmonary artery.

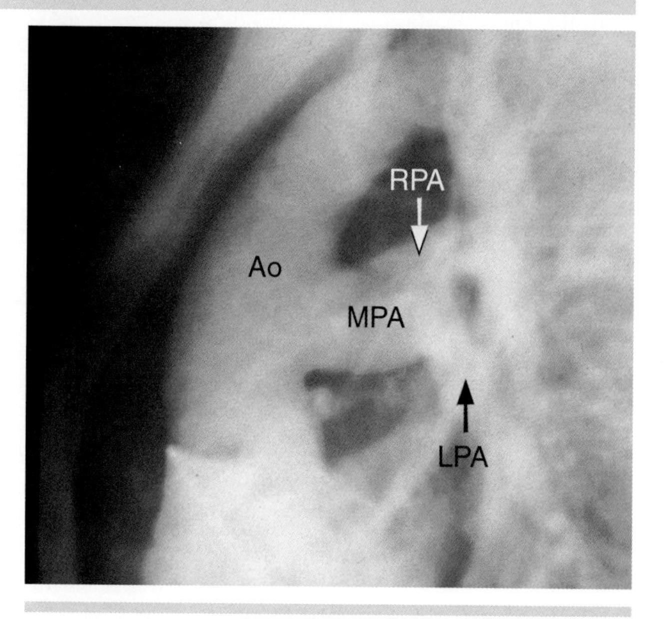

incompetence, or both. There is little or no cyanosis because of the high pulmonary blood flow and complete mixing of the circulation. The vast majority of unoperated patients will not survive, but a few will develop pulmonary vascular disease and live into late childhood or even into adult life. Rarely, an infant will have naturally occurring stenosis of the pulmonary arteries, limiting pulmonary blood flow to the degree that pulmonary pressure is normalized in the presence of adequate pulmonary blood flow. Such patients will survive infancy without symptoms.

Surgical Repair

Cardiac surgery usually is required in the first weeks of life. In the years prior to successful neonatal open-heart surgery, bilateral pulmonary artery banding was performed on some patients to restrict pulmonary blood flow. Although mortality was high, a few patients survived into late childhood or even into adult life. In recent years, primary repair of truncus arteriosus is carried out. The ventricular septal defect is closed by means of a patch incorporating the truncal valve into the left ventricle. The truncal valve thus serves as the aortic valve. An outlet to the right ventricle may be constructed by placement of a homograft or conduit from the right ventricular body to the main pulmonary artery, which has been separated from the ascending aorta (Fig. 13-2). More extensive pulmonary arterioplasty is required if the left and right pulmonary arteries arise separately. The homografts and xenografts eventually must be replaced, and this is most likely to be required on more than one occasion by the time a patient with truncus arteriosus reaches adulthood. Some surgeons avoid the use of a conduit by directly anastomosing the main pulmonary artery segment directly to the right ventricular outlet. This technique results in pulmonary insufficiency, and will also need late surgical modification.

Truncus Arteriosus in the Adult

Most adults who have had early surgery for truncus arteriosus have had a homograft or xenograft repair; it is rare to encounter an unoperated patient. A few patients will be seen with either natural pulmonary artery stenosis or pulmonary vascular obstructive disease. Major late problems include (1) various types of progressive homograft or conduit dysfunction, most often stenosis requiring replacement; (2) truncal valve insufficiency, which may require valve replacement (Fig. 13-3*A* and *B*); (3) residual ventricular septal defect; (4) varying degrees of left and right ventricular dysfunction, which may be secondary to residual abnormalities of the left and right ventricular outflow tracts as well as the cumulative effects of multiple operations on the myocardium; and (5) pulmonary vascular disease.

Patients who reach adulthood after a nonconduit repair with direct anastomosis of the pulmonary artery to the right ventricle may show the effects of long-standing severe pulmonary insufficiency, and may ultimately benefit from insertion of a pulmonary valve. However, virtually all patients with this type of repair are presently in the first decade of life. Associated congenital abnormalities, either unoperated or previously repaired, are unusual but can be seen with truncus arteriosus. Cardiac arrhythmias are not specific for truncus arteriosus, but may be present due to long-standing ventricular dysfunction. Heart block requiring a pacemaker only occasionally occurs.

FIGURE 13-2

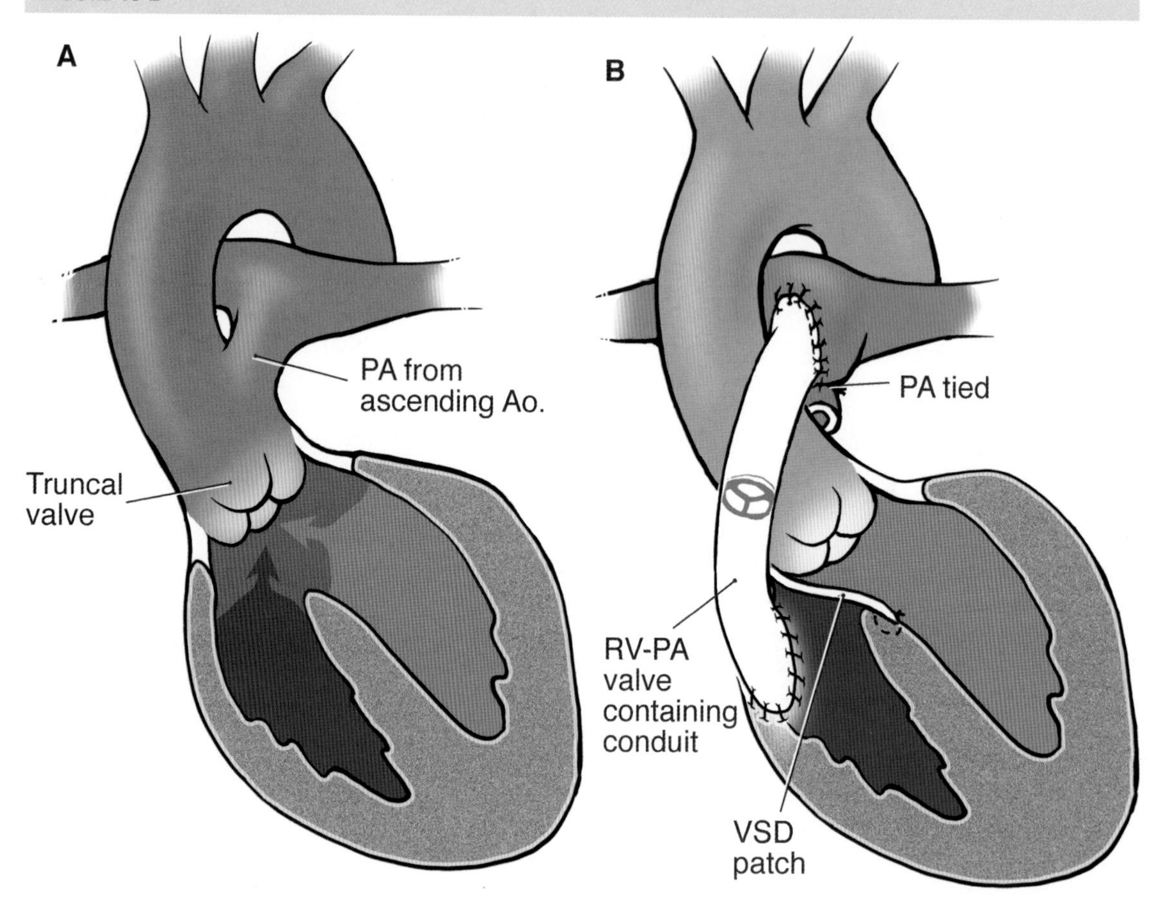

Repair of truncus arteriosus. *A*. In type I truncus arteriosus, the pulmonary artery arises from the single trunk from the posterior portion of the ascending aorta. The truncal valve may have four cusps. Both deoxygenated and oxygenated blood enters the truncus from the ventricles. *B*. Repair of truncus arteriosus includes closure of the ventricular septal defect so that the truncal valve arises entirely from the left ventricle. A homograft or valve containing conduit is placed between the right ventricle and pulmonary artery after it is removed from the ascending aorta.

Physical Examination

Physical examination is similar to that for other patients who have had a homograft xenograft conduit repair; typical systolic and diastolic murmurs are audible along the left mid- and upper sternal border consistent with varying degrees of pulmonary stenosis and insufficiency. A loud pansystolic murmur may indicate the presence of a residual ventricular septal defect. The diastolic murmur typical for aortic insufficiency may be present, indicating truncal valve insufficiency. Truncal valve stenosis does not occur in adults with truncus arteriosus.

FIGURE 13-3*A*

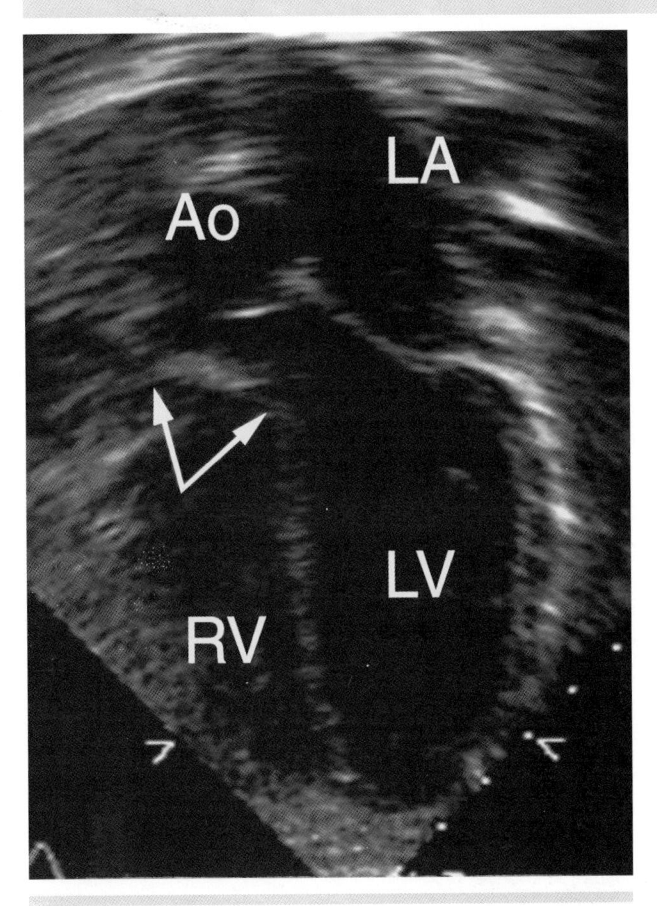

An apical four-chamber view following repair of truncus arteriosus. The aorta overrides the ventricular septum. There is an angled patch which closes a large malalignment ventricular septal defect (VSD). The arrows define the extent of the VSD patch. LV, left ventricle; RV, right ventricle; LA, left atrium; Ao, aorta.

Noninvasive Evaluation and Cardiac Catheterization

The *electrocardiogram* usually shows right bundle branch block or biventricular hypertrophy or both. The *chest x-ray* shows various degrees of cardiac enlargement. *Echocardiography* provides information regarding ventricular function, estimation of right ventricular pressure by tricuspid regurgitation jet or by a gradient within a conduit, and the degree of pulmonary insufficiency. A flow gradient across the homograft is usually noted. The frequency of studies such as Holter monitoring and exercise testing will depend on the status of the individual patient. *Cardiac catheterization* may be required to delineate important hemodynamic and angiographic data. Assessment should include measurements of pulmonary artery pressure and vascular resistance, left and right ventricular function, and the status of the right ventricular–pulmonary artery connections regarding restenosis or insufficiency, or both.

FIGURE 13-3*B*

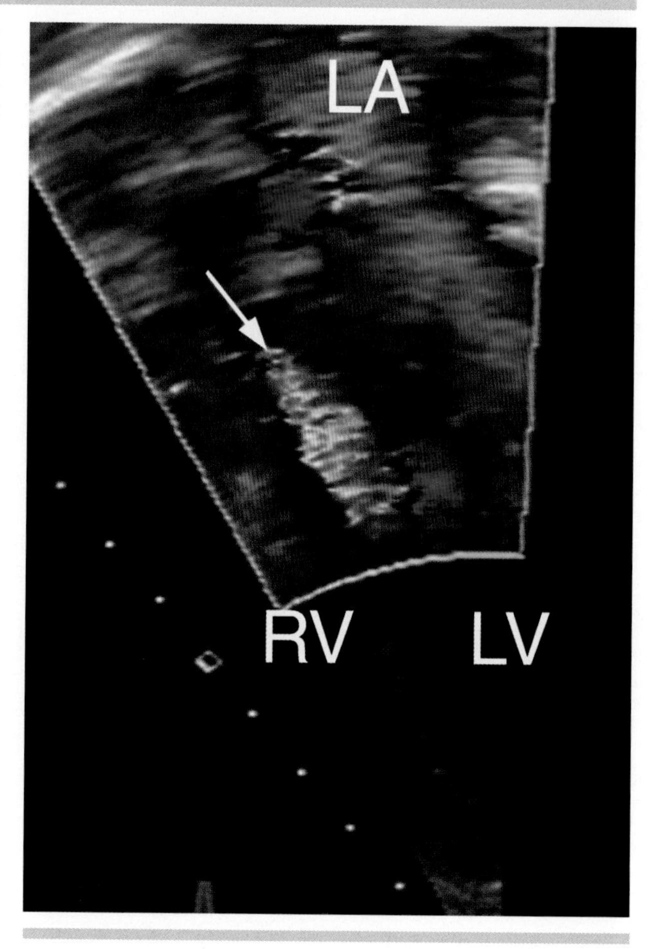

Color Doppler from an apical four-chamber view in the same patient which shows moderate truncal valve insufficiency. The arrow points to the origin of the regurgitant jet. LA, left atrium; LV, left ventricle; RV, right ventricle.

LONG-TERM FOLLOW-UP

Cardiac surgery may be required during adulthood to replace an RV-PA homograft or an insufficient truncal valve with an aortic valve prosthesis, or to insert a pulmonary valve. Conduits typically calcify and often are adherent to the sternum. Reoperation should be performed by surgeons familiar with the difficulties of conduit replacement. Conduit or homograft replacement is generally indicated when the right ventricular pulmonary artery gradient is 65 mm Hg or more, but intervention for a lower gradient may be indicated in the presence of right ventricular dysfunction or low cardiac output, or both. In recent years, a narrowed homograft became acceptable for interventional techniques utilizing ballooning and stents, thereby avoiding or delaying the need for reoperation. Knowledge of the specific issues will allow proper timing of such procedures.

SUMMARY

The adult with truncus arteriosus most often presents to the cardiologist with a homograft or xenograft conduit from the right ventricle to the pulmonary artery. Evaluation of the effectiveness of this connection and the status of right ventricular function are important areas of assessment. Severe stenosis of the conduit or homograft generally requires replacement surgery; however, some of these patients may be successfully treated with a stent. When right ventricular function is significantly affected as a result of long-standing pulmonary insufficiency, insertion of a pulmonary valve may be required to reduce right ventricular preload, especially if tricuspid insufficiency ensues. Truncal valve replacement may be necessary if insufficiency is severe. Residual ventricular septal defect, associated

Algorithm 13–1
Truncus Arteriosus—Unoperated

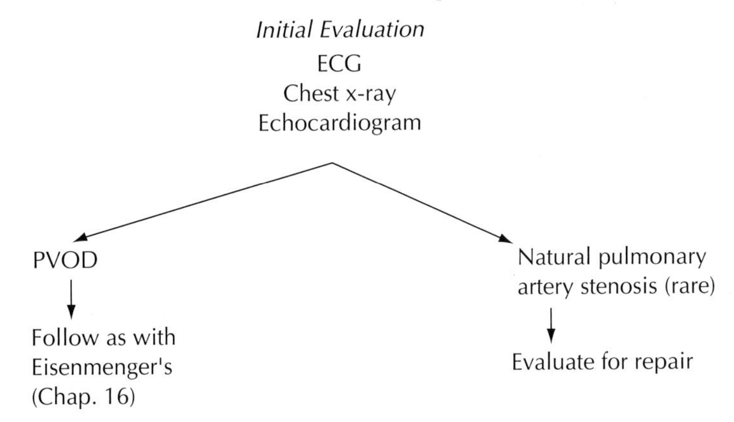

KEY: ECG, electrocardiogram; PVOD, pulmonary vascular obstructive disease.

Algorithm 13–2
Truncus Arteriosus—Operated

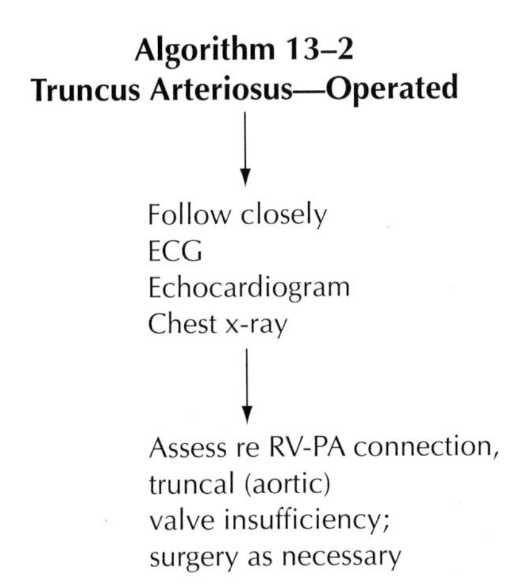

KEY: ECG, electrocardiogram; PA, pulmonary artery; RV, right ventricle.

atrioventricular valve abnormalities, and other congenital cardiac lesions are less likely to be encountered. Patients should be monitored for cardiac arrhythmias.

BIBLIOGRAPHY

Behrendt DM, Dick M: Truncus repair with a valveless conduit in neonates. *J Thorac Cardiovasc Surg* 110:1148, 1995.

Besson WT, Kirby ML, Van Mierop LHS, Teabeaut JR: Effects of the size of lesions of the cardiac neural crest at various embryonic ages on incidence and type of cardiac defects. *Circulation* 73:360, 1986.

Bull C, Macartney FJ, Horvath P, et al: Evaluation of long term results of homograft and heterograft valves in extracardiac conduits. *J Thorac Cardiovasc Surg* 94:12, 1987.

Calder L, Van Praagh R, Van Praagh S, et al: Truncus arteriosus communis: Clinical, angiographic and pathologic findings in 100 patients. *Am Heart J* 92:23, 1976.

DiDonato RM, Ryfe DA, Puga FJ, et al: Fifteen-year experience with surgical repair of truncus arteriosus. *J Thorac Cardiovasc Surg* 89:414, 1984.

Gelband H, Van Meter S, Gersony WM: Truncal valve abnormalities in infants with persistent truncus arteriosus: A clinicopathologic study. *Circulation* 45:397, 1972.

Lacour-Gayet F, Serraf A, Komiya T, et al: Truncus arteriosus repair: Influence of techniques of right ventricular outflow tract reconstruction. *J Thorac Cardiovasc Surg* 111:849, 1996.

Mair DD, Ritter DG, Danielson GK, et al: Truncus arteriosus with unilateral absence of a pulmonary artery. Criteria for operability and surgical results. *Circulation* 55:641, 1977.

Patterson DF, Pexieder T, Schnarr WR, et al: A single major gene defect underlying cardiac conotruncal malformations interferes with myocardial growth during embryonic development: Studies in the CTD line of keeshond dogs. *Am J Hum Genet* 52:388, 1993.

Scambler PJ, Kelly D, Linsay E, et al: Velo-cardio-facial syndrome associated with chromosome 22 deletions encompassing the DiGeorge locus. *Lancet* 339:1138, 1992.

Stark J, Weller P, Leanage R, et al: Late results of surgical treatment of transposition of the great arteries. *Adv Cardiol* 27:254, 1988.

Van Praagh R, Van Praagh S: The anatomy of common aorticopulmonary trunk (truncus arteriosus communis) and its embryologic implications. A study of 57 necropsy cases. *Am J Cardiol* 16:406, 1965.

Wilson DJ, Burn J, Scambler P, Goodship J: DiGeorge syndrome. Part of CATCH 22. *J Med Genet* 30:852, 1993.

CHAPTER 14

TOTAL ANOMALOUS PULMONARY VENOUS CONNECTIONS

Total anomalous pulmonary venous connection (TAPVC) is an uncommon anomaly that accounts for 1.5% to 3% of all congenital heart disease. This lesion is characterized by complete drainage of the pulmonary veins into the systemic venous system or directly into the right atrium. The embryologic defect results from failure of incorporation of the common pulmonary vein into the left atrium. Partial incorporation results in various degrees of obstruction from the common vein to the left atrium without anomalous pulmonary venous connections (cor triatriatum).

In the absence of a pulmonary venous connection to the left atrium, the pulmonary veins return to the right side of the heart via persistent primitive communications. The dominant pathway that remains patent will determine the course of pulmonary venous return. Vena caval and pulmonary venous blood mix in the right atrium before passing through the tricuspid valve into the right ventricle and across the atrial septal defect into the left heart. A patent foramen ovale or atrial septal defect is always present. Associated congenital cardiac abnormalities occur in one-third of patients with TAPVC.

The simplest classification of this disease is to divide the various types by location of the anomalous connection: supracardiac, cardiac, and infradiaphragmatic. The common pulmonary vein may connect with either the innominate vein or the right superior vena cava—superior connection (Figs. 14-1*A* and 14-2); directly enter the coronary sinus—intracardiac (Fig. 14-1*B*); or the portal system—infracardiac. In rare instances, the pulmonary veins drain directly into the right atrium. Mixed connections through more than one of these routes may also occur, but they are rare.

The most important determinant in the natural history of this disease is the presence of pulmonary venous obstruction caused by (1) intrinsic abnormalities in the pulmonary veins, (2) extrinsic compression from adjacent structures, or (3) drainage into a high-

FIGURE 14-1

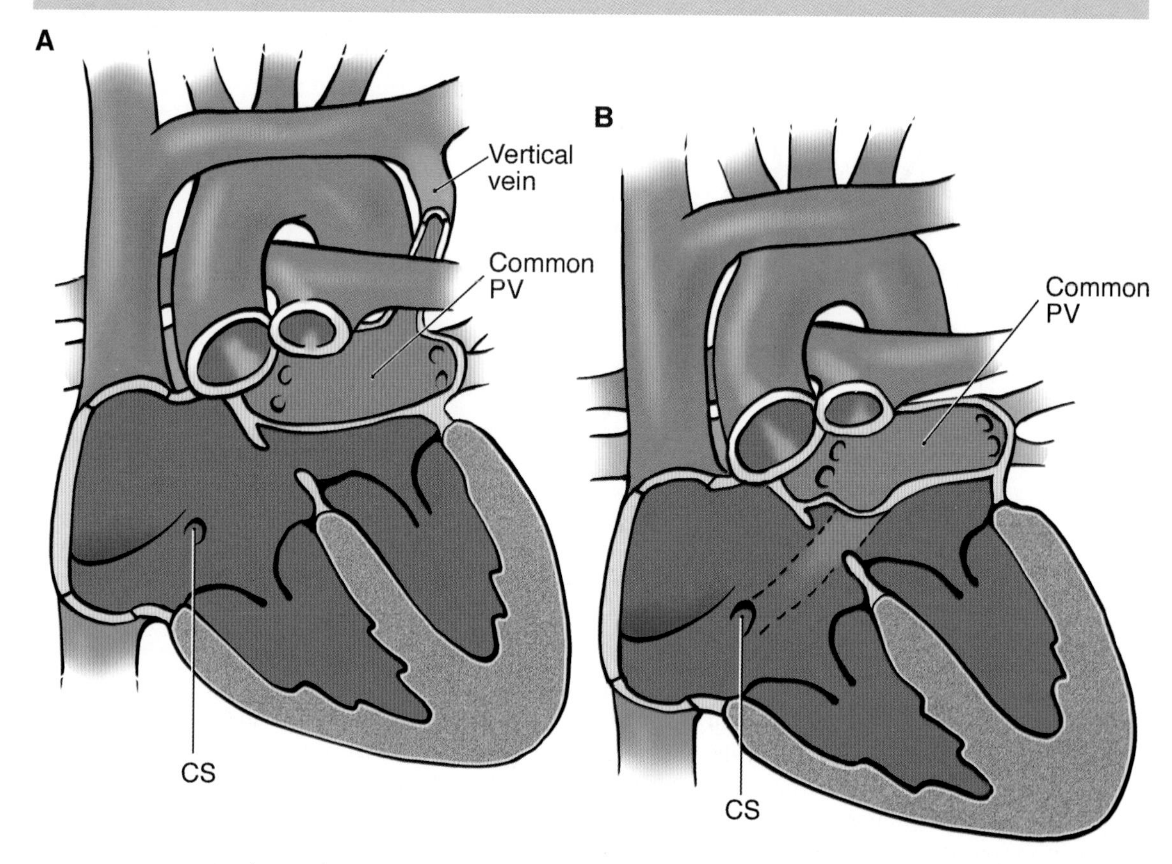

Total anomalous pulmonary venous connections. The superior-type connection is shown in panel *A*. The common pulmonary vein, which has no connection to the left atrium, carries pulmonary venous return superiorly through the vertical vein (persistent left superior vena cava) across the innominate vein into the right atrium. Blood flow to the left heart is via a dilated foramen ovale or atrial septal defect. Total anomalous pulmonary venous drainage to the coronary sinuses (CS) is shown in panel *B*. Oxygenated blood from the common pulmonary vein enters the right atrium directly through the coronary sinus (CS). The inferior type connection is not shown.

resistance channel such as the portal system. The incidence of pulmonary venous obstruction is related to the site of anomalous drainage. For example, pulmonary venous obstruction is uniformly present in the infradiaphragmatic forms, whereas anomalous drainage into the coronary sinus almost never is obstructed.

Extrinsic compression of the anomalous pulmonary vessel (vertical vein) is not uncommon and may occur as it passes through the esophageal hiatus as it ascends between the left pulmonary artery and bronchus to join the left innominate vein, or as it passes between the trachea and the right pulmonary artery to connect to the right superior vena cava. Obstruction at the site of connection of the vertical vein to the innominate vein or right superior vena cava also may be seen.

FIGURE 14-2

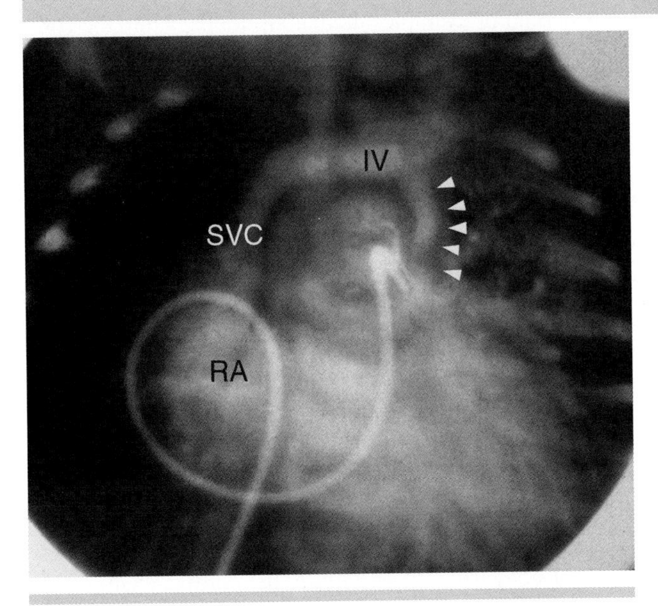

Angiographic study of an infant with total anomalous pulmonary venous connection—superior type. The levophase of a pulmonary angiogram shows no filling of the left atrium; rather, blood flows superiorly through the vertical vein (series of small arrows) to the innominate vein, superior vena cava, and right atrium. IV, innominate vein; RA, right atrium; SVC, superior vena cava.

CLINICAL FEATURES

The clinical manifestations of this disease are most often noted in early infancy and are related to (1) the presence of pulmonary venous obstruction, (2) the size of the atrial septal communication, and (3) pulmonary vascular resistance.

Infants with severe pulmonary venous obstruction have marked pulmonary hypertension and low pulmonary blood flow. The physiology is similar to that of severe mitral stenosis. These infants display cyanosis and marked tachypnea in the first few days of life. A large number of such patients have subdiaphragmatic venous connections. The chest x-ray often shows a small heart with diffuse pulmonary edema, and has classically been mistaken for severe lung disease.

The majority of infants with TAPVC will present somewhat later, although still within the first few months of life, with mild-to-moderate pulmonary venous obstruction, pulmonary vascular resistance that is slightly elevated (although having fallen since birth), and markedly increased pulmonary blood flow. Significant pulmonary hypertension is present. The resultant clinical state is that of congestive heart failure, manifested by striking tachypnea, hepatomegaly, and only mild cyanosis. The chest x-ray shows a large cardiac image with markedly increased pulmonary vascularity.

Finally, there are patients with TAPVC who do not have pulmonary venous obstruction, and also have extremely low pulmonary resistance. Pulmonary blood flow is increased, but pulmonary artery pressure is normal. This results in a clinical state much like that of a patient with a large atrial septal defect. A large left-to-right shunt is tolerated very well in the absence of pulmonary artery hypertension, and very few signs or symptoms are noted in the first years of life. Such patients may present in late childhood, adolescence, or even adulthood.

It is usually possible to predict the clinical manifestations based on the site of the anomalous pulmonary venous connection. For example, anomalous drainage into the coronary sinus is rarely obstructed and, therefore, presents later in infancy with heart failure caused by high pulmonary blood flow and right ventricular volume overload. Most infants with supracardiac pulmonary venous drainage usually have only mild obstruction, and present similarly. In contrast, anomalous drainage of the pulmonary veins below the diaphragm is invariably obstructed, resulting in respiratory distress and pulmonary edema in the neonatal period. TAPVC directly to the right superior vena cava and the mixed-return type communication also are often markedly obstructed.

Significant obstruction of blood flow to the left heart at the site of the atrial communication is rare, because the natural direction of flow is from the right to the left atrium. However, even mild impedance can result in a further increase in pulmonary hypertension and increased symptoms of right heart failure.

Physical Examination

The diagnosis of TAPVC must be considered in any neonate who presents with respiratory distress. A murmur is often not heard in infants with severe obstruction to pulmonary venous return. In infants with signs of congestive heart failure, the cardiac examination usually demonstrates a low-intensity systemic ejection murmur along the left sternal border secondary to increased blood flow across the right ventricular outflow tract. A diastolic flow rumble across the tricuspid valve may be appreciated.

In older children and adults, the physical findings are similar to those of the patient with a large atrial septal defect. As long as the pulmonary vascular resistance has remained normal, pulmonary blood flow is high and the degree of cyanosis is minimal.

Noninvasive Evaluation and Cardiac Catheterization

The *electrocardiogram* may show right atrial enlargement and right ventricular hypertrophy in patients with pulmonary hypertension. The *chest x-ray* in the neonate with pulmonary venous obstruction shows a small heart with diffuse pulmonary edema. In contrast, the older infant, child, or adult with increased pulmonary blood flow has a large heart and pulmonary overcirculation. The site of the anomalous connection may be suspected radiographically. Drainage into the right superior vena cava may show prominence of the right-sided cardiac border. Anomalous drainage to the left innominate vein results in the "snowman" or "figure-of-eight" configuration of the heart. However, the thymic image often obscures these findings during the newborn period.

Echocardiography has greatly simplified the diagnosis and management of these patients and has generally replaced cardiac catheterization for delineation of anatomy. The study should visualize the site of the anomalous pulmonary venous connection in addition to ruling out the presence of associated congenital cardiac lesions.

Cardiac catheterization is not routinely performed in infants with this lesion and is generally reserved for the patient in whom the clinical picture is complicated by coexisting lesions or uncertainty about the degree of pulmonary venous obstruction, pulmonary artery pressure, and/or size of the atrial septal defect.

In older patients, the exact anatomy may be more difficult to visualize with transthoracic echocardiography, and ancillary studies such as transesophageal echocardiography, cardiac magnetic resonance imaging, or cardiac catheterization may be helpful in delineating the anomalous connections. In addition, pulmonary artery pressure should be measured in older patients to determine the pulmonary vascular resistance.

Patients with TAPVC have abnormally high right atrial saturation with similar saturations throughout the right- and left-sided cardiac chambers. A pulmonary angiogram delineates the site of the anomalous pulmonary venous connection, which in unoperated older patients is almost always to the coronary sinus or innominate vein.

MANAGEMENT

Total anomalous pulmonary venous drainage always requires surgical correction. Natural history studies of this lesion have demonstrated an extremely high mortality rate during the first year of life without surgery. The timing of surgery is dependent on the clinical presentation, which is usually related to the presence of pulmonary venous obstruction.

If pulmonary venous obstruction is present, surgery must be performed in the neonatal period because of intractable pulmonary edema and pulmonary hypertension. Delay in surgery usually results in rapid clinical deterioration. Surgical mortality is related to the critical condition of these infants preoperatively as well as the presence of increased pulmonary vascular resistance in the early postoperative period. However, the vast majority of anomalies can be successfully repaired. Patients presenting with congestive heart failure later in infancy also require urgent surgical repair, and the results are good. When the diagnosis of TAPVC is made during childhood or early adulthood, the anatomy is almost invariably favorable for surgical correction. There is no pulmonary venous obstruction or restriction of blood flow at the atrial level.

During surgery, the pulmonary venous return is redirected to the left atrium, and the atrial septal defect is closed. The nature of the repair depends on the site of the anomalous pulmonary venous drainage. When the pulmonary veins drain into the left innominate vein, a side-to-side anastomosis is constructed between the common pulmonary venous chamber and the left atrium. The vertical vein is ligated, and the atrial septal defect is closed. A similar type of anastomosis is performed when the pulmonary veins drain below the diaphragm or into the right superior vena cava. Often the left atrium must be enlarged by moving the atrial septum rightward.

When the pulmonary veins drain into the coronary sinus, the coronary sinus is opened within the left atrium through a right atriotomy. The atrial septal defect and the os of the coronary sinus are both closed, thereby redirecting all of the coronary sinus blood flow into the left atrium. These patients will be mildly desaturated postoperatively from desaturated coronary artery blood flow into the coronary sinus.

Pulmonary venous obstruction is the most common cause of surgical failure in infancy. Anastomotic strictures between the common pulmonary venous chamber and the left atrium are uncommon with good surgical technique, but have been described after repair of the infradiaphragmatic and supracardiac forms, especially when the left atrium is small. Recurrent pulmonary venous obstruction may be difficult to relieve surgically. If surgical correction is not successful, these patients generally will not reach adulthood. Obstruction caused by small pulmonary veins or venules may result in persistent pulmonary hypertension, and, although rare, patients with this anatomy have a poor prognosis. These patients usually have persistent signs of pulmonary venous obstruction despite an apparently successful surgical procedure.

LONG-TERM FOLLOW-UP

The long-term prognosis for this disease depends on the adequacy of the surgical repair. For the vast majority of patients, hemodynamics will be normal if pulmonary venous obstruction has been relieved and there are no residual shunts. Possible residual abnormalities include residual pulmonary venous obstruction at the site of the pulmonary venous left atrial anastomosis, small pulmonary veins, unilateral obstruction presenting with increased pulmonary blood flow to one lung, or pulmonary vascular disease. Also, a residual atrial septal defect may be present or a persistent anomalous vein may have been overlooked at the time of surgery. Late arrhythmias occurring in these patients are most often supraventricular tachycardia and sinus node dysfunction, similar to the sequellae for patients with a history of other types of atrial surgery, such as atrial septal defect or Mustard operation.

COR TRIATRIATUM

Cor triatriatum defines an anomaly that results from partial failure of the common pulmonary vein to incorporate into the left atrium, causing potential obstruction. There are no anomalous pulmonary venous connections. The physiology of this lesion is similar to that of mitral stenosis, and there is a broad spectrum of severity. Critical narrowing of the common pulmonary vein–left atrium (CPV-LA) connection results in critical obstruction during infancy, and, if not relieved, may lead to early demise. Because there may be no defining features on physical examination, less severe stenosis may go unobserved for many years or even decades. Many patients are thought to have chronic lung disease because of persistent pulmonary congestion. In rare instances, nonobstructed cor triatriatum may be seen in an adult.

The diagnosis is made with echocardiography, which identifies the site and degree of obstruction (Fig. 14-3*A* and *B*). Pulse Doppler is used to measure the gradient between the common pulmonary vein and the distal portion of the left atrium. The size of the CPV-LA opening defines the hemodynamics as determined by cardiac catheterization. With severe stenosis there is elevation of pulmonary venous and capillary wedge pressure, and pulmonary artery hypertension will be present, similar to the finding in patients with mitral stenosis.

Surgical repair consists of removal of the wall between the common pulmonary vein and the left atrium. The operative result is usually excellent, and in most cases there will be regression of pulmonary vascular changes and pulmonary pressure will revert to normal levels. As is the case with mitral stenosis, severe long-standing obstruction may not respond promptly.

A supramitral web produces a similar picture to cor triatriatum, but in this anomaly, the obstruction is virtually at the mitral valve annulus rather than in the mid-atrium. Sur-

FIGURE 14-3A

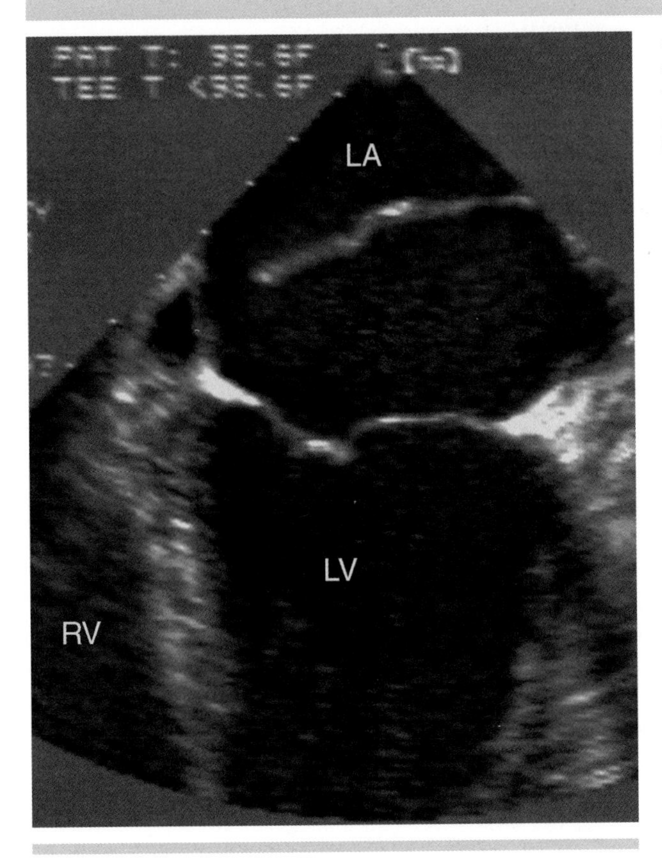

An apical four-chamber view in an adult with a nonobstructive form of cor triatriatum. The membrane divides the left atrium into a posterior chamber, which receives the pulmonary veins, and an anterior chamber, which gives rise to the left atrial appendage.

gical excision may not be possible without injury to the mitral valve apparatus. Thus, mitral valve replacement may be necessary in some cases, a consideration that is not an issue for patients with cor triatriatum.

SUMMARY

Total Anomalous Pulmonary Venous Connections: Unoperated Large Left-to-Right Shunt

The patient is often suspected of having an atrial septal defect, but the echocardiogram or cardiac catheterization study, or both, indicate the presence of total anomalous pulmonary venous drainage to the coronary sinus or via a vertical vein to the innominate vein and superior vena cava. These patients have minimal or no symptoms. Pulmonary artery hypertension is absent, but large left-to-right shunts are noted by imaging techniques and documented by hemodynamic calculations if the patient is catheterized. Open-heart surgical repair is indicated in such patients, just as for those with large septal defects. In the

FIGURE 14-3*B*

Color Doppler imaging in the same patient as Figure 14-3*A* shows mildly turbulent flow around the membrane, indicating minimal obstruction.

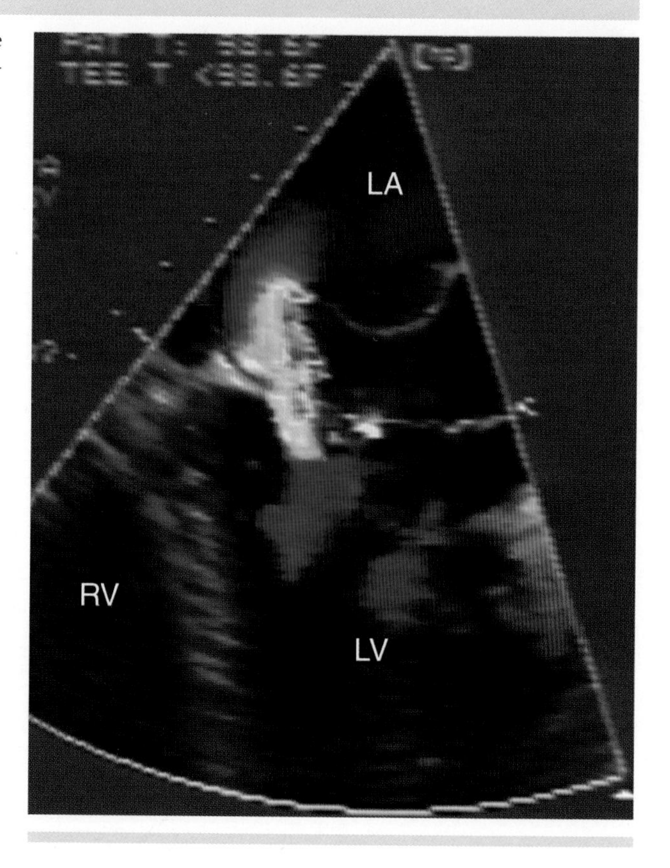

case of drainage to the innominate vein, the common pulmonary vein is incorporated into the left atrium. When connections are noted to the coronary sinus or enter directly into the right atrium, an intra-atrial repair is carried out to direct all pulmonary venous return to the left atrium. The surgical risk is low and the prognosis is excellent.

Patients with pulmonary venous obstruction do not survive childhood without surgical intervention.

Postoperative Total Anomalous Pulmonary Venous Connections

Following surgery in infancy or childhood, most patients are asymptomatic and have a normal hemodynamic result. However, such patients should be followed for the possibility of (1) pulmonary artery hypertension secondary to intrapulmonary arteriolar or venule disease, (2) obstruction at the site of an inadequate anastomosis of the common pulmonary vein into the left atrium at the time of surgery, (3) postoperative cardiac arrhythmias, including supraventricular tachyarrhythmias and sick sinus syndrome, and (4) a persistent pulmonary vein returning to the right heart via the cava or directly into the right atrium. Noninvasive imaging with MRI can be useful in delineating the pulmonary veins in older patients with anatomic questions.

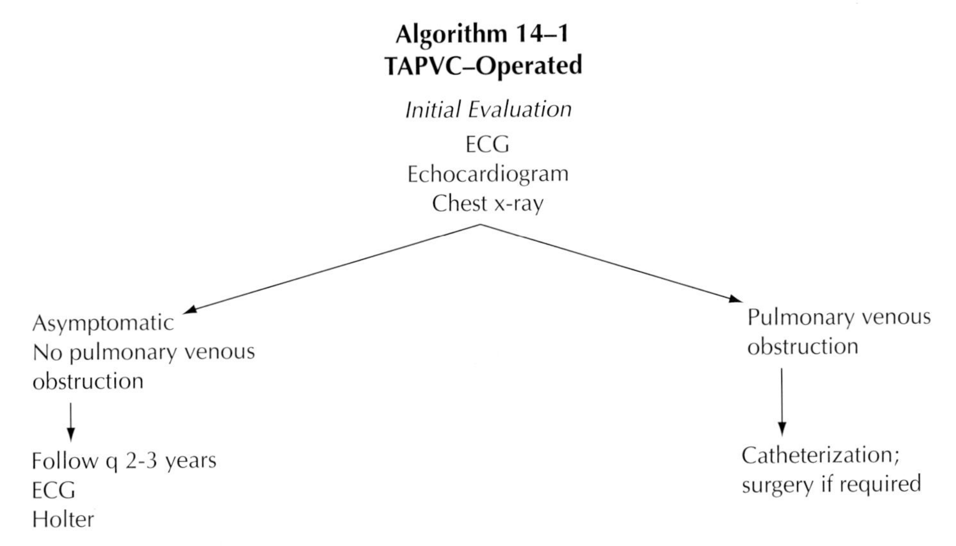

KEY: ECG, electrocardiogram; TAPVC, total anomalous venous connection.

BIBLIOGRAPHY

Ammash NM, Seward JB, Warnes CA, et al: Partial anomalous pulmonary venous connection: Diagnosis by transesophageal echocardiography. *J Am Coll Cardiol* 29:1351, 1997.

Delisle G, Ando M, Calder AL, et al: Total anomalous pulmonary venous connection. Report of 93 autopsied cases with emphasis on diagnostic and surgical considerations. *Am Heart J* 91:99, 1976.

Jonas RA, Smolinsky A, Mayer JE, Castaneda AR: Obstructed pulmonary venous drainage with total anomalous pulmonary venous connection to the coronary sinus. *Am J Cardiol* 59:431, 1987.

Sano S, Brawn WJ, Mee RB: Total anomalous pulmonary venous drainage. *J Thorac Cardiovasc Surg* 97:886, 1989.

Sreeramo N, Walsh K: Diagnosis of total anomalous pulmonary venous drainage by Doppler color flow imaging. *J Am Coll Cardiol* 19:577, 1992.

CHAPTER 15

EBSTEIN'S ANOMALY

Ebstein's anomaly is an uncommon defect that consists of an abnormality of the tricuspid valve in which the septal and posterior leaflets of the valve are downwardly displaced into the right ventricular cavity. In addition, the normally placed anterior leaflet is most often larger than normal and frequently associated with abnormal leaflet attachments. These abnormalities result in partitioning of the right side of the heart into a right atrium, an atrialized portion of the right ventricle, and a right ventricular cavity. A large foramen ovale is present in most of the patients. As a consequence of these abnormalities, right ventricular compliance is abnormal and varying degrees of tricuspid regurgitation and right-to-left intra-atrial shunts are often present.

CLINICAL FEATURES

The clinical manifestations of Ebstein's anomaly are extremely variable and are related to the severity of the tricuspid valve abnormalities, atrial communication, right ventricular function, and the presence of right ventricular outflow obstruction as well as rhythm disturbances. The most severe form of the disease may present in utero with signs of fetal hydrops, followed by severe congestive heart failure and cyanosis in the neonatal period. In contrast, patients with mild forms of this defect may not be discovered until adulthood.

When severe Ebstein's anomaly presents in the neonatal period, the combination of elevated pulmonary vascular resistance with poor right ventricular compliance and severe tricuspid regurgitation limits antegrade flow across the pulmonary valve into the pulmonary artery. As a result, there is massive right-to-left shunting at the atrial level, producing severe cyanosis. Because a widely patent foramen ovale is almost invariably present, right-sided "failure" is most often manifested by increased right-to-left shunting and hypoxemia rather than liver congestion, ascites, and peripheral edema. Patients with less severe tricuspid regurgitation and adequate right ventricular function may display only transient right-to-left shunting in the neonatal period. Symptomatic neonates with Ebstein's anomaly improve as pulmonary vascular resistance falls in the first weeks of life; cyanosis diminishes, and patients will remain stable for various periods of time, some for decades.

Patients who are not diagnosed until late childhood, or beyond, present with a cardiac murmur, cardiomegaly on a chest x-ray, arterial oxygen desaturation, a decline in exercise capacity, or an arrhythmia. Whereas some patients may have progressive tricuspid regurgitation with age, a significant number of patients develop cardiac decompensation with the onset of arrhythmia such as atrial flutter or atrial fibrillation. The arrhythmia may be caused by progressive right atrial enlargement or specifically related to Wolff-Parkinson-White syndrome. Patients with normal sinus rhythm and stable hemodynamics may live for many decades without symptoms.

In one series, 9% of patients with Ebstein's anomaly were diagnosed during the fetal period, 40% as neonates, 10% as infants, 23% as children, and 17% during adolescence and adulthood. Patients younger than 2 years of age generally presented with symptoms related to hemodynamic abnormalities, whereas those older than 10 years of age most often presented with arrhythmias. Arrhythmias appeared in one-third of patients during late follow-up, including junctional tachycardia, atrial flutter or fibrillation, and ventricular tachycardia.

Physical Examination

Most cases of Ebstein's anomaly can be diagnosed by a careful physical examination in conjunction with an electrocardiogram (ECG) and chest x-ray. Before the era of echocardiography, Ebstein's anomaly was suspected by the presence of cyanosis, a widely split second sound, a systolic murmur, a "scratchy" diastolic murmur along the left sternal border, abnormal chest x-ray, and ECG. One or more clicks are usually heard during the cardiac cycle; these are related to the abnormal timing of tricuspid valve opening and closure. The intensity of the cardiac murmur of tricuspid regurgitation does not correlate with the severity of regurgitation. While the degree of tricuspid regurgitation is typically determined by inspection of the jugular venous pulse and by palpation of the liver for pulsatility the extent may be underestimated by a compliant, markedly dilated right atrium.

Noninvasive Evaluation

The *chest x-ray* is abnormal in nearly all cases and usually shows marked right atrial enlargement along the right cardiac border (Fig. 15-1). The right heart is enlarged, but the pulmonary vascularity is normal. The *electrocardiogram* typically shows right atrial enlargement, low-voltage, right bundle branch block, and occasionally first-degree atrioventricular block (Fig. 15-2). In 20% of patients, Wolff-Parkinson-White syndrome is present, manifested by a short PR interval and a delta wave. The majority of the accessory pathways in patients with Ebstein's anomaly are located on the right side of the heart.

Echocardiography provides precise definition of the anatomic abnormalities of Ebstein's anomaly and screens for the presence of associated cardiac defects. The echocardiogram is essential in assessing the degree of septal leaflet displacement, the morphology of the anterior leaflet and its chordal attachments, the severity of tricuspid regurgitation, the extent of right ventricular and right atrial enlargement, and the presence of shunting across the foramen ovale (Fig. 15-3).

A consistent feature of Ebstein's anomaly is the downward displacement of the septal and posterior leaflets of the tricuspid valve resulting in an atrialized portion of the right ventricle. The anterior leaflet is usually enlarged and elongated. The chordal attachments

FIGURE 15-1

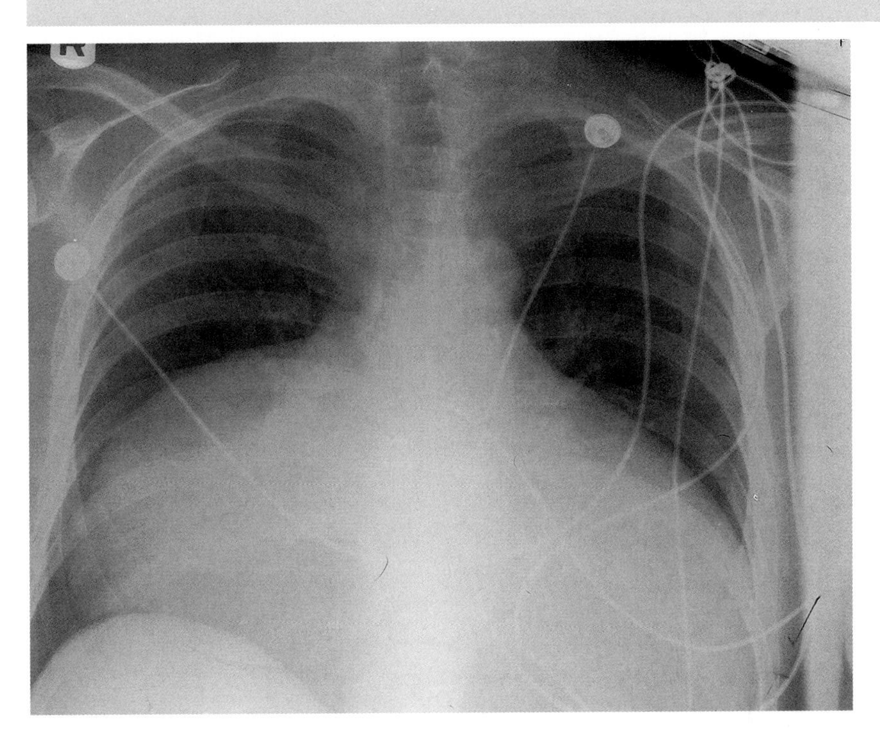

A chest x-ray in an adult with Ebstein's anomaly, showing massive enlargement of the right heart.

may be abnormal, affecting whether valve repair is possible. The tricuspid valve annulus is often dilated. A markedly dilated right atrium is to be expected, and often there is marked tricuspid regurgitation. A variable portion of the right ventricle is atrialized; often there is only a small, dysfunctional right ventricular outflow tract is variable in size. The foramen ovale is widely patent in the majority of patients. In rare instances, the margins of the valve are adherent to the right ventricle and result in tricuspid obstruction. The left ventricle often appears compressed by the right ventricle. Occasional associated anomalies may be encountered, most often right ventricular outflow obstruction. Ventricular septal defects may occur but are uncommon.

Cardiac Catheterization

Echocardiography has made cardiac catheterization less important today in the management of patients with Ebstein's anomaly. In the pre-echocardiography era, Ebstein's anomaly was diagnosed during cardiac catheterization by simultaneously recording a ventricular electrogram and right atrial pressure within the atrialized portion of the right ventricle, as well as by angiography. In arrhythmia-prone patients, the risk of the procedure was high. Although no longer necessary for diagnostic purposes, cardiac catheterization may

FIGURE 15-2

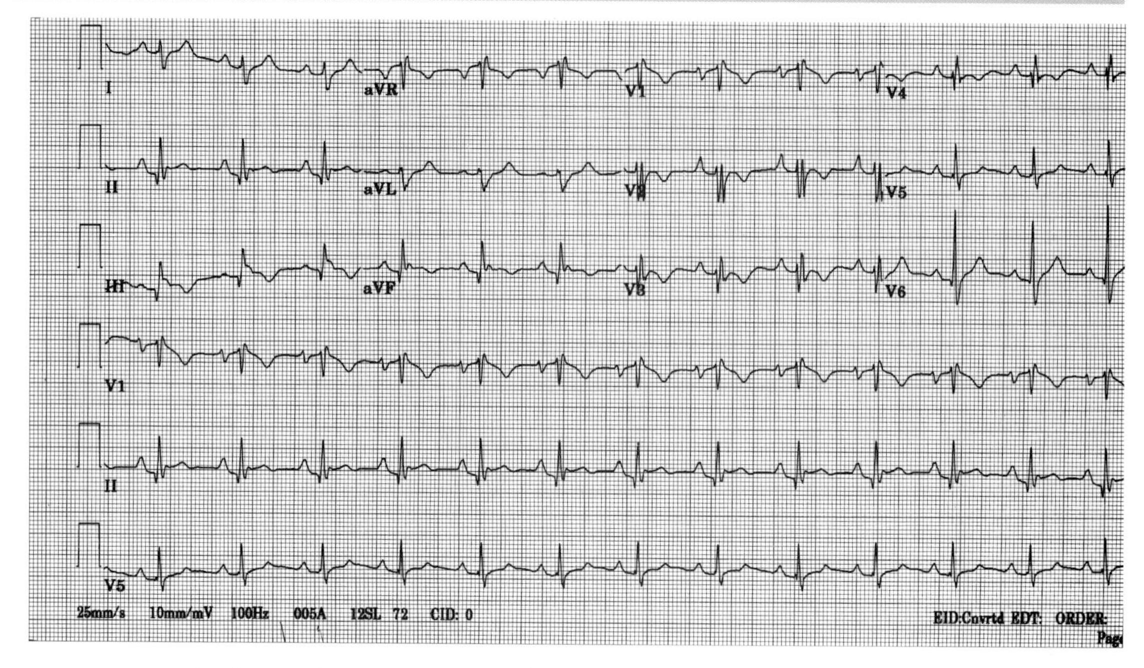

An electrocardiogram in a patient with Ebstein's anomaly shows right atrial enlargement and right bundle branch block.

FIGURE 15-3

An apical four-chamber view in an adult with Ebstein's anomaly. There is severe right atrial and right ventricular dilatation. The proximal attachment of the septal leaflet of the tricuspid valve is displaced downward along the ventricular septum. The atrialized portion of the right ventricle lies between the true tricuspid valve annulus and the tricuspid valve. The left ventricle is compressed by the right ventricle. RA, right atrium; RV, right ventricle; LA, left atrium; LV, left ventricle.

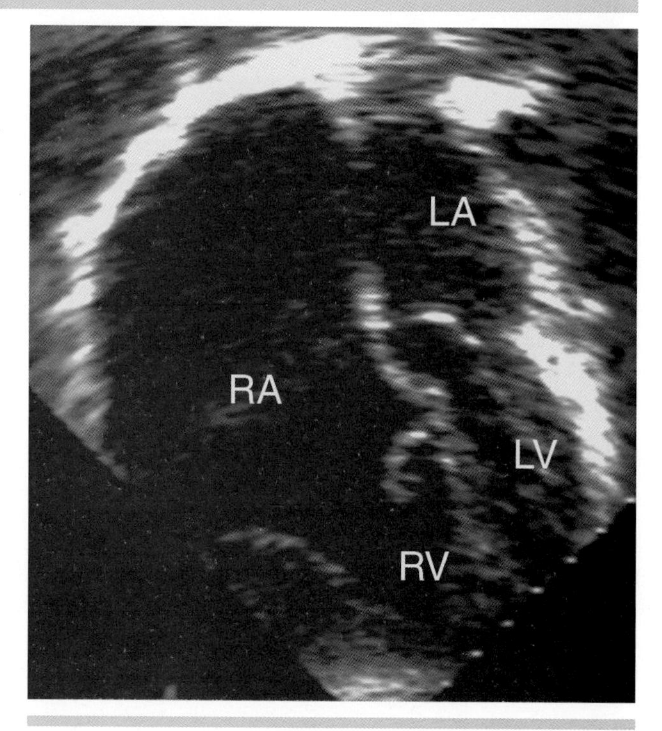

be useful in some patients to assess hemodynamics as well as right ventricular morphology and tricuspid valve function. However, the hemodynamic and saturation data obtained during a resting study may not reflect the clinical findings that occur with activity and exertion. For example, a patient with Ebstein's anomaly may have a small left-to-right shunt across the atrial septum during cardiac catheterization, but develop significant right-to-left shunting even at low levels of exercise.

Cardiac catheterization and angiography is now generally performed for the preoperative assessment of right and left ventricular function and tricuspid valve regurgitation in adult patients. When indicated, these studies may be combined with electrophysiologic studies to demonstrate and evaluate an accessory pathway. Right ventricular anatomy can also be delineated with cardiac MRI.

MANAGEMENT

The management of Ebstein's anomaly depends on the presence and type of symptoms, the age of the patient, and the anatomic abnormalities. Although surgery is indicated for symptomatic patients, there is less certainty about the timing of surgery in asymptomatic patients with apparent similar degrees of anatomic abnormalities. It is important to realize that the echocardiographic abnormalities may be very dramatic even in an asymptomatic patient.

Symptomatic neonates with massive right-to-left shunting from inadequate forward flow through the pulmonary valve have a poor prognosis. Valve repair at this age is rarely feasible, and closure of the atrial communication may result in low cardiac output and massive right heart failure. One treatment option involves closure of the tricuspid valve, excision of the atrial septum, and placement of a systemic to pulmonary artery shunt as a first stage toward the ultimate creation of a Fontan-type repair. Cardiac transplantation may be a consideration in some cases.

Older patients who have symptoms of exercise intolerance or congestive heart failure should be considered candidates for cardiac surgery. Exercise testing with pulse oximetry is often useful to determine functional capacity and degree of arterial desaturation with exercise. Significant desaturation during exercise would indicate inadequate right heart function, usually with tricuspid insufficiency and increasing right-to-left shunting through the foramen ovale as right atrial pressure rises. Surgical repair is indicated in such patients.

Some patients with Ebstein's anomaly are first noted to be symptomatic with the onset of supraventricular tachyarrhythmias, such as recurrent supraventricular tachycardia, or persistent atrial flutter or fibrillation. Pre-excitation may be present. These patients may be candidates for both surgical repair as well as specific treatment of the arrhythmia. In such cases, treatment of supraventricular tachycardia may be approached with either radiofrequency ablation prior to surgery, or with operative ablation of the accessory pathway in conjunction with surgical repair.

Surgical Repair

There are several different surgical approaches in the treatment of Ebstein's anomaly. The type of surgery is related to the clinical presentation and age of the patient. Presentation during the neonatal period is nearly always associated with a critically ill infant having little or no antegrade flow through the pulmonary valve. If spontaneous improvement does not occur as neonatal pulmonary vascular constriction diminishes, palliative surgery (e.g., systemic arterial-pulmonary shunt for associated right ventricular outflow obstruction) may be required, possibly in anticipation of a future Fontan repair.

Tricuspid valve repair and closure of an atrial septal defect in children and adults is often feasible for symptomatic patients. The atrialized portion of the right ventricle is plicated, the foramen ovale or atrial septal defect closed, and either valve repair or tricuspid valve replacement is performed (Fig. 15-4). The techniques for plication of the atrialized portion of the right ventricle vary among centers and include both a longitudinal and a vertical plication. The goal is to create a competent monocusp anterior valve leaflet. Plication of the atrialized portion of the right ventricle results in a marked reduction in the diameter of the tricuspid valve annulus. The anterior leaflet of the tricuspid valve is incised and reanastomosed along the newly established tricuspid valve annulus to produce a monocusp tricuspid valve (Fig. 15-5*A* and *B*). Closure of an atrial septal defect or patent foramen ovale eliminates the potential for right-to-left shunting. Some surgeons use an annuloplasty ring in the repair. Valve replacement is often reserved for nonrepairable valves.

The results of surgery for Ebstein's anomaly are good when performed at an experienced center. Beyond infancy, the operative mortality and morbidity are low in appropriate, selected patients. Successful reconstruction of the tricuspid valve is associated with a decrease in tricuspid regurgitation, relief of cyanosis in patients with a right-to-left shunt, and an improvement in exercise capacity. Postoperative patients may still be at risk for sudden death, presumably due to ventricular tachyarrhythmias.

LONG-TERM FOLLOW-UP

Asymptomatic patients with mild-to-moderate Ebstein's anomaly may live for decades before the onset of complications. Rarely, a patient with unrecognized Ebstein's anomaly may be encountered late in life, and the anomaly has been described as an unexpected autopsy finding in late middle age or even old age. The majority of patients who are diagnosed beyond the neonatal period are symptomatic as adults due to either arrhythmias and/or the development of congestive heart failure. With some restriction in activities and careful attention to management of rhythm disorders, mildly symptomatic patients often remain stable for many years. Thus, the clinical spectrum for Ebstein's anomaly varies from a lethal lesion in a symptomatic newborn to a near-normal life expectancy. It is important to realize that the degree of x-ray and echocardiographic abnormalities does not always correlate well with the clinical course, although in general patients with minimal anatomic abnormalities do better than those with severe structural lesions. The least predictable variable appears to be rhythm disorders, which can be associated with sudden death. Various forms of atrial tachyarrhythmias commonly occur in patients with severely dilated right atria. However, the presence of Wolff-Parkinson-White syndrome clearly predisposes the patient to AV reciprocating tachycardia.

Management approaches for the asymptomatic patient with Ebstein's anomaly differ. Some centers advocate operative repair based on anatomic factors even among asymptomatic patients, whereas others are more conservative, reserving surgery for the sympto-

FIGURE 15-4

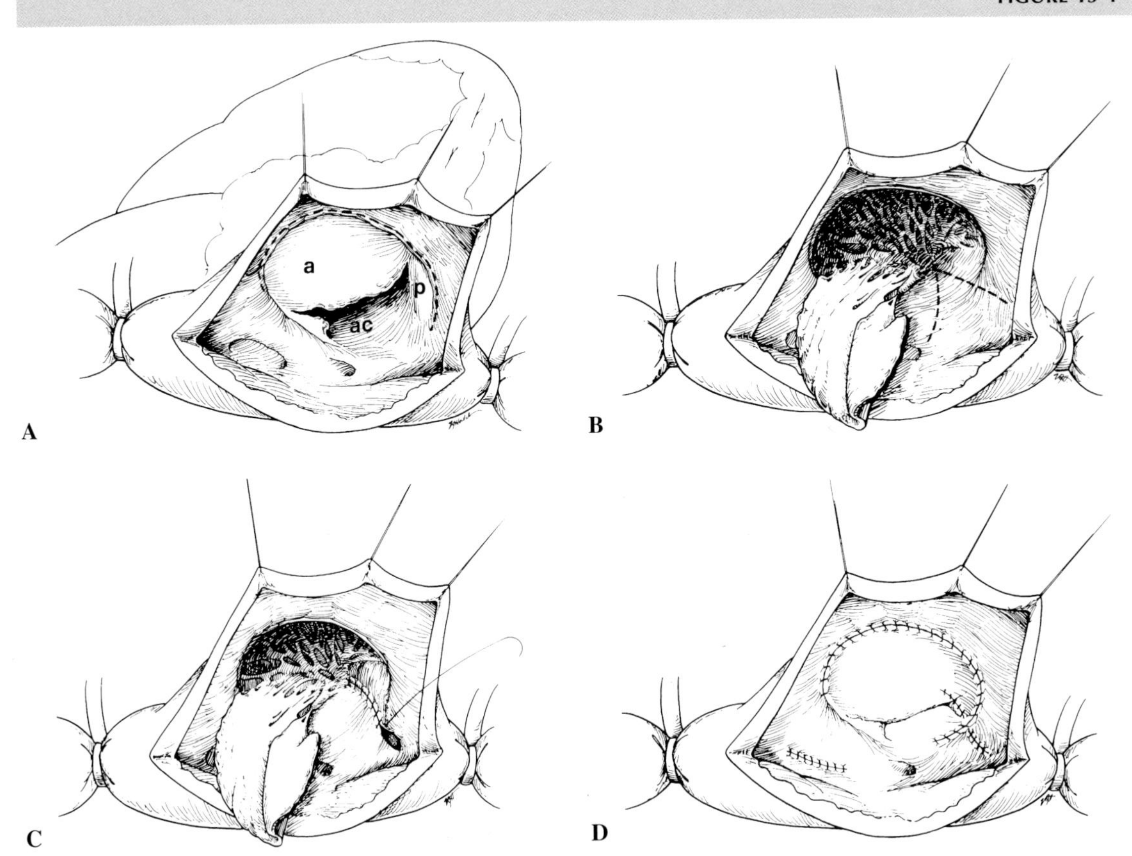

These four drawings outline the steps in surgical reconstruction of the tricuspid valve in Ebstein's anomaly. *A.* Surgeon's view after opening the right atrium (a, anterior leaflet of the tricuspid valve; ac, atrialized ventricular chamber; p, posterior leaflet). *B.* Detachment of the anterior and posterior tricuspid valve leaflets and their muscular attachments to the ventricular wall. The dashed lines denote the suture insertion points to exclude the atrialized portion of the RV. *C.* Longitudinal plication of the atrialized portion of the right ventricle. *D.* Clockwise rotation of the anterior and posterior leaflets on the newly created tricuspid valve annulus; direct closure of the atrial septal defects without atrial reduction. (Reprinted with permission from Surgery for Ebstein's anomaly: the clinical and echocardiographic evaluation of a new technique. Quagebeur JM, Sreeram N, Fraser AG et al. *J Am Coll Cardiol,* 1991, Vol. 17; pp. 722–728.)

matic patient. The latter approach is based on the lack of evidence that surgical repair changes the incidence of rhythm abnormalities or sudden death. However, as surgical techniques improve, the rationale for intervention is becoming less rigid.

After successful repair, the postoperative patient most often becomes asymptomatic; exercise capacity improves, and cyanosis disappears. The vast majority of postoperative patients are in New York Heart Association class I or II. Even patients who have required

FIGURE 15-5A

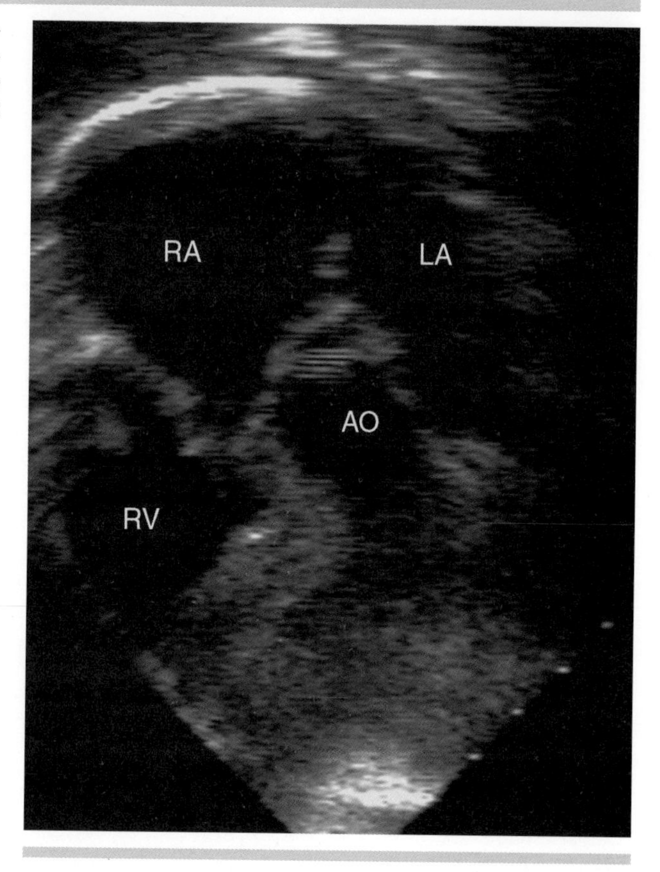

Apical chamber view in a patient with Ebstein's anomaly following tricuspid valve reconstruction as described in Fig. 15-4. The inferior displacement of the tricuspid valve leaflets has been eliminated. RA, right atrium; LA, left atrium; RV, right ventricle; Ao, aorta.

tricuspid valve replacement remain stable for decades, although some will require future replacement for degeneration of a bioprosthetic valve. Women with Ebstein's anomaly have had successful pregnancies, but patients with severe disease are at high risk for both maternal and fetal complications (see Chap. 17). In some cases, surgical repair should be carried out before a woman becomes pregnant, and careful observation in a high-risk obstetric program is indicated.

SUMMARY

Ebstein's anomaly is a congenital heart disorder that is seen with some frequency in adult patients. Patients with the most severe abnormalities may not survive childhood, but in the modern era, there is an increasing population of patients who have undergone repair later in life. Most adults with Ebstein's anomaly have milder abnormalities and have not had a surgical procedure.

FIGURE 15-5*B*

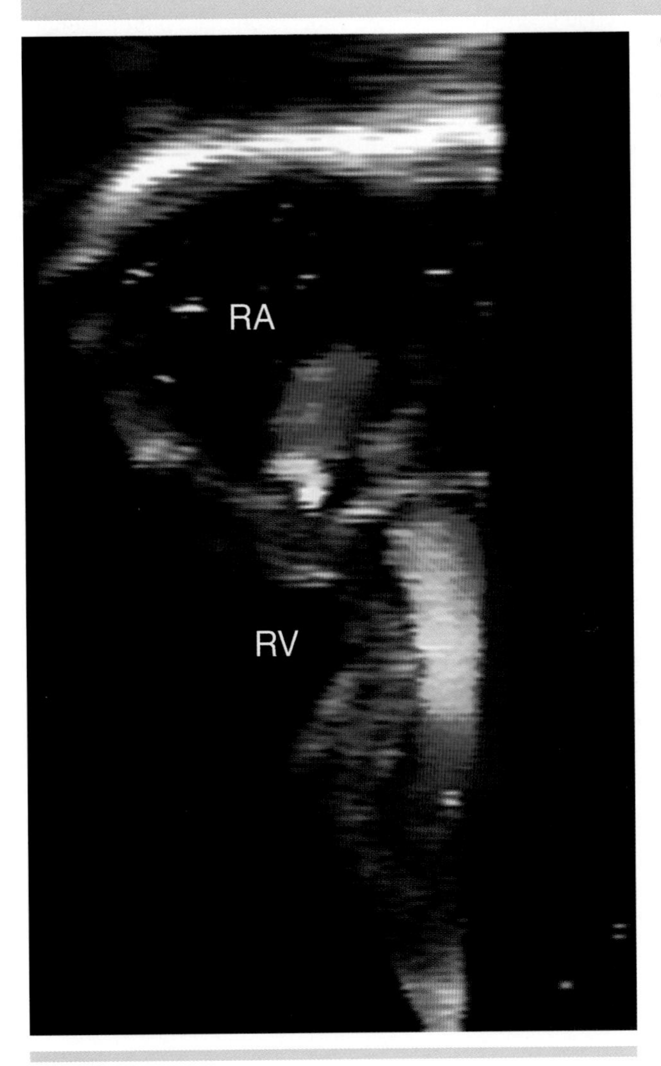

Color Doppler from the same patient as in Fig. 15-5*A* showing good coaptation of the tricuspid valve with only mild tricuspid regurgitation.

Fetal diagnosis of Ebstein anomaly usually identifies a subset of patients who have a poor outcome. After birth, some patients will improve as the normally high pulmonary vascular resistance diminishes over the first weeks of life, and pulmonary blood flow improves. However, severely symptomatic patients will rarely survive early infancy despite attempts at surgical palliation. Older symptomatic children and adults benefit from newer operative techniques that eliminate significant tricuspid insufficiency and close the atrial communication to prevent cyanosis even with exercise. The indications for surgery vary among medical centers, but there is general agreement that symptomatic patients should undergo an operative intervention.

Physical examination of a patient with Ebstein's anomaly usually reveals mild cyanosis. On auscultation, the second heart sound may be widely split, and multiple clicks may be present. A pansystolic murmur may be heard along the left sternal border, indicative of tricuspid regurgitation, and a "scratchy" diastolic murmur is also often audible in the same region. The ECG is almost always abnormal. Almost half of the patients fulfill the criteria for right atrial enlargement, and almost all will exhibit low-voltage right bundle branch block in the right precordial leads. Pre-excitation will be noted in approximately 20% of cases. Echocardiography shows downward displacement of the septal leaflet of the tricuspid valve, right atrial enlargement, and an atrialized portion of the right ventricle. In the modern era, cardiac catheterization has a limited role in the diagnosis of Ebstein's anomaly. However, invasive studies may be indicated for hemodynamic assessment of ventricular function and electrophysiologic evaluation.

Supraventricular arrhythmias are common in Ebstein's anomaly due to the dilated right atrium as well as the presence of Wolff-Parkinson-White syndrome or a concealed bypass tract. Arrhythmia control may be accomplished in the electrophysiology laboratory with radiofrequency ablation, but in some cases surgical ablation may be carried out in conjunction with tricuspid repair and closure of an atrial septal defect.

Operative repair usually includes tricuspid valve reconstruction with plication of the atrialized portion of the right ventricle, whereas some methods utilize tricuspid valvuloplasty, others may require tricuspid valve replacement. Postoperative patients are in an improved functional class. Nonoperated patients with mild disease often remain stable for many decades but most will develop late rhythm disorders almost to the same degree as individuals with more severe anatomic abnormalities. The spectrum of Ebstein's anomaly is perhaps the widest of all congenital heart defects, ranging from nonsurvival in fetal life to a young asymptomatic adult. Patients with Ebstein's anomaly must be followed carefully by cardiologists who must be alert for early symptoms of fatigue, cyanosis, or rhythm disorders.

Algorithm 15–1
Ebstein's Anomaly—Unoperated

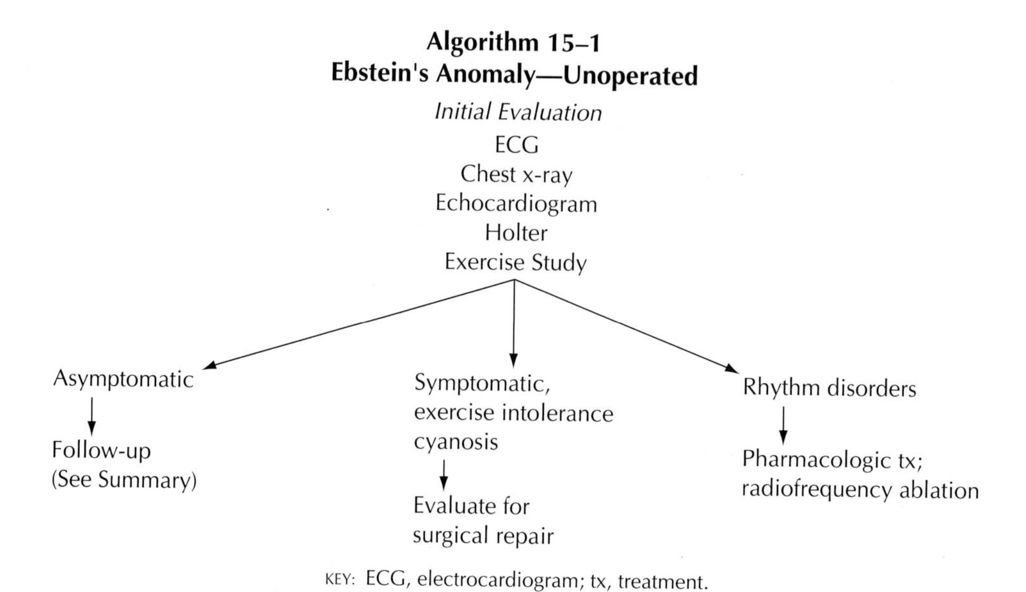

KEY: ECG, electrocardiogram; tx, treatment.

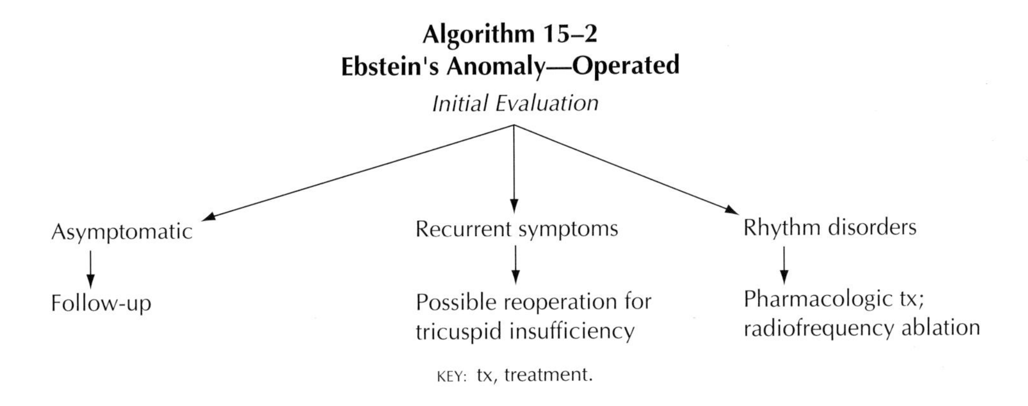

BIBLIOGRAPHY

Anderson KR, Zuberbuhler JR, Anderson RH, et al: Morphologic spectrum of Ebstein's anomaly of the heart: A review. *Mayo Clin Proc* 54:174, 1979.

Augustin N, Schmidt-Habelmann P, Wottke M, et al: Results after surgical repair of Ebstein's anomaly. *Ann Thorac Surg* 63:1650, 1977.

Cappato R, Schluter M, Weiss C, et al: Radiofrequency current catheter ablation of accessory atrioventricular pathways in Ebstein's anomaly. *Circulation* 94:376, 1996.

Carpentier A: A new reconstructive operation for Ebstein's anomaly of the tricuspid valve. *J Thorac Cardiovasc Surg* 96:92, 1988.

Celermajer DS, Bull C, Till JA, et al: Ebstein's anomaly: Presentation and outcome from fetus to adult. *J Am Coll Cardiol* 23:170, 1994.

Connolly HM, Warnes CA: Ebstein's anomaly: outcome of pregnancy. *J Am Coll Cardiol* 23:1194, 1998.

Danielson GK, Driscoll DJ, Mair DD, et al: Operative treatment of Ebstein's anomaly. *J Thorac Cardiovasc Surg* 104:1195, 1992.

Gentles TL, Calder AL, Clarkson PM, Neutze JM: Ebstein's anomaly of the tricuspid valve: A clinical review with long term follow up. *Am J Cardiol* 69:377, 1992.

Giuliani ER, Fuster V, Brandenburg RO, Mair DD: Ebstein's anomaly: The clinical features and natural history of Ebstein's anomaly of the tricuspid valve. *Mayo Clin Proc* 54:163, 1979.

Kiziltan HT, Theodoro DA, Warnes CA, et al: Late results of bioprosthetic tricuspid valve replacement in Ebstein's anomaly. *Ann Thorac Surg* 66:1539, 1998.

MacLellan-Tobert SG, Driscoll DJ, Mottram CD, et al: Exercise tolerance in patients with Ebstein's anomaly. *J Am Coll Cardiol* 29:1615, 1997.

Mair DD: Ebstein's anomaly: Natural history and management. *J Am Coll Cardiol* 19:1047, 1992.

Mair DD, Seward JB, Driscoll DJ, Danielson GK: Surgical repair of Ebstein's anomaly: Selection of patients and early and later operative results. *Circulation* 72(Suppl 2):II-70, 1985.

Olsen TM, Porter CJ: Electrocardiographic and electrophysiologic findings in Ebstein's anomaly, pathophysiology, diagnosis and management. *Prog Pediatr Cardiol* 2:38, 1993.

Quaegebeur JM: Surgery for Ebstein's anomaly: The clinical and echocardiographic evaluation of a new technique. *J Am Coll Cardiol* 17:722, 1991.

Shiina A, Seward JB, Edwards WD, et al: Two-dimensional echocardiographic spectrum of Ebstein's anomaly: Detailed anatomic assessment. *J Am Coll Cardiol* 3:356, 1984.

Smith WM, Gallagher JJ, Kerr CR, et al: The electrophysiologic basis and management of symptomatic recurrent tachycardia in patients with Ebstein's anomaly of the tricuspid valve. *Am J Cardiol* 49:1223, 1982.

Vargas FJ, Mengo G, Granja MA, et al: Tricuspid annuloplasty and ventricular plication for Ebstein's malformation. *Ann Thorac Surg* 65:1755, 1998.

CHAPTER 16

EISENMENGER'S SYNDROME

Eisenmenger's syndrome classically refers to patients with a ventricular septal defect (VSD) and pulmonary vascular obstructive disease. High pulmonary resistance causes right-to-left shunting at the ventricular level, resulting in cyanosis. The eponym evolved from the original description of a high-positioned large VSD that was thought to increase the possibility of late pulmonary vascular obstructive disease due to direct high-pressure volume flow from the left ventricle into the pulmonary artery. The term *Eisenmenger's syndrome* no longer refers to the anatomic position of the VSD, but to the association of pulmonary vascular disease with a VSD in any position. In common usage, the Eisenmenger syndrome also describes pulmonary vascular obstructive disease with other types of left-to-right shunts, such as atrioventricular (AV) canal, patent ductus arteriosus, truncus arteriosus, and single ventricle anomalies. The term is generally not used for patients with isolated atrial septal defect and pulmonary vascular disease.

CLINICAL FEATURES

The evolution to Eisenmenger's syndrome begins with a large, unrestrictive VSD with high pulmonary blood flow and only minimal pulmonary arteriolar vasoconstriction. An infant with this defect has hyperkinetic pulmonary hypertension secondary to the large left-to-right shunt, and presents in congestive heart failure at a few weeks of age. The natural history of untreated surviving patients with this physiology may be the gradual development of pulmonary arteriolar injury secondary to sheer stress, leading to muscular hypertrophy, intimal proliferation, and, eventually, obliteration of arterioles. A surviving infant with an unrepaired VSD who originally presents with a large left-to-right shunt may first evolve to a balanced shunt and improve clinically. However, as vascular disease progresses and the level of pulmonary vascular resistance approaches systemic resistance, a right-to-left shunt develops, and the patient becomes cyanotic and polycythemic. Although the pulmonary vascular injury begins in infancy, clinical manifestations of Eisenmenger's syndrome may not be recognized until the second decade of life or later.

Before the advent of open-heart surgery to repair VSD in infancy, pulmonary artery banding was utilized to protect the pulmonary vascular bed from high pressure until the patient was a candidate for debanding and VSD closure. In the modern era, VSDs are repaired at any age. Infants who have a VSD repaired by the end of the second year of life do not develop pulmonary vascular disease. It should be noted that children with a restrictive VSD in which pulmonary blood flow is increased, but pulmonary pressure is normal, do not develop Eisenmenger's syndrome, and early surgery is not indicated on the basis of this rationale (see Chap. 3). Furthermore, patients with "pretricuspid defects," such as atrial septal defect and partial anomalous pulmonary venous return, almost never develop pulmonary vascular disease, with the exception of a few cases that present in adult life.

There appears to be a subgroup of patients with VSD and pulmonary vascular obstructive disease who did not have a history of early hyperkinetic pulmonary hypertension symptoms or failure to thrive secondary to large left-to-right shunts. Normally, pulmonary vascular resistance is elevated at birth and falls over the first few weeks of life, but these individuals appear to have had unabated constriction of pulmonary vascular arterioles during infancy which evolved to pathologic medial and intimal disease, without the usual phase of high-flow hyperkinetic pulmonary hypertension. There may be a genetic component for this unusual sequence of events. Among this subgroup of patients whose pulmonary resistance never fell after birth, blood flow across the VSD is minimal over the years. Thus, the patient may never have been diagnosed with congenital heart disease, and only when symptoms of fatigue or cyanosis appear, is heart disease suspected. As with pulmonary hypertension with ASD, patients who live at high altitudes are more likely to evolve in this way.

The clinical course of Eisenmenger's syndrome is variable; cyanosis may not be recognized until the second or even third decade of life, and the patient remains stable well into adult life. This is determined by the severity and rate of progression of pulmonary vascular disease. The course of other left-to-right shunts may differ from isolated VSD. Patients with transposition of the great arteries and VSD, AV canal, truncus arteriosus, and various forms of complex single ventricles without pulmonary stenosis often develop vascular disease earlier and progress more rapidly. At the other side of the spectrum, there are rare patients, despite many years of large left-to-right shunts and hyperkinetic pulmonary hypertension, who do not develop irreversible pulmonary vascular changes. Our understanding of the vascular biology of the lungs remains limited.

Clinical Presentation of the Adult

Patients with classic Eisenmenger's syndrome usually have not had a previous operation. A patient may present with irreversible pulmonary hypertension because of inadequate banding of the pulmonary artery, but this is an extremely rare occurrence in recent years. Often, at the time of diagnosis, the pulmonary vascular resistance is already markedly elevated, and VSD closure would be detrimental, merely shifting the patient into the anatomic equivalent of "primary pulmonary hypertension." If a VSD is inappropriately closed, the right ventricle is not decompressed, right heart failure ensues, and cardiac output falls; the patient's prognosis is worse than for Eisenmenger's syndrome. A patient with a VSD, right-to-left shunt, and normal cardiac output, although cyanotic, fares better than when pulmonary vascular obstruction limits cardiac output with no augmentation by right-to-left blood flow.

If pulmonary vascular disease remains relatively stable, and shunting at the ventricular level remains balanced, the patient may have adequate functional capacity. However, as vascular disease progresses, the patient becomes more cyanotic and debilitated. Ultimately, tricuspid regurgitation develops, RV function declines, and signs of systemic congestion contribute to the clinical deterioration. Symptoms include exercise intolerance, syncope, chest pain, and hemoptysis. Sudden death may occur, presumably secondary to an arrhythmia.

Physical Examination

Patients who present to the cardiologist as young adults have variable clinical symptoms. Mild to moderate cyanosis and digital clubbing are usually present, and often the patient does not appear to be debilitated. Cardiac examination reveals a substernal right ventricular heave. The second heart sound is loud and single at the left upper sternal border. A pulmonary artery ejection click may be present. A minimal short- to medium-length systolic ejection murmur is audible along the left mid-sternal border. A high-pitched diastolic murmur representing pulmonary insufficiency (Graham Steell murmur) may be present in severe cases. Because the right ventricle is vented to the left, there may be no evidence on physical examination of either right or left ventricular failure. Signs of systemic venous congestion occur late. The subsequent development of tricuspid regurgitation may portend an acceleration in clinical symptoms. Patients with pulmonary vascular obstructive disease and other types of communications between the two circulations have physical examination findings related to the original lesion (e.g., valvar regurgitation or stenosis) although none will have findings of a large left-to-right shunt.

Noninvasive Evaluation and Cardiac Catheterization

The *chest x-ray* reveals a normal or slightly enlarged cardiac silhouette with a prominent main pulmonary artery segment and large pulmonary vessels at the hilum, decreasing rapidly in size distally (Fig. 16-1). The *electrocardiogram* typically shows severe right ventricular hypertrophy, occasionally associated with right bundle branch block, especially if an early operation had been attempted. Cardiac arrhythmias may be present. Echocardiography reveals a large VSD, most often in a perimembranous position with evidence of *bidirectional* shunting, but predominately right to left. The main pulmonary artery is markedly enlarged. Right ventricular hypertrophy is striking.

Patients with still-predominant left-to-right shunts in the context of early pulmonary vascular obstructive disease may require a *cardiac catheterization* to be certain that the left-to-right shunt is not large enough to warrant surgical closure of the ventricular septal defect. Patients whose P_{AO_2} is normal in room air and whose pulmonary vascular resistance is less than 50% of systemic resistance with a significant left-to-right shunt (1.8 to

FIGURE 16-1

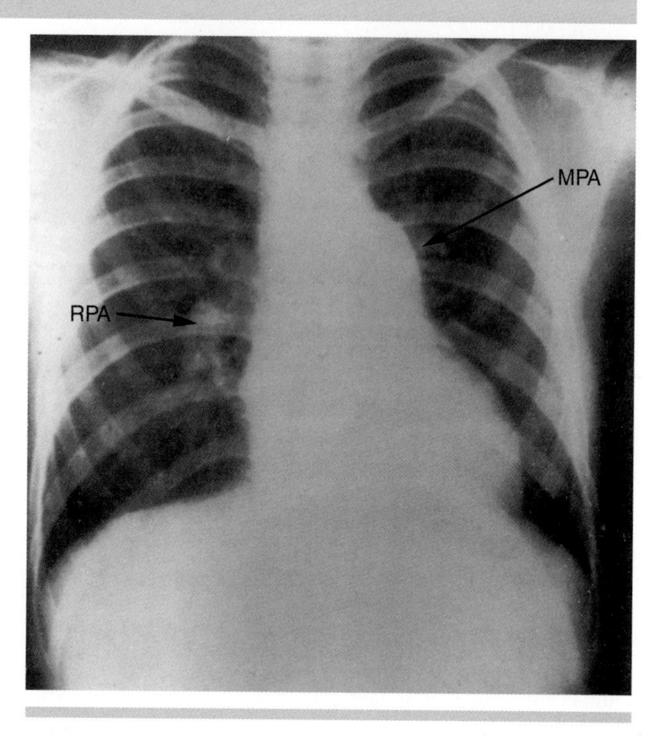

Chest x-ray of a patient with Eisenmenger's syndrome. Note the dilated main pulmonary artery and prominent right pulmonary artery at the hilum. MPA, main pulmonary artery; RPA, right pulmonary artery.

1 or more) almost always benefit from surgical closure. Angiography may be useful to delineate the septal defect and shunting pattern at the ventricular level, but a power injection in either ventricle may distort the findings by overestimating the degree of shunting. The typical "tree in winter" angiographic appearance of the pulmonary branch arteries can be displayed (Fig. 16-2). Angiograms are generally avoided because of increased risk in patients with advanced pulmonary vascular disease.

Natural History

Patients with Eisenmenger's syndrome may live for many decades. In the Natural History Study of VSD, 40% of those who were enrolled with established Eisenmenger's disease at an average age of 20 years were alive 25 years later. The median survival rate in a recent large series from Toronto, which included both VSD and more complex lesions, was 53 years. Most patients die suddenly. Autopsy studies have revealed massive intrapulmonary hemorrhage, rupture of the pulmonary trunk, stroke, as well as in situ thromboses of dilated proximal pulmonary arteries. Patients may also succumb to heart failure and arrhythmias, which is the etiology for most of the remaining deaths.

Bleeding tendencies are increased in patients with polycythemia and include both hemoptysis, which is common, as well as minor bleeding from dental procedures. Aspirin and nonsteroidal anti-inflammatory drugs should be avoided, if possible. Cholecystitis may

FIGURE 16-2

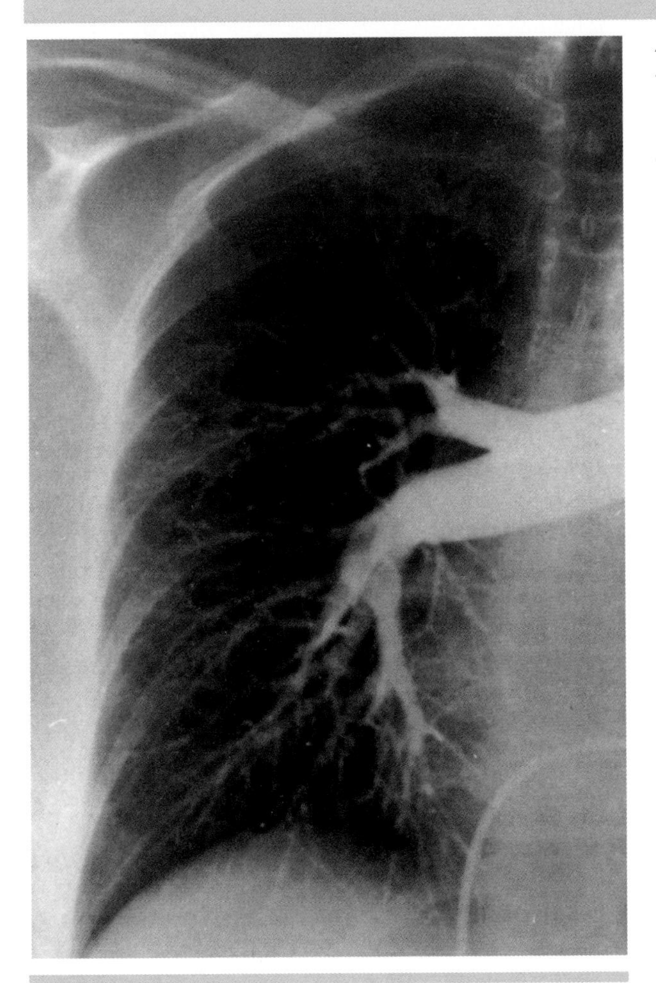

Angiogram showing a large right pulmonary artery in a patient with Eisenmenger's syndrome. Small pulmonary arteries taper markedly as they emerge from larger branches with a paucity of peripheral vessels, giving the impression of a "tree in winter."

be seen in patients with Eisenmenger's syndrome and may require cholecystectomy. The gallstones are typically calcium bilirubinate and formed from the increased breakdown of heme in patients with erythrocytosis. Hyperuricemia is commonly seen in these patients; the incidence of gout is approximately 20%. Hypertrophic osteoarthropathy may occur in approximately one third of patients with cyanotic heart disease and may cause pain and tenderness in the long bones of the arms and legs.

MANAGEMENT

In Eisenmenger's syndrome, pulmonary blood flow depends on the relationship between pulmonary and systemic resistance. When pulmonary resistance is high, systemic resistance must rise even further to allow acceptable pulmonary blood flow despite the large right-to-left shunt at the ventricular level. If systemic vascular resistance falls quickly, severe hypoxemia may occur acutely, leading to death. Thus, most of the lifestyle measures suggested to patients relate to the avoidance of this sequence of events. The patient should be advised to (1) avoid dehydration by exposure to prolonged high ambient temperature without sufficient fluids, (2) avoid high altitudes, and (3) be aware of certain hazards (which may not always be obvious) that could acutely change the relationship between systemic and pulmonary vascular resistance. Among others, these include diving into cold water, sustained external heat, prolonged fever, anesthesia, contrast angiography, drug ingestion, and pregnancy (see Chap. 17). General management measures include aggressive antibiotic therapy for pulmonary infections, flu vaccine, antipyretic treatment for fever, and supplemental oxygen for high-altitude exposure. Noncardiac surgery may be required in patients with Eisenmenger's syndrome, sometimes as a complication of the underlying problem, such as cholecystectomy, urologic and gynecologic procedures, and neurosurgery. Management of such patients requires specific expertise to minimize the risks of these procedures.

Medical management of a stable patient with Eisenmenger's syndrome should consist of periodic follow-up evaluations. It is especially important to monitor the hemoglobin and hematocrit. When a hematocrit exceeds 65 to 70%, phlebotomy with plasma or crystalline exchange may be considered to lower the hematocrit to the 55 to 60% range. This must be done carefully, because simply removing blood can, in adults, decrease systemic vascular resistance and result in a sudden hypoxic event. In recent years, the practice of phlebotomy in an asymptomatic polycythemic patient has been challenged because a clear-cut relationship between elevated hemoglobin and stroke has not been demonstrated. Cerebrovascular events more often may be related to iron-deficiency anemia. However, an exchange procedure appears to provide symptomatic relief for patients with severe polycythemia. Fortunately, many patients with Eisenmenger's syndrome tend to have stable hematocrit in the 60 to 65% range for many years or even decades. Brief periods of iron supplementation may be used carefully in iron-deficient patients; it is important to avoid an abrupt rise in hemoglobin levels.

Some patients with extremely severe Eisenmenger's syndrome have been treated with newer pulmonary vasodilatory agents, but experience with these drugs in this context is limited. Heart-lung transplantation or lung transplantation with repair of VSD or other intracardiac communications has been offered to some patients with advanced Eisenmenger's syndrome. These are high-risk procedures, and careful patient selection should be exercised. Heart transplantation alone is not beneficial to patients with severe pulmonary vascular obstructive disease (PVOD). Chronic pulmonary vasodilator therapy has been used as a bridge to transplantation, and in some younger patients, stability has been sufficient to delay transplantation.

SUMMARY

Eisenmenger's syndrome generally refers to patients with large VSDs and pulmonary vascular obstructive disease of sufficient severity to initially reduce left-to-right shunting, and eventually cause right-to-left shunts and polycythemia. Pulmonary vascular obstructive disease is also associated with other forms of intracardiac or great vessel communications between the left and right heart circulations. Most patients with Eisenmenger's syndrome had significant left-to-right shunts during infancy, and in the absence of surgical correction, hyperkinetic pulmonary hypertension results in sheer stress damage to the pulmonary vascular bed, causing irreversible medial and intimal vascular changes in pulmonary arterioles. Thus, although patients are often first recognized to have Eisenmenger's syndrome as late as the second or third decade of life, the problem begins in early childhood. In a patient with a large nonrestrictive VSD, the defect must be repaired before the end of the second year of life to prevent pulmonary vascular disease. Patients with other forms of heart disease, such as transposition of the great vessels and VSD, AV canal, and truncus arteriosus may require even earlier surgical repair to eliminate the risk of Eisenmenger's syndrome later in life. A few patients, some of whom live at high altitude, do not have a history of heart failure in infancy, which is the clinical course expected with a large left-to-right shunt. Symptoms related to PVOD in such patients may appear later; often after the opportunity has passed for intracardiac repair to prevent pulmonary vascular changes. Intrinsic pulmonary vascular pathology on a genetic basis may be a prominent part of the disease process of these patients in that the elevated pulmonary vascular resistance normally present in the neonatal period fails to regress.

The natural history of Eisenmenger's syndrome is that of gradual increase in cyanosis and polycythemia, resulting in progressive symptoms of fatigue and dyspnea. Sudden death may occur with acute hypoxia or a lethal arrhythmia, or both. However, most often the clinical course is extended over several decades; many patients live productive lives despite the presence of this disease. The prognosis is more favorable than for patients with primary pulmonary hypertension in which there is no augmentation of systemic output from right to left shunting as pulmonary vascular obstruction progresses. The latter group has a more progressive decline in cardiac output and is more symptomatic than patients with Eisenmenger's syndrome.

Physical examination reflects the presence of right ventricular hypertrophy and pulmonary hypertension manifested by a right ventricular heave and a loud single second heart sound. A short systolic ejection murmur is present along the left sternal border in most cases, and a short, high-pitched protodiastolic murmur of pulmonary valve insufficiency also may be audible. The ECG shows right ventricular hypertrophy, and the chest x-ray reveals a large main pulmonary artery and tapering of distal pulmonary vessels. The echocardiogram shows the intracardiac anatomy with bidirectional shunting by color Doppler examination and marked pulmonary artery dilatation.

Management includes avoidance of activities that suddenly decrease systemic vascular resistance, because changes in the relationship between pulmonary and systemic vascular resistance may result in a sudden marked increase in right-to-left shunting, severe hypoxemia, and sudden arrhythmias. Phlebotomy with volume replacement may be utilized for patients with extremely high hematocrits, and will relieve symptoms of hyperviscosity. The use of new vasodilator agents such as prostacyclin is investigational and experience is extremely limited. Heart-lung transplantation or lung transplantation with intracardiac repair are the only viable options for some patients, but the risks are high and the long-term survival is limited.

Algorithm 16–1
Eisenmenger's Syndrome

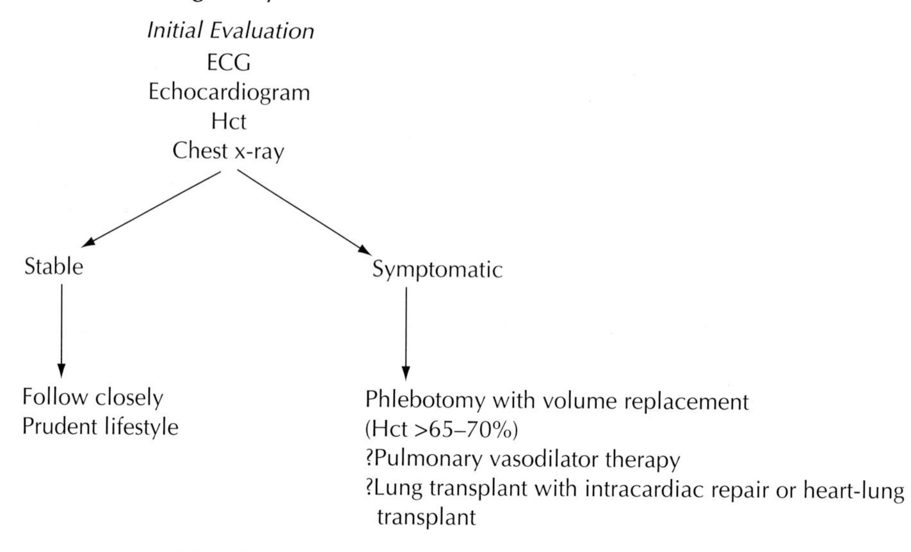

KEY: ECG, electrocardiogram; Hct, hematocrit; VSD, ventricular septal defect.

BIBLIOGRAPHY

Ammash NM, Connolly HM, Abel MD, Warnes CA: Noncardiac surgery in Eisenmenger syndrome. *J Am Coll Cardiol* 33(1):222, 1999.

Arcasoy SM, Kotloff RM: Lung transplantation. *N Engl J Med* 340:1081, 1999.

Barst RJ, Long W, Gersony W: Long-term vasodilator treatment improves survival in children with primary pulmonary hypertension. *Cardiol Young* (Suppl I):89, 1993.

Barst RJ, Rubin LJ, McGood MD, et al: Survival in primary pulmonary hypertension with long-term continuous intravenous prostacyclin. *Ann Intern Med* 121:409, 1994.

Bowyer JJ, Busst CM, Denison DM, Shinebourne EA: Effect of long term oxygen treatment at home in children with pulmonary vascular disease. *Br Heart J* 55:385, 1986.

Cantor WJ, Harrison DA, Moussadji JS, et al: Determinants of survival and length of survival in adults with Eisenmenger syndrome. *Am J Cardiol* 84:677, 1999.

Corpne S, Davido A, Lang T, Corone P: [Outcome of patients with Eisenmenger syndrome. Apropos of 62 cases followed-up for an average of 16 years (review)]. [French]. *Arch Mal Coeur Vaiss* 85:521, 1992.

Gleicher N, Midwall J, Hochberger D, Jaffin H: Eisenmenger's syndrome and pregnancy. *Obstet Gynecol Surv* 34:721, 1979.

Harinck E, Hutter PA, Hoorntje TM, et al: Air travel and adults with cyanotic congenital heart disease. *Circulation* 93:272, 1996.

Heath D, Edwards JE: The pathology of hypertensive pulmonary vascular disease: A description of six grades of structural changes in the pulmonary arteries with special reference to congenital cardiac septal defects. *Circulation* 18:533, 1958.

Jones P, Patel A. Eisenmenger's syndrome and problems with anaesthesia. *Br J Hosp Med* 54:214, 1996.

Linderkamp O, Klose HJ, Betke K, et al: Increased blood viscosity in patients with cyanotic congenital heart disease and iron deficiency. *J Pediatr* 95:567, 1979.

Newman JH, Sinclair-Smith BC: Risk of high-altitude travel in a patient with Eisenmenger's syndrome. *South Med J* 77:1057, 1984.

Niwa K, Perloff JK, Kaplan S, et al: Eisenmenger syndrome in adults: ventricular septal defect, truncus arteriosus, univentricular heart. *J Am Coll Cardiol* 34(1):223, 1999.

Perloff JK, Rosove MH, Child JS, Wright GB: Adults with cyanotic congenital heart disease: Hematologic management. *Ann Intern Med* 109:406, 1988.

Rosenthal A, Nathan DG, Marty AT, et al: Acute hemodynamic effects of red cell volume reduction in polycythemia of cyanotic congenital heart disease. *Circulation* 42:297, 1970.

Rosenzweig EB, Kerstein D, Barst RJ: Long-term prostacyclin for pulmonary hypertension with associated congenital heart defects. *Circulation* 99:1858, 1999.

Saha A, Balakrishnan KG, Jaiswal PK, et al: Prognosis for patients with Eisenmenger syndrome of various aetiology. *Int J Cardiol* 45:199, 1994.

Sondel PM, Tripp ME, Ganick DJ, et al: Phlebotomy with iron therapy to correct the microcytic polycythemia of chronic hypoxia. *Pediatrics* 67:667, 1981.

Vongpatanasin W, Brickner ME, Hillis LD, Lange RA: The Eisenmenger syndrome in adults. *Ann Intern Med* 128:745, 1998.

Young D, Mark H: Fate of the patient with the Eisenmenger syndrome. *Am J Cardiol* 28:658, 1971.

PART III

PREGNANCY AND GENETICS

CHAPTER 17

MATERNAL CONGENITAL HEART DISEASE AND PREGNANCY

Severe maternal heart disease is associated with risk for both the mother and the fetus during pregnancy and at the time of labor and delivery. In the past only women with mild to moderate congenital heart disease became pregnant. Patients with severe lesions did not survive childhood, or would be too ill to even consider pregnancy. However, with a marked increase in survival of women with complex congenital heart disease due to surgical intervention, a significant increase in pregnancy is to be expected.

Pregnancy represents a unique problem for the patient with congenital heart disease that must be approached by a physician with particular knowledge of the specific defects, the effects of pregnancy, and sensitivity to the desires of the patient. The risks of pregnancy and childbirth must be balanced against a woman's strong desire to have a child. The cardiologist must be certain that the patient understands the complex issues involved, including both maternal and fetal risk and the likelihood of a successful outcome. If a decision to carry a pregnancy to term is made, the cardiologist must maintain a continuous role in reevaluation and management.

Major changes occur in the circulation during pregnancy, which can markedly affect the hemodynamic status of a woman with previously stable unoperated or operated congenital heart disease. Whereas some severe forms of congenital cardiac defects are not compatible with a successful pregnancy or may be associated with high maternal mortality, other conditions may not cause significant cardiac issues during late gestation and childbirth. In situations where pregnancy must be avoided, the various forms of contraception must be tailored to the type of congenital heart disease and pulmonary vascular physiology.

CIRCULATORY PHYSIOLOGY OF NORMAL PREGNANCY

In a normal pregnancy, cardiac output increases 30 to 50%; this is achieved by an increase in stroke volume and heart rate. The increase in cardiac output is associated with low-resistance placental blood flow, a fall in pulmonary and systemic vascular resistance, and a widening of the pulse pressure. Blood volume increases by up to 50%. A discrepancy in the increase in plasma volume, which is approximately 50%, and the total red cell mass, which increases 25%, results in a mild physiologic anemia.

The changes in maternal circulation reach their peak at different times during gestation. Heart rate and cardiac output increase rapidly late in the first trimester, peaking during the fifth to sixth months, whereas maternal plasma volume reaches its peak levels in the seventh to eighth months. During the third trimester, stroke volume declines because of decreased venous return secondary to uterine compression of the inferior vena cava. This decrease is maximal in the supine position. Supine hypotension is normal in late pregnancy and may result in symptoms even in women without cardiovascular disease.

During labor, uterine contractions result in increased circulating blood volume with increased stroke volume and cardiac output. After delivery, intravascular volume increases transiently, probably as a result of relief of caval compression. Over the first month postpartum, circulatory hemodynamics and cardiac output gradually return to normal.

MATERNAL CONGENITAL HEART DISEASE: RISK ASSESSMENT

Cardiac risk assessment for congenital heart disease patients during pregnancy can be a complex issue. In most situations, guidelines can be developed that utilize functional capacity and the status of prior surgical repair. However, in certain complex situations, where experience with pregnancy is quite limited or not known, advice becomes more difficult. The patient's decision to embark upon pregnancy should include a thorough understanding of the complexities of the situation both for herself and the fetus. In addition, problems such as arrhythmias and the need for cardiovascular drugs not previously evaluated during pregnancy can increase the level of uncertainty.

General recommendations concerning pregnancy risk in maternal congenital heart disease may be made according to the patient's NYHA classification. Most patients with acyanotic congenital heart disease in functional class I or II can tolerate pregnancy without significant complications. However, risks increase proportionately in patients with Class III and IV symptoms, associated with congestive heart failure, unrelieved cyanotic heart disease, and significant pulmonary hypertension. Fetal outcome may also be related to maternal functional capacity and the presence of cyanosis. The probability of delivering a live-born infant is significantly reduced in cyanotic mothers. In addition, the incidence of prematurity and small-for-gestational-age infants is increased in mothers who are cyanotic. Pregnancy is also associated with a hypercoagulable state caused by increased clotting factors. Thus, management of anticoagulation therapy in patients with prosthetic valves is especially important.

In addition to assessment by functional capacity, specific lesions in maternal congenital heart disease can usually be classified as high-, medium- and low-risk. High-risk patients in whom pregnancy is contraindicated include those with severe obstruction involving the left or right side of the heart, severe pulmonary hypertension (Eisenmenger's syndrome), forms of uncorrected cyanotic heart disease, and those with decompensated large left-to-right shunts with elevated pulmonary artery pressure.

Medium-risk patients are those in whom symptoms may develop during the latter course of pregnancy, while low-risk patients are those with repaired forms of cyanotic and acyanotic congenital heart disease in whom pregnancy should be well-tolerated.

SPECIFIC LESIONS

High-Risk Group

Pulmonary Hypertension and Eisenmenger's Disease
Pulmonary hypertension associated with congenital heart disease may portend a poor prognosis during pregnancy, although less so than for women with primary pulmonary hypertension. Patients with Eisenmenger's disease are at the highest risk for maternal mortality, which is currently estimated in the range of 30 to 40%.

The increased intravascular volume that is present during pregnancy may result in heart failure in women whose cardiac output is limited by pulmonary vascular disease and associated ventricular dysfunction. Furthermore, if pregnancy is carried past the first trimester, the decrease in systemic vascular resistance will increase right-to-left ventricular septal defect shunting and cyanosis in patients with Eisenmenger's disease. Both of these problems are exacerbated during labor and delivery. While women with mild pulmonary hypertension may have uncomplicated pregnancies, in general, interruption of pregnancy must be strongly considered in patients with severe pulmonary vascular obstructive disease (PVOD).

Aortic Stenosis
All forms of left ventricular outflow tract obstruction have the potential to be symptomatic during pregnancy. The most commonly encountered lesion in this group is valvar aortic stenosis. The risks of pregnancy are related to the severity of aortic stenosis, which can be assessed by valve gradient and calculation of the aortic valve area. Mortality rates for pregnant women with aortic stenosis have been reported to be as high as 17%, but this is undoubtedly dependent on severity, and in the modern era, a pregnant woman with severe unrepaired aortic stenosis is rarely encountered. If at all possible, surgical or interventional treatment for severe aortic stenosis should be carried out prior to contemplation of pregnancy. However, insertion of a prosthetic valve with requirements for anticoagulation creates a new set of problems that require careful management. Balloon valvuloplasty without valve replacement, pulmonary autograft procedure (Ross operation), or a tissue valve do not require anticoagulation, and elimination of left ventricular outflow tract obstruction reduces the risks during gestation, labor, and delivery.

Asymptomatic patients with moderate aortic stenosis may be encountered in whom symptoms may develop during the second and third trimester of pregnancy. These patients pose the greatest difficulty in decision making prior to pregnancy. Balloon valvuloplasty prior to pregnancy should probably be considered in such patients when there is a resting gradient in the range of 50 mm Hg. When valvuloplasty is not feasible and the degree of aortic stenosis is sufficient enough to warrant cardiac surgery, then valve replacement with a Ross operation may be the best option. Patients with mild aortic stenosis can generally tolerate pregnancy without adverse effects.

Marfan Syndrome

Pregnancy in patients with Marfan syndrome may be complicated by the development of an aortic dissection. The risks of this complication are increased in patients with significant cardiovascular involvement and an aortic root diameter exceeding 40 mm.

Single Ventricle/Tricuspid Atresia

Pregnancy is associated with major risks in the patient with single ventricle or tricuspid atresia. The unoperated adult with a single ventricle usually has balanced hemodynamics, with just enough pulmonary stenosis to maintain an adequate O_2 saturation without significant pulmonary hypertension. Some patients may also be encountered with PVOD. In either case, pregnancy carries major risks for cardiovascular complications and should be strongly discouraged.

In the postoperative patient with single ventricle atresia who has undergone a Fontan repair, a small number of successful pregnancies have been reported. The largest published series in Fontan patients reported 33 pregnancies with 15 live births from 14 mothers, 13 spontaneous abortions and 5 elective terminations. One patient developed supraventricular tachycardia during pregnancy and had conversion to sinus rhythm. No maternal cardiac complications were reported during labor, delivery, or the immediate puerperium.

While in the past, patients with a Fontan operation were uniformly advised against pregnancy, these recent studies would suggest that highly motivated women with satisfactory hemodynamics, normal rhythm, good ventricular function and exercise capacity may be considered for pregnancy. Unfortunately, such patients represent only a small minority of the present-day adult Fontan population.

Moderate-Risk Group

Coarctation of the Aorta

Severe unoperated coarctation of the aorta is infrequently discovered in pregnant women; surgical correction usually had been carried out during childhood. Nevertheless, an occasional patient may present during pregnancy with symptomatic coarctation characterized by severe upper extremity hypertension and diminished lower extremity pulses. The cardiovascular risks during pregnancy for a woman with unrepaired severe aortic coarctation are similar to those for other forms of left ventricular outflow obstruction in that increased blood volume and necessity for increased cardiac output may result in heart failure. Early reports cite a 3.5% maternal mortality associated with coarctation of the aorta; the risks of aortic rupture or dissection are increased especially if there is a bicuspid aortic valve which is present in up to 70% of patients. Coarctation of the aorta may also be associated with cerebrovascular events, a complication which has been reported to occur during pregnancy.

The patient who has undergone repair of coarctation of the aorta also requires special consideration during pregnancy, since some late complications can be potentially serious. This includes the development of an aneurysm at the repair site, dilatation of the ascending aorta, residual aortic obstruction, aortic regurgitation, and potential hemodynamic consequences of other associated lesions. The risk of aneurysm formation is highest in patients in whom patch aortoplasty was used. Patients who underwent balloon angioplasty or stenting for treatment of either native or residual coarctation should also be assessed for aneurysm formation or residual obstruction. Cardiac MRI provides excellent visualization of the aorta and can detect unsuspected residual problems related to this lesion. Hypertension may persist after late coarctation repair even in the absence of a residual gradient.

Ebstein's Anomaly

Ebstein's anomaly has an extremely variable clinical presentation, and only a portion of these patients reaches adulthood sufficiently well compensated to contemplate pregnancy. Asymptomatic or mildly symptomatic women of childbearing age have had successful pregnancies. In a study of 111 pregnancies in 44 women, there were 23 premature births and 19 spontaneously unsuccessful pregnancies, but no serious pregnancy-related maternal complications. The birth weight of the infants born to cyanotic mothers was significantly lower as compared with that of infants born to acyanotic women. The outcome of pregnancy was related to the presence of cyanosis, arrhythmias, and evidence of right-sided congestive heart failure. Thus, these problems need to be carefully evaluated to determine the likelihood of a successful pregnancy and whether cardiac surgery should be considered prior to pregnancy. Postoperative patients with Ebstein's anomaly who are doing well without symptoms should be able to tolerate pregnancy.

Congenitally Corrected Transposition of the Great Vessels

Congenitally corrected transposition of the great vessels (L-TGA) is only rarely encountered without additional cardiac lesions. Some of these patients develop left AV valve regurgitation, dysfunction of the systemic ventricle, and heart block. When this occurs, the risks of pregnancy may be similar to patients with chronic mitral regurgitation and varying degrees of ventricular dysfunction. In the postoperative patient with L-TGA associated with VSD and pulmonary stenosis, a conduit has usually been placed from the pulmonary ventricle to the pulmonary artery. Prior to pregnancy, these patients should undergo conduit evaluation in addition to assessment of ventricular function, AV valve regurgitation, and rhythm.

The results of pregnancy with L-TGA depend on the status of ventricular function and the presence of associated lesions. In a study of 22 women with L-TGA, there were 60 pregnancies resulting in 50 live births; one patient developed congestive heart failure and required valve replacement early postpartum. Cardiac risks are increased in patients with cyanotic forms of this lesion. In another study of 45 pregnancies in 19 patients, 36% involving cyanotic women, there was a 26% incidence of cardiovascular complications.

D-Transposition of the Great Vessels

D-transposition of the great arteries without repair is not compatible with adult survival. The postoperative adult of childbearing age has usually undergone surgical repair using an *atrial* switch operation such as the Mustard or Senning repairs. Patients who have undergone the *arterial* switch operation have not yet reached adulthood but will do so over the next five years. It is expected that the cardiac risk for pregnancy in these patients should be low.

As a consequence of the Mustard and Senning operations, the morphologic right ventricle is the systemic pumping chamber. Ventricular dysfunction and AV valve regurgitation may develop in some young adults. These patients also may be prone to atrial flutter and sick sinus syndrome.

Published data for pregnancy following the Mustard and Senning operations is limited. Recommendations must be individualized, based on an assessment of the patient's clinical status. In one study, there were 12 successful pregnancies among asymptomatic patients.

Low-Risk Group

Bicuspid Aortic Valve

Among patients with an isolated bicuspid aortic valve, there is a small incidence of progressive dilatation of the ascending aorta. This can lead to the development of an ascending aortic aneurysm and, in rare instances, aortic dissection secondary to cystic medial necrosis. Although the incidence of this complication is quite small, it may be prudent in the patient with a bicuspid aortic valve to obtain an echocardiogram prior to or at the onset of pregnancy to determine aortic root dimensions. Some patients with a bicuspid aortic valve develop aortic regurgitation, which is usually well tolerated during pregnancy, provided that left ventricular function is preserved. The fall in systemic vascular resistance during pregnancy generally improves the hemodynamics of aortic regurgitation.

Atrial Septal Defect

Most women of childbearing age with unoperated atrial septal defect (ASD) are asymptomatic. Many are first discovered to have an ASD during pregnancy after an echocardiogram is performed to evaluate a prominent murmur. Closure of an atrial septal defect prior to pregnancy is advised to eliminate the potential for paradoxical embolism as well as the small possibility of heart failure from the combination of a large left-to-right shunt and the additional blood volume of pregnancy. Patients with a primum ASD may be more symptomatic during pregnancy if there is significant coexisting mitral regurgitation with the left-to-right shunt. Supraventricular arrhythmias may complicate any of these forms of ASD. In rare instances, pulmonary hypertension may be discovered at this early stage in a woman with an ASD.

Ventricular Septal Defect

The patient with a small or moderate-size ventricular septal defect, as well as the well-repaired postoperative patient, should have no adverse hemodynamic problems related to pregnancy. Patients with a large VSD and severe elevation of pulmonary vascular resistance (Eisenmenger's disease) should be strongly counseled against pregnancy.

Patent Ductus Arteriosus

The patient with a small or moderate-size patent ductus arteriosus with normal pulmonary artery pressure or the postoperative patient with no residual hemodynamic abnormalities should tolerate pregnancy without difficulty. Pregnancy in a patient with a large patent ductus arteriosus with PVOD (Eisenmenger's disease) is associated with a high maternal mortality and should be avoided.

Pulmonary Stenosis

Patients with significant pulmonary stenosis are usually treated during childhood with either surgery or balloon valvuloplasty; thus, pregnant patients with untreated severe pulmonary stenosis are rarely encountered today. The cardiac risks of pregnancy following the uncomplicated repair of pulmonary stenosis should be no different from the risks to the general population.

Tetralogy of Fallot

Tetralogy of Fallot is the most common form of cyanotic congenital heart disease. As such, the issue of pregnancy is commonly encountered in these patients, many of whom have reached childbearing age. Nearly all patients with this lesion have undergone surgical correction during childhood, although in rare instances, an uncorrected well-balanced patient may present with only minimal cyanosis in conjunction with a significant left-to-right shunt at the VSD level. Surgical repair prior to pregnancy is recommended for such patients to prevent additional complications related to excess volume on both right and left ventricles as well as the potential for a paradoxical embolism.

The well-repaired patient with tetralogy of Fallot will generally tolerate pregnancy without hemodynamic problems. Most of these patients have only mild to moderate right ventricular outflow tract obstruction in conjunction with pulmonary regurgitation. The occasional patient with severe residual right ventricular outflow tract obstruction should be evaluated for intervention prior to pregnancy. Cardiac arrhythmias may occasionally be seen and should be appropriately treated.

Prosthetic Heart Valves

The optimal management of anticoagulation in the pregnant woman with a mechanical valve remains controversial. Although treatment with warfarin has a low incidence of thromboembolic complications, the drug crosses the placenta and can result in an embryopathy in approximately 4–10% of fetuses when taken during the first trimester. The abnormality is related to bone development and can cause nasal hypoplasia and chondrodysplasia punctata. Warfarin has also been associated with CNS abnormalities when taken during the second and third trimester, as well as with spontaneous abortion, prematurity, stillbirth, and fetal cerebral hemorrhage during vaginal delivery. A recent study showed that adverse fetal effects appear to be dose-related and occurred predominantly in woman taking >5 mg/day of warfarin.

Heparin has been used as an alternative to warfarin. It does not cross the placenta and is generally considered safer. However, long-term use may be complicated by osteoporosis and thrombocytopenia. In addition, there are numerous instances of thromboembolic complications, including fatal valve thrombosis, in pregnant women treated with subcutaneous heparin. While most of these complications have occurred in women with first-generation prosthetic valves in the mitral position, it has not been clearly shown that these risks are prevented in patients with newer mechanical valves and a more rigorous anticoagulation protocol.

Thus, the precise anticoagulation regimen for pregnancy continues to be controversial. Many patients find the fetal risks of warfarin to be unacceptable and choose to begin heparin at the onset of conception, continuing it through the first trimester or sometimes until the 36th week of pregnancy. However, it is important that the patient understand that heparin incurs an increased risk of prosthetic valve thrombosis as compared to warfarin.

The current guidelines for anticoagulation, which have been adopted by the European Society of Cardiology, American Heart Association, and American College of Cardiology, vary according to the perceived risk for thromboembolic complications. In high-risk patients, warfarin is currently considered the anticoagulant of choice for the first 35 weeks of pregnancy in patients with a mechanical valve. However, these recommendations have been problematic and have not necessarily been adopted by many physicians or patients due to the concern about warfarin embryopathy.

Guidelines for Prevention of Thromboembolic Events in Valvular Heart Disease*

- *Recommendations for anticoagulation during pregnancy: weeks 1 through 35 in patients with mechanical prosthetic valves*
  1. The decision whether to use heparin during the first trimester or to continue oral anticoagulation throughout pregnancy should be made after full discussion with the patient and her partner; if she chooses to change to heparin for the first trimester, she should be made aware that heparin is less safe for her, with a higher risk of both thrombosis and bleeding, and that any risk to the mother also jeopardizes the baby. (*Class I*)
  2. High-risk women (a history of thromboembolism or an older-generation mechanical prosthesis in the mitral position) who choose not to take warfarin during the first trimester should receive continuous unfractionated heparin intravenously in a dose to prolong the midinterval (6 hours after dosing) aPTT to 2 to 3 times control. Transition to warfarin can occur thereafter. (*Class I*)
  3. In patients receiving warfarin, INR should be maintained between 2.0 and 3.0 with the lowest possible dose of warfarin, and low-dose aspirin should be added. (*Class IIa*)
  4. Women at low risk (no history of thromboembolism, newer low-profile prosthesis) may be managed with adjusted-dose subcutaneous heparin (17 500 to 20 000 U BID) to prolong the midinterval (6 hours after dosing) aPTT to 2 to 3 times control. (*Class IIb*)
- *Recommendations for anticoagulation during pregnancy: after the 36th week in patients with mechanical prosthetic valves*
  1. Warfarin should be stopped no later than week 36 and heparin substituted in anticipation of labor. (*Class IIa*)
  2. If labor begins during treatment with warfarin, a cesarean section should be performed. (*Class IIa*)
  3. In the absence of significant bleeding, heparin can be resumed 4 to 6 hours after delivery and warfarin begun orally. (*Class IIa*)

*From the European Society of Cardiology Guidelines for Prevention of Thromboembolic Events in Valvular Heart Disease.

Class I: Conditions for which there is evidence and/or general agreement that a given procedure or treatment is useful and effective
Class II: Conditions for which there is conflicting evidence and/or a divergence of opinion about the usefulness/efficacy of a procedure or treatment
IIa. Weight of evidence/opinion is in favor of usefulness/efficacy
IIb. Usefulness/efficacy is less well established by evidence/opinion.

The development of low-molecular-weight heparin adds an additional drug in the management of anticoagulation. It has the advantages over heparin of better bioavailability and a lower incidence of thrombocytopenia and osteoporosis. It is administered subcutaneously on a bid schedule which is based on body weight. However, there is only limited experience with this drug in patients with a mechanical valve and studies will be necessary to define its role in this situation.

Cardiovascular Drug Therapy During Pregnancy

Drug therapy should be avoided or limited during pregnancy unless absolutely necessary to avoid adverse effects on both the mother and fetus. The cardiologist should become familiar with the potential adverse effects of any cardiac drugs contemplated for use in a pregnant woman. For many older agents, sufficient data are available so that reasonable risk-versus-benefit assessments can be made. As new drugs appear, decisions may be based on knowledge of the effects of other agents in a particular family but with the understanding that untoward responses are possible. Dosages generally should be at the lower end of the recommended normal range, but the increased volume of distribution of various agents during pregnancy also may be a consideration.

Digoxin is an agent that has been demonstrated to be well tolerated by gravid women when serum levels are appropriate. Although digoxin crosses the placenta, the gestational use of this drug also has been found to be safe for the fetus. The fetus may be digitalized by administering digoxin to the mother. Diuretics are utilized for the treatment of maternal heart failure and, occasionally, hypertension. There have been very few reports of adverse fetal effects at normal maternal dosages.

Antiarrhythmic therapy is occasionally necessary for management of maternal arrhythmias. Although quinidine crosses the placenta, reports of toxic effects are extremely rare, and the agent is generally considered to be safe. Procainamide, on the other hand, is best avoided because of the development of antinuclear antibodies, and possible inducement of maternal lupus erythematosus. Maternal lupus can result in complete heart block in the fetus.

Low doses of lidocaine are also safe for mother and fetus, but a high dosage may result in fetal central nervous system effects. A multitude of side effects in the fetus have been individually reported with the use of amiodarone; these include hypothyroidism, hypotonia, and bradycardia, although the overall prevalence of such fetal effects is not known. Both maternal and fetal thyroid function should be monitored in any pregnant patient who must be treated with this agent. Data are limited regarding the effects on the fetus of other antiarrhythmic medications, such as verapamil, disopyramide, mexiletine, and calcium channel blockers. Therefore, these drugs should be used with great care. High-dose beta-blocker therapy may result in fetal uterine growth retardation, bradycardia, jaundice, and hypoglycemia. An increased risk for premature delivery and neonatal renal failure has been reported with the use of angiotensin-converting enzyme inhibitors, but the prevalence of these findings is unknown. These agents are generally not recommended for a gravid woman.

Antibiotic prophylaxis for dental and surgical procedures should be utilized appropriately for patients with congenital heart defects as recommended by the American Heart Association. Routine antibiotic prophylaxis at the time of normal vaginal delivery is recommended only for patients with prosthetic valves.

Surgical Intervention During Pregnancy

It is rare that cardiac surgery must be contemplated for a gravid woman. When surgical intervention is absolutely necessary, such procedures are best performed between 16 and 20 weeks of gestation. The risks to the fetus increase when cardiac surgery is performed later. When surgery is deemed to be absolutely necessary, measures must be taken to protect the fetus from the effects of maternal low cardiac output during surgery. Mean arterial pressure during surgery should be higher for a gravid woman than for other patients, and the fetal heart rate should be monitored closely. Flow rate should be adjusted in keeping with fetal heart rate. Deep hypothermia should be avoided, but moderate hypothermia has been utilized successfully. In the presence of fetal distress or persistent bradycardia during an operation carried out in the last trimester, emergency cesarean delivery may be necessary—in some cases during, but in most instances immediately after, maternal heart surgery. For optimal fetal survival, maternal uterine contractions should be monitored and carefully controlled because inappropriate labor during cardiopulmonary bypass is associated with fetal loss. Despite all preventive efforts, fetal mortality in the context of maternal open-heart surgery is reported in the 15 to 20% range.

CONTRACEPTION

Gynecologists and cardiologists should work together to define the most appropriate method of contraception for the congenital heart disease patient. For most patients with mild congenital heart defects, or well-repaired defects, contraceptive techniques can be chosen with no specific precautions related to heart disease. However, some patients with severe congenital heart disease who are advised to avoid pregnancy must also face increased risks for certain methods of contraception. These risks must be balanced against the effectiveness of the technique. There is sufficient information about specific risks of various contraceptive methods for women with congenital heart disease so that reasonable advice can be provided by the knowledgeable physician.

The first step in providing consultation is to determine for each individual case whether pregnancy is advisable. It is best that the patient be aware, prior to conception, of the risks to herself and the fetus during gestation. Some women may elect to go forward despite advice to the contrary, and the physician must be sensitive to the patient's needs in this regard. If conception is achieved, a specific management regimen is recommended, including the risks involved with medications, and in the case of women with mechanical prosthetic valves, a specific plan for anticoagulation throughout pregnancy, labor, and delivery. A high-risk obstetrical service is advisable for some patients.

If the patient decides to avoid pregnancy, there are a number of contraceptive options, each with various degrees of effectiveness and associated hazards.

Methods of Contraception

Barrier Methods

Barrier methods are simple to use, with no adverse effects on either the male or female. However, despite multiple combinations of condom, diaphragm, cervical cap, and spermicidal creams, this method has the lowest efficacy, with failure rates as high as 20% or more.

Intrauterine Devices

Intrauterine devices are an effective form of contraception. These devices are safe and may be left in place for a number of years. The pregnancy rate is 2 to 4%. The use of an intrauterine device may be associated with bleeding, and local infection has been reported to be associated with bacterial endocarditis. However, the risk of this complication is extremely low. This method should probably be avoided in patients at high risk for infective endocarditis.

Hormonal Methods

Oral contraceptives are the most widely used contraceptive method in the United States. For most women, safety, efficacy, and convenience of use have been well documented and complications are few. The three primary hormonal methods are (1) oral estrogen and progesterone therapy, (2) low-dose oral progesterone alone, and (3) depoprogesterone, administered by either intramuscular injection or subdermal, slow-released capsules. Failure rate is in the range of 3% for oral estrogen/progesterone methods, but is virtually zero for depoprogesterone injection.

The most important adverse effects of hormonal therapy for women with significant congenital heart disease are the cardiovascular complications. The risk of venous thromboembolic disease for both women with pulmonary hypertension and cyanotic patients is formidable. Hazards are also higher in patients with congestive heart failure and low cardiac output states. The use of hormonal methods for this group of patients should be avoided.

Tubal Ligation and Vasectomy

These forms of contraception are usually permanent and advised for patients in whom pregnancy is associated with a substantial risk of maternal mortality such as Eisenmenger's disease.

For the vast majority of women with mild-to-moderate or repaired congenital heart disease, advice concerning contraception should be similar to that for the general population. Careful and meticulous use of barrier methods probably is the safest option for most patients, but because the failure rate is high, personal decisions related to other contraceptive techniques or early interruption of an unplanned pregnancy will be important considerations for some women, and they will require advice and support from their physicians.

BIBLIOGRAPHY

Anderson RA, Fineron PW: Aortic dissection in pregnancy: Importance of pregnancy-induced changes in the vessel wall and bicuspid aortic valve in pathogenesis. *Br J Obstet Gynaecol* 101:1085, 1994.

Ando M, Okita Y, Morota T, Takamoro S: Thoracic aortic aneurysm associated with congenital aortic valve. *Cardiovasc Surg* 6(6):629, 1998.

Barash PG, Hobbins JC, Hook R, et al: Management of coarctation of the aorta during pregnancy. *J Thorac Cardiovasc Surg* 69:781, 1975.

Bhagwat AR, Engel PJ: Heart disease and pregnancy. *Cardiol Clin* 13:163, 1995.

Bonow RO, Carabello B, de Leon AC Jr, et al: ACC/AHA guidelines for the management of patients with valvular heart disease: A report of the American College of Cardiology/American Heart Association Task Force on Practice Guidelines (Committee on the Management of Patients with Valvular Heart Disease). *J Am Coll Cardiol* 5:1486, 1998.

Braunwald E: Cardiovascular diseases and pregnancy, in *Heart Disease: A Textbook of Cardiovascular Medicine*, 4th ed, E Braunwald (ed). Philadelphia, Saunders, 1992.

Canobbio MM, Mair DD, van der Velde MVD, Koos BJ: Pregnancy outcomes after the Fontan repair. *J Am Coll Cardiol* 28:763, 1996.

Chan WS: What is the optimal management of pregnant women with valvular heart disease in pregnancy. *Haemostasis Suppl* S1:105, 1999.

Chan WS, Anand O, Ginsberg JS: Anticoagulation of pregnant woman with mechanical heart valves: a systematic review of the literature. *Arch Intern Med* 160(2): 191, 2000.

Chesebro JH, Adams PC, Fuster V: Antithrombotic therapy in patients with valvular heart disease and prosthetic valves. *J Am Coll Cardiol* 8:41B, 1986.

Clarkson PM, Wilson NJ, Neutze JM: Outcome of pregnancy after the Mustard operation for transposition of the great arteries with intact ventricular septum. *J Am Coll Cardiol* 24:190, 1994.

Cobbs CG: IUD and endocarditis. *Ann Intern Med* 78:451, 1973.

Connolly HM, Grogan M, Warnes CA: Pregnancy among women with congenitally corrected transposition of the great arteries. *Am J Cardiol* 82(6):786, 1999.

Connolly HM, Warnes CA: Ebstein's anomaly: Outcome of pregnancy. *J Am Coll Cardiol* 23:1194, 1994.

de Swiet M, et al: Bacterial endocarditis after insertion of intrauterine contraceptive device. *Br Med J* 3:76, 1975.

Elkayam U, Gleicher N: Cardiac problems in pregnancy. I. Maternal aspects: The approach to the pregnant patient with heart disease. *JAMA* 251:2838, 1984.

Elkayam U, Ostrzega E, Shotan A, Mehra A: Cardiovascular problems in pregnant women with the Marfan syndrome (review). *Ann Intern Med* 123:117, 1995.

Genoni M, Jenni R, Hoerstrup SP, Vogt P, Tarna M: Pregnancy after atrial repair for transposition of the great arteries. *Heart* 81(3):276, 1999.

Gersony WM, Hayes CJ, Driscoll DJ, et al: Second natural history study of congenital heart defects: Quality of life in patients with aortic stenosis, pulmonary stenosis, or ventricular septal defect: Long-term follow-up of congenital aortic stenosis, and ventricular septal defect. *Circulation* 87:I-52, 1993.

Hall J, et al: Maternal and fetal sequelae of anticoagulation during pregnancy. *Am J Med* 68:122, 1980.

Kjeldsen J: Hemodynamic investigations during labor and delivery. *Acta Obstet Gynecol Scand* 89(Suppl):252, 1979.

Mane SV, Gharpure VP, Merchant RH: Maternal heart disease and perinatal outcome. *Indian Pediatr* 30:1407, 1993.

McFaul PB, Dornan JC, Lamki H, Boyle D: Pregnancy complicated by maternal heart disease. A review of 519 women. *Br J Obstet Gynaecol* 95:861, 1988.

Montalescot G, Polle V, Collet JP, et al: Low molecular weight heparin after mechanical heart valve replacement. *Circulation* 101(10):1083, 2000.

Neumayer U, Somerville J: Outcome of pregnancies in patients with complex pulmonary atresia. *Heart* 78:16, 1997.

Nissenkorn A, Friedman S, Schonfeld A, Ovadia J: Fetomaternal outcome in pregnancies after total correction of the tetralogy of Fallot. *Int Surg* 69:125, 1984.

Oakley CM: Anticoagulants in pregnancy. *Br Heart J* 74:107, 1995.

Parry AJ, Westaby S: Cardiopulmonary bypass during pregnancy. *Ann Thorac Surg* 61:1865, 1996.

Perloff JK: Epidemiology of heart disease and pregnancy, in *Progress in Cardiology*, D Zipes, D Rowlands (eds). Philadelphia, Lea & Febiger, 1992.

Pumphrey CW, et al: Aortic dissection during pregnancy. *Br Heart J* 55:106, 1986.

Roberts CS, Roberts WC: Dissection of the aorta associated with congenital malformation of the aortic valve. *J Am Coll Cardiol* 17:712, 1991.

Roberts SL, Chestnut DH: Anesthesia for the obstetric patient with cardiac disease. *Clin Obstet Gynecol* 30:601, 1987.

Sanson BJ, Lensing AW, Prins MH, et al: Safety of low-molecular-weight heparin in pregnancy: A systematic review. *Thromb Haemost* 81:668, 1999.

Sbarouni E, Oakley CM: Outcome of pregnancy in women with valve prosthesis. *Br Heart J* 71:196, 1994.

Shime J, Mocarski EJ, Hastings D, et al: Congenital heart disease in pregnancy: Short- and long-term implications. *Am J Obstet Gynecol* 156:313, 1987.

Snabes MC, Poindexter AN: Laparoscopic tubal sterilization under local anesthesia in women with cyanotic heart disease. *Obstet Gynecol* 78:437, 1991.

Szekely P, Julian DG: Heart disease and pregnancy (review). *Curr Probl Cardiol* 4:1, 1979.

Tahir H: Pulmonary hypertension, cardiac disease and pregnancy. *Int J Gynecol Obstet* 51:109, 1995.

Vitale N, De Feo M, De Santo LS, et al: Dose-dependent fetal complications of warfarin in pregnant women with mechanical heart valves. *J Am Coll Cardiol* 33(6):1637, 1999.

Vuerrien J, Barnes I, Somerville J: Outcome of pregnancy in patients with congenitally corrected transposition of great arteries. *Am J Cardiol* 84(7):820, 1999.

Whittemore R, Hobbins JC, Engle MA: Pregnancy and its outcome in women with and without surgical treatment of congenital heart disease. *Am J Cardiol* 50:641, 1982.

CHAPTER 18

GENETICS OF CONGENITAL HEART DISEASE

Kwame Anyane-Yeboa

Advances in the detection, surgical treatment, and management of infants with congenital heart disease have contributed to survival into adulthood of over 85% of affected individuals. Information regarding the genetic basis of congenital heart disease is rapidly accumulating. Basic knowledge in this arena is important for the internist and cardiologist in order to select the adults with congenital heart disease for genetic consultation, genetic screening, and special counseling regarding education, career planning, and pregnancy.

The understanding of the genetic basis of most congenital heart disease has been greatly enhanced by discoveries of new cytogenetic and molecular genetic techniques. Chromosome banding techniques, which are now universal in all laboratories, have improved detection of chromosome deletions and translocations. The technique of fluorescence in situ hybridization (FISH) is now used routinely for detection of subtle chromosome rearrangements, microdeletions, duplications, and the characterization of marker chromosomes. In addition, advances in molecular genetics have led to the identification of a number of genetic mutations responsible for certain genetic disorders, such as Holt-Oram syndrome and the long QT syndrome.

Congenital heart disease is caused by genetic and environmental factors. The contributions of teratogens such as alcohol, maternal rubella, and maternal diabetes mellitus to congenital heart disease are well established, but the number of teratogens that can potentially cause congenital heart disease is unknown. The genetic defects fall into three major categories: multifactorial or polygenic, monogenic, and chromosomal. Previous studies have suggested that 3% of all congenital heart disease, both syndromic and isolated, is caused by single gene mutations, 7% by chromosome aberrations, and the rest by multifactorial and environmental factors. Further advances in genetic research almost certainly will lead to the ability to detect subtle changes in the chromosomes that current cytogenetic and molecular cytogenetic techniques are unable to detect. Application of these techniques will detect minute changes, mostly microdeletions, in additional families with congenital heart disease, particularly in those families in which the heart disease is associated with mental retardation and dysmorphic features. Many additional families with single gene mutations will also be identified. It should be expected over time that the proportion of congenital heart disease caused by chromosomal and single gene mutations will increase, with a corresponding decrease in the proportion thought to be caused by multifactorial and environmental factors.

It is quite likely that most teratogens interact with certain genes to cause congenital disease and other malformations. It is known, for example, that only about 10% of chronic alcoholic mothers will give birth to an infant with fetal alcohol syndrome (FAS). These infants are generally microcephalic, growth and developmentally delayed, and have some form of congenital heart disease, usually tetralogy of Fallot. Another 30 to 40% of alcoholic mothers will give birth to infants with milder features associated with FAS, and the offspring of the remaining 50 to 60% will be healthy. It is possible that the first two groups have genes that increase the susceptibility to the effects of alcohol. The third group may have other genes that are "protective" and modify the effects of alcohol on the fetus. Susceptibility genes have now been described for a wide variety of human diseases. It is known, for example, that individuals with sickle cell trait (AS) are less susceptible to falciprum malaria than AA and SS individuals, but individuals who have certain polymorphisms of tumor necrosis factor alpha (TNFα) gene are at high risk for development of cerebral malaria, a condition with a very high mortality rate.

INHERITANCE OF CONGENITAL HEART DISEASE

Congenital heart disease may occur as either isolated defects or as a component of a genetic syndrome.

ISOLATED CONGENITAL HEART DISEASE

Empiric observation about recurrence and transmission risks of most forms of congenital heart disease indicates that they are usually much below those observed in classical mendelian inheritance (Table 18-1). The theory of polygenic inheritance was proposed to explain this finding. In this model, the recurrence risks should be equal in siblings and offspring and should be approximately equal to the square root of the population incidence. The risk is decreased in more distant relatives (second- and third-degree relatives) and increased when many family members are affected or when the disorder is more severe. When there is an unequal sex incidence, the risk is greater among relatives of the more rarely affected sex. The actual incidence figures are altered by environmental factors. Risks can be underestimated by lack of detection in family members who may be mildly affected, especially for small ventricular septal defects (VSDs) and mild pulmonary stenosis.

TABLE 18-1

Recurrence Risks in Offspring and Siblings of Individuals with Congenital Heart Defects (%)

Defect	Offspring[a]	Father Affected	Mother Affected	One Affected Sibling	Reference
Ventricular septal defect		2	6–10	3	Nora and Nora, 1988
		3	9.5	2.5	Nora, Nora, and Berg, 1991
				3	Burn and Goodship, 1997[b]
	4			6	Hoffman, 1990
Atrial septal defect		3	4–4.5	2.5	Nora and Nora, 1988
		1.5	6	2.5	Nora, Nora, and Berg, 1991
		0	11.1	3	Burn and Goodship, 1997
	4			3	Hoffman, 1990
Patent ductus arteriosus		2.5	3.5–4	3	Nora and Nora, 1988
		2.5	4	3	Nora, Nora, and Berg, 1991
				2.5	Burn and Goodship, 1997
	3			2.5	Hoffman, 1990
Atrioventricular canal defect		1	14	3	Nora and Nora, 1988
		1	14	2.5	Nora, Nora, and Berg, 1991
		0.83	10.5–13.9	2	Burn and Goodship, 1997
	5–10			2	Hoffman, 1990
Tetralogy of Fallot		1.5	2.5	2.5	Nora and Nora, 1988
		1.5	2.5	2.5	Nora, Nora, and Berg, 1991
		0–1.6	3.1–4.7	2	Burn and Goodship, 1997
	4			2	Hoffman, 1990
Pulmonary stenosis		2	4–6.5	2	Nora and Nora, 1988
		2	6.5	2	Nora, Nora, and Berg, 1991
				2	Burn and Goodship, 1997
	6			2	Hoffman, 1990
Coarctation of aorta		2	4	2	Nora and Nora, 1988
		2.5	4	2	Nora, Nora, and Berg, 1991
				2	Burn and Goodship, 1997
	3			2	Hoffman, 1990
Aortic stenosis		3	13–18	2	Nora and Nora, 1988
		5	18	2	Nora, Nora, and Berg, 1991
				3	Burn and Goodship, 1997
	5–10			3	Hoffman, 1990
Transposition of the great arteries				1.5	Nora, Nora, and Berg, 1991
	5			2	Hoffman, 1990
		0	0	2	Burn and Goodship, 1997
				1.5	Nora and Nora, 1988

(Continued)

TABLE 18-1 (*Continued*)

Recurrence Risks in Offspring and Siblings of Individuals with Congenital Heart Defects

Defect	Offspring[a]	Father Affected	Mother Affected	One Affected Sibling	Reference
Hypoplastic left heart	5			1–2	Hoffman, 1990
				3	Nora, Nora, and Berg, 1991
				2	Nora and Nora, 1988
TAPVC	5			3	Hoffman, 1990
Truncus arteriosus				1	Nora and Nora, 1988
				1	Nora, Nora, and Berg, 1991
				1	Burn and Goodship, 1997
Double outlet right ventricle	4			2	Hoffman, 1990
Atrial isomerism	1			5	Hoffman, 1990
				5	Burn and Goodship, 1997
Single ventricle	5			3	Hoffman, 1990
Ebstein's anomaly	5			1	Nora and Nora, 1988
				1	Burn and Goodship, 1997

[a]Offspring—independent of sex of the affected parent.
[b]Compilation of numerous studies, with recurrence risks assigned by Burn and Goodship (in Emery and Rimoin, 1997).
ABBREVIATION: TAPVC, total anomalous pulmonary venous connections.

The phenotype in the polygenic model is assumed to be due to the additive effect of multiple genes, interaction with other genes and the environment, and random (stochastic) effects. Recurrence in siblings and offspring of affected individuals is generally 3% to 5%. Patent ductus arteriosus (PDA) is the only lesion that fits this model. In one study, recurrence risk was found to be 2.5% for siblings and 0.6% in second- and third-degree relatives. Those with the largest ductus had a higher risk of 4.8%, compared with 1.8% for those with a small ductus. Recurrence risks for other types of congenital heart disease may be higher or lower than would be expected based on the polygenic model alone. Most recent studies suggest that the risk of transmission to the offspring is higher if the mother is affected rather than the father. In general, there appear to be low recurrence risks for defects resulting from abnormal migration and high risks for defects resulting from flow disturbances. In many recent studies the transmission rate for the lesions is 1.9 to 3.5% higher if the affected parent is the mother rather than the father. The higher recurrence rate reported by recent studies, and the fact that recurrence risks do not seem to fit the polygenic model, strongly suggest genetic heterogeneity as a possible explanation.

MENDELIAN INHERITANCE OF CONGENITAL HEART DISEASE

Secundum Atrial Septal Defect

This malformation accounts for 10% of all isolated congenital heart malformations. The majority of cases are presumed to be caused by polygenic or multifactorial factors, but autosomal dominant transmission has been observed in some families. In such families, affected relatives have secundum atrial septal defect (ASD), or other congenital heart lesions. Coexisting heart block has been observed in some of the affected relatives.

A gene mutation for one form of autosomal dominant secundum ASD has been mapped to chromosome 5p and has been designated ASD1. Genetic studies in families with this mutation revealed skipped generations, indicating incomplete penetrance. Secundum ASD is the most common lesion among affected family members, but PDA, VSD, atrial septal aneurysm, left superior vena cava, tetralogy of Fallot, bicuspid aortic valve, valvar or subaortic stenosis, and atrioventricular (AV) conduction defects were also observed. Overall, 40% of affected individuals had additional or other cardiac anomalies. The penetrance of this gene was estimated to be about 45%. Many reported families with autosomal dominant secundum ASD do not map to this locus, suggesting that other as yet unidentified genes play a role in the causation of secundum ASD. Further genetic heterogeneity is suggested by a family with multiple affected individuals in a typical autosomal dominant pattern in which some affected individuals also have cleft lip and palate.

Ebstein's Anomaly

Ebstein's anomaly is rare and accounts for only 0.5% of all congenital heart malformations, with an incidence of 0.12 per 1000 live births. The cause of Ebstein's anomaly is heterogeneous with most cases thought to be a multifactorial trait. Thus, although the frequency of congenital heart disease in first-degree relatives was higher than in the general population, recurrence of Ebstein's anomaly in the same family is rare. Autosomal dominant and autosomal recessive forms have been described. In some cases extracardiac malformations were reported. Ebstein's anomaly has also been associated with in utero exposure to lithium.

Patent Ductus Arteriosus

Most cases of PDA are multifactorial. In those families where a single gene is suspected, however, the inheritance pattern has been interpreted as showing autosomal dominant and, in some cases, autosomal recessive inheritance. Recurrence for offspring in autosomal dominant cases is 50% and, in recessive cases, 25%.

Coarctation of the Aorta

Isolated coarctation of the aorta can be attributed to multifactorial inheritance, but a few families have been reported in which the transmission is autosomal dominant. In one reported family, for instance, coarctation of the aorta, interrupted aortic arch, and hypoplastic left heart syndrome were seen in five members in three generations. Four of them were born with mild to severe aortic coarctation, either isolated or in association with other cardiac lesions. The fifth was detected, through fetal echocardiography, to have hypoplastic left heart syndrome. In such families, the recurrence risk is 50%.

Valvar Pulmonary Stenosis

Most types of valvar pulmonary stenosis fall into the multifactorial category, but a few families have been described with autosomal dominant transmission. In one family, a mother and her three children were affected. Two of the three affected children had other congenital heart lesions as well.

Total Anomalous Pulmonary Venous Connections

Many families have now been reported in which total anomalous pulmonary venous connections (TAPVC) occurs as an isolated autosomal dominant trait. In 1960, the disorder was described in a father and daughter and referred to as the "Scimitar syndrome," because of the radiologic appearance created by the anomalous vein draining the right lower lung and connecting the inferior vena cava.

A large Utah-Idaho family was described in 1994, in which nonsyndromic TAPVC occurred as an autosomal dominant trait with incomplete penetrance and variable expression. There were 14 affected family members. The gene for TAPVC in this family has been mapped to 4p13-q12. Other Utah families have not mapped to this chromosome locus, suggesting genetic heterogeneity in TAPVC. In an affected adult, recurrence in offspring is 50%, but reduced penetrance makes actual recurrence less than 50%.

ATRIOVENTRICULAR CANAL DEFECT

AV canal defects account for 7.4% of all cardiac defects. Overall, 76% of cases are associated with genetic syndromes and 24% are sporadic. Down syndrome is associated with AV canal defect, accounting for 78% of syndromic cases and 60% of all AV canal defects. Isomerism accounts for 8.3% of the total, with AV canal defect present in 60% of cases of isomerism. AV canal defects are occasionally seen in Noonan syndrome, Ellis-Van Creveld syndrome, and the VACTERL association (see later discussion). Recurrence in each of these syndromes depends on the genetic basis for that syndrome and the frequency of association of the syndrome with AV canal defect.

Nonsyndromic AV canal defects account for about 24% of all cases. This group is autosomal dominant with incomplete penetrance and 10% recurrence. An autosomal gene for AV canal defect has been mapped to chromosome 1p31-p21. Direct DNA mutation analysis is not yet available.

Holt-Oram Syndrome

Holt-Oram syndrome is characterized by autosomal dominant inheritance with over 90% penetrance, congenital heart disease, and radial ray defects. It has a prevalence of 1 per 100,000 live births. The characteristic hand malformation is a finger-like thumb, so that the thumb is attached in the same plane as other fingers. In some cases the thumb may be hypoplastic or completely absent. The radius may be severely hypoplastic. The ulna and humerus also may be affected. The most common heart lesions are ASD, VSD, and PDA. ASD alone or in combination with other heart lesions occurs in about 60% of patients. In addition, 17% have more complicated heart malformations such as tetralogy of Fallot or AV canal defect, and 6% have severe defects, including TAPVC, DORV, and HLHS. Recurrence in offspring is 50%. Mutations in the TBX5 gene, a transcription factor located on chromosome 12q24.1, underlie this disorder.

Noonan Syndrome

This is an autosomal dominant disorder characterized by short stature, facial anomalies, webbed neck, congenital heart disease, mild mental retardation, and other anomalies. Short stature is present in about 60% of individuals with Noonan syndrome and webbed neck in 80% of recognized cases. About 35 to 40% of affected males have cryptorchidism. Pectus excavatum and wide-set nipples are present in about 80%. Microcephaly is present in most individuals with Noonan syndrome, but macrocephaly may also be present. Frequently found facial anomalies are hypertelorism, epicanthic folds, upper eyelid ptosis, proptosis, and down-slanted palpebral fissures. The hair tends to be short, curly, and woolly in texture.

Hypertrophic cardiomyopathy is one of the most important heart problems in Noonan syndrome and is present in 20 to 30% of affected individuals. The obstructive form of hypertrophic cardiomyopathy is observed in about 40% of cardiomyopathic patients with Noonan syndrome. The typical morphology of hypertrophic cardiomyopathy is asymmetrical septal hypertrophy, but some cases exhibit symmetric (concentric) hypertrophy. Significant stenosis in nondysplastic pulmonary valves is present in about 20% of individuals and dysplastic valves in about 10%. Recent studies indicate that aortic coarctation is present in about 8.7%. The Noonan syndrome phenotype in females overlaps greatly with that of Turner's syndrome; therefore, chromosome studies must be ordered in all patients with suspected Noonan syndrome. This is especially true in females with coarctation of the aorta. The clinical features of Noonan syndrome vary from very mild to severe and overlap with other genetic syndromes as well. Approximately 50% of cases are suspected to be fresh dominant mutations. Recurrence in the offspring of individuals with Noonan syndrome is 50%. A Noonan syndrome gene has been mapped to chromosome 12q22, and efforts to clone the gene are still in progress; however, many families do not map to this locus, indicating genetic heterogeneity.

Alagille Syndrome

The main features of Alagille syndrome are intrahepatic cholestasis, congenital heart disease, and skeletal and ocular anomalies. In about 90% of patients, there is a history of prolonged neonatal jaundice resulting from paucity of intrahepatic and occasionally extrahepatic bile ducts. Cardiac lesions, which occur in about 85% of patients, are predominantly peripheral pulmonary stenosis but might include pulmonary valve stenosis, partial anomalous venous drainage, ASD, or VSD. About 90% of Alagille patients have anterior segment dysgenesis, particularly posterior embryotoxon, as well as pigmentary retinopathy. Bilateral optic disc drusen is found in 80% and unilateral drusen in 95%. Skeletal manifestations include hemivertebrae or butterfly vertebrae in about 90% of patients and short stature in 50%. In general, the liver abnormalities resolve with age, but occasional individuals can have more severe hepatic problems leading to death.

Alagille syndrome is an autosomal dominant trait with incomplete penetrance. Mutations have been detected in the Jagged 1 gene in the majority of patients. The Jagged 1 gene, which maps to chromosome 20p11, encodes a ligand for the notch receptor. An inadequate amount of Jagged 1 protein during morphogenesis (haploinsufficiency) leads to the Alagille phenotype. In a small proportion of patients, a microchromosome deletion is present on chromosome 20. DNA testing is currently available and should be offered to affected individuals who wish to have a child.

VATER Association

VATER is a useful acronym for a condition presenting as ***v***ertebral defects, ***a***nal atresia, ***t***racheoesophageal fistula with ***e***sophageal atresia, and ***r***adial dysplasia. The VATER association has been expanded to include VACTERL, which is an acronym for ***v***ertebral defects, ***a***nal atresia, ***c***ardiac malformations, ***t***racheoesophageal fistula with ***e***sophageal atresia, ***r***enal anomalies, and ***l***imb anomalies. Nearly all described cases are sporadic, with no associated chromosomal abnormality or teratogen exposure. VATER association should be differentiated from Fanconi anemia by chromosome breakage and diepoxybutane (DEB)-induced chromosome studies.

Other conditions that overlap with the VATER phenotype include Holt-Oram syndrome and the Müllerian duct aplasia, renal aplasia, cervicothoracic somite dysplasia (MURCS) association. A few cases of parent-to-child transmission have been recorded with the VATER association. Thus, although the recurrence risk for offspring is less than 1%, it is prudent to use ultrasound to monitor at-risk pregnancies.

CHROMOSOMAL SYNDROMES

Numerous chromosome abnormalities are associated with congenital abnormalities. Some, such as trisomies 13 and 18, are lethal in the first few years of life. Others lead to severe mental retardation precluding reproduction in the affected individuals. The discussion here is restricted to chromosome and microchromosome syndromes, which are not lethal; are associated with mild, moderate, or no retardation; and occur frequently in adult cardiac patients.

Down Syndrome

The major features of Down syndrome are well described in most standard texts and will not be described here in detail. Down syndrome is caused by the presence of three copies of chromosome 21 (trisomy 21) or three copies of the Down syndrome–determining region on chromosome 21. The mean intelligence quotient (IQ) is usually in the 30 to 70 range, but there are occasional exceptions. The pathologic, metabolic, and neurochemical changes of Alzheimer's disease are present in the brains of almost all individuals with Down syndrome explaining a progressive loss of cognitive function.

AV canal defects and VSD occur in about 30 to 40% of individuals with Down syndrome. Furthermore, Down syndrome individuals are 10 to 20 times more likely to develop acute leukemia than normal individuals. Hematologic abnormalities, autoimmunity, immunologic dysfunction, and thyroid disease are common.

Many pregnancies have been reported in women with Down syndrome; these frequently are the result of sexual abuse. About one-third of the offspring have Down syndrome but for reasons that are not clear, one-third of the offspring with normal chromosomes are abnormal. Prenatal diagnosis using chorionic villus sampling on amniocentesis will detect the trisomy 21 fetus, but not the abnormalities in the one-third of fetuses with normal chromosomes. Termination of pregnancy as an option should be discussed with a guardian. Males with Down syndrome have normal spermatogenesis but usually do not reproduce owing to their low IQ; however, a few individuals have fathered children.

Turner Syndrome

Turner syndrome is associated with short stature; short, webbed neck (60% of cases); broad chest with wide-spaced nipples; cubitus valgus; perception hearing loss (50% of cases); and cardiovascular malformations, primary amenorrhea, and infertility as a result of streak gonads. The syndrome is associated with a substantial increase in the prevalence of cardiovascular malformations, with reported prevalence rates that vary from 17 to 47%. In a large Danish study in 1994, Gotzsche and associates reported a prevalence of 26%. They detected bicuspid aortic valves in 14% of participants with Turner's syndrome. Other studies cite a prevalence of 9 to 34% for bicuspid aortic valves. If one includes women with aortic stenosis and/or regurgitation without a bicuspid valve, a total of 18% are found to have abnormal aortic valves. It is generally agreed that bicuspid aortic valve predisposes to valvar stenosis and/or insufficiency with advancing age, and, indeed, 32% of patients in the Danish study were found to have stenosis, or insufficiency, or both. The prevalence of aortic coarctation varies from 2 to 19%. In the Danish study, 10% of females with Turner's syndrome were detected to have coarctation.

There is a higher incidence of cardiovascular disease among 45,X females than among mosaics; in the Danish study, the incidence was 38% of those with 45,X versus 11% for mosaics. In a study by Lin and colleagues, aortic dilation and dissection occurred in at least 6% of affected individuals, 13% of whom had aortic dissection. An associated cardiovascular malformation or hypertension is present in about 90% of those with dilation and dissection, and about 10% have no predisposing factors.

Pregnancy has been achieved in many Turner's patients through in vitro fertilization using donor eggs. There is no risk for Turner's syndrome in the offspring from this method of assisted pregnancy.

Microdeletion Chromosome Syndromes

In recent years, an increasing number of genetic syndromes have been associated with microdeletions in various chromosomes. The common examples are Prader-Willi syndrome, Angelman's syndrome, DiGeorge and velocardiofacial syndromes, Miller-Dieker syndrome, multiple osteochondromatosis, Williams syndrome, Alagille syndrome, and ***W***ilms tumor–***a***niridia–***a***mbiguous ***g***enitalia–mental ***r***etardation (WAGR) syndrome. Significant congenital malformations are present in DiGeorge/velocardiofacial, Williams, and Alagille syndromes only.

DiGeorge Syndrome and Velocardiofacial Syndrome

Chromosome 22q11 microdeletion is a well-established genetic origin of DiGeorge syndrome, conotruncalfacial syndrome, and velocardiofacial syndrome. These syndromes have been incorporated into a group under the acronym CATCH 22 (***c***onotruncal cardiac defect, ***a***bnormal face, ***t***hymic hypoplasia, ***c***left palate, ***h***ypocalcemia, microdeletion ***22***q11). Estimated prevalence of the deletion is 1 in 4500 live births.

The phenotypic spectrum is quite broad. Facial anomalies include a broad nasal root with a bulbous tip, and small rounded ears. Cardiovascular malformations, hypocalcemia, T-cell abnormalities, velopharyngeal incompetence, and renal malformations are common. Autoimmune disease has been reported in a small fraction of patients. Learning disabilities have been reported in 80 to 100% of cases, and in another study, intellectual disability (IQ below 70) was reported in 45%. Schizophrenia, major depression, and bipolar disease have been reported in adults with chromosome 22q11 deletion.

About 80% of patients with DiGeorge syndrome have a congenital heart malformation, usually including a conotruncal heart lesion, including tetralogy of Fallot, DORV, truncus arteriosus communis, and interrupted aortic arch. VSD and other malformations have also been documented. About 17.5% to 22.5% of patients with conotruncal heart lesions have chromosome 22q11 deletions. Table 18-2 provides risk estimates from a study by Goldmuntz and associates. Right aortic arch as an isolated defect is present in 9 to 12% of patients with deletions. Other types of isolated arch defects in chromosome 22q11 deletion include cervical aorta, vascular ring, aberrant origin of the left subclavian artery, retroesophageal arch, and Komnerell's diverticulum. Individuals with tetralogy of Fallot and chromosome 22q11 deletion have a significantly higher incidence of associated aortic arch anomalies. The arch anomalies frequently found are right aortic arch, aberrant origin of the subclavian artery, isolation of the subclavian artery, and isolation and connec-

TABLE 18-2

Frequency of 22q11 Deletions in Patients with Conotruncal Defects

Defect	Percent
Interrupted aortic arch	50
Type A	—
Type B	57
Truncus arteriosus	34
Type A_1	25
Type A_2	33
Type A_3	—
Type A_4	50
Posterior malalignment type	33
Ventricular septal defect with coarctation	25
Tetralogy of Fallot	15
Double outlet right ventricle	5
Double outlet left ventricle	0
Transposition of the great arteries	0
Total	**17.5**

SOURCE: Modified from Goldmuntz et al, 1993.

tion of the ductus arteriosus to the pulmonary artery. Tetralogy of Fallot with pulmonary atresia or VSD with PA is associated in 32% of cases with chromosome 22q11 deletion.

The spectrum of parathyroid gland dysfunction in 22q11 deletion has not been well characterized. Absent parathyroid tissue with hypocalcemia is well recognized in patients with DiGeorge syndrome. Hypocalcemic hypoparathyroidism has been described in adolescents with DiGeorge syndrome and velocardiofacial syndrome. Infants with chromosome 22q11 deletion have presented with hypocalcemic hypoparathyroidism that spontaneously improves in childhood and then recurs in adolescence or young adulthood. Furthermore, normocalcemia has been shown to evolve to hypocalcemic hypoparathyroidism in some patients. Insidious onset of parathyroid gland dysfunction has been documented as late as the fourth decade in a patient with DiGeorge syndrome. Adult physicians must continue to monitor parathyroid function in patients with DiGeorge syndrome periodically throughout their lives and during periods of stress.

Schizophrenia has been repeatedly ascertained in 25 to 30% of patients with DiGeorge syndrome and chromosome 22q11 deletion, suggesting a risk 25% greater than for the normal populations. Studies also suggest that 2 to 9% of patients with schizophrenia have chromosome 22q11 deletions. Routine psychiatric evaluations should be considered for all patients with chromosome 22q11 deletion.

The majority of chromosome 22q11 deletions are sporadic, with a recurrence rate of 7% in siblings. Transmission of chromosome 22q11 deletion from a parent to offspring is theoretically 50%, but there is inadequate information on parent-to-offspring transmission at the present. It is suspected that fewer parents with chromosome 22q11 deletions have children because of their reduced intellectual function and the frequency of psychiatric illness in this group. In a few patients with DiGeorge syndrome, deletions of chromosome 10p13, 18q21.3, and 4q21–q25 have been detected. These sites are not considered major loci for DiGeorge syndrome. The DiGeorge phenotype has been described in FAS and fetal isotretinous syndrome. Those cases are not associated with chromosome abnormalities.

Williams Syndrome

This condition was described initially by Williams in 1961. The main features are a characteristic face, heart defects, mental retardation with an outgoing personality, and, sometimes, hypercalcemia in infancy. The facial features consist of periorbital fullness, medial eyebrow flare, a flat malar region with full cheeks and hips, and a wide mouth with a long, smooth philtrum. Mild mental retardation and hyperactivity are frequent manifestations. Personality is usually described as friendly, outgoing, and talkative. Many adults are capable of holding simple supervised jobs, but independent living is usually restricted more by mental and adaptive limitations than by physical limitations. Hypercalcemia may be difficult to document in infancy, but when present, may persist. In other individuals, hypercalcemia may disappear and reappear later in life. Nephrocalcinosis may be a complication in a few patients. Renal malformations are found in about 18% of individuals with Williams syndrome and include renal agenesis or hypoplasia, duplicated kidney, and renal artery stenosis.

The characteristic of heart defect is supravalvar aortic stenosis or a peripheral pulmonary artery stenosis (see Chap. 6), but valvar aortic stenosis, bicuspid aortic valve, and mitral valve prolapse are also common. One report describes 19 cases of sudden death in children and adolescents with Williams syndrome, most of them associated with anesthesia administered for catheterization. Although some fatalities were associated with catheter manipulation, others occurred before the procedure had begun or after apparently successful completion. Myocardial ischemia from coronary insufficiency has been the likely mechanism of sudden death in most cases reported. Coronary artery stenoses or severe biventricular outflow tract obstruction have been documented in most cases. In a series of 104 patients with Williams syndrome followed for about 30 years, a 3% incidence of sudden death was documented. Hypertension is uncommon in children but quite common in adults with Williams syndrome. Many adults have a progression of their cardiovascular complications and high blood pressure. Other complications include inguinal hernias, obesity, short stature, lordosis, and progressive scoliosis.

Sudden death is a well-recognized complication of nonsyndromic supravalvar aortic stenosis. This is a dominantly inherited condition that shares similar cardiovascular characteristics with Williams syndrome but lacks the cognitive behavior and phenotypic abnormalities of the latter.

A microdeletion of chromosome 7q11 can be demonstrated in 96% of all cases of Williams syndrome. This deletion removes the elastin gene and other genes in that region of the chromosome. Except for a few cases that are caused by balanced chromosome translocations, all microdeletion cases are sporadic. Transmission of the deletion from parents to their offspring is limited by their intellectual capacity. When Williams syndrome is suspected, confirmation is achieved by chromosome studies and FISH using a probe specific for this region. This test is currently standard in most cytogenetic laboratories. Intragenic deletions and translocations disrupting the elastin gene have been documented in dominant supravalvar aortic stenosis.

GENETIC COUNSELING

Genetic counseling should be a routine part of the care provided to adults with congenital heart disease and their families. This counseling can be provided by the patient's primary physician, a medical geneticist, or a genetic counselor. To provide accurate information, the physician must first determine if the patient's condition is isolated or syndromic and if other relatives have similar congenital heart malformations. The closer the degree of relationship between the patient and the affected relative, the more significant the information. It is also important to differentiate all syndromic types from nonsyndromic types. All individuals with a history of conotruncal heart malformation should be tested for DiGeorge and velocardiofacial syndromes.

In certain syndromic types, DNA tests may be available. The primary physician can order tests for such disorders through a medical geneticist or genetic counselor. If the physician orders any of these laboratory tests directly, all individuals who are identified as having a microchromosome deletion or mutation must be adequately counseled. Efforts should be made to contact and inform at-risk relatives. The recurrence risk estimates provided in this chapter are the best current estimates, but these are likely to change as the genes responsible for most cardiac malformations are identified.

BIBLIOGRAPHY

Balaj S, Dennis NR, Keeton BR: Familial Ebstein's anomaly: A report of six cases in two generations associated with mild skeletal anomalies. *Br Heart J* 66:26, 1991.

Bassett A, Chow W: 22q11 deletion syndrome: A genetic subtype of schizophrenia. *Biol Psychiatry* 46:882, 1999.

Bassett AS, Hodgkinson K, Chow EWC, et al: 22q11 deletion syndrome in adults with schizophrenia. *Am J Med Genet* 81:328, 1999.

Basson CT, Bachinsky DR, Lin RC, et al: Mutations in human cause limb and cardiac malformation in Holt-Oram syndrome. *Nat Genet* 15:30, 1997.

Benson DW, Sharkey A, Fatkin D, et al: Reduce penetrances, variable expressivity, and genetic heterogeneity of familial atrial septal defects. *Circulation* 97:2043, 1998.

Bleyl S, Nelso L, Odelberg SJ, et al: A gene for familial total anomalous pulmonary return maps to chromosome 4p13-q12. *Am J Hum Genet* 56:408, 1995.

Braunwald E: *Heart Disease: A Textbook of Cardiovascular Medicine*, 5th ed. Philadelphia, Saunders, 1997, p 896.

Burch M, Sharland M, Shinebourne E, et al: Cardiologic abnormality in Noonan syndrome: Phenotypic diagnosis and echocardiographic assessment of 118 patients. *J Am Coll Cardiol* 20: 1189, 1993.

Burn J and Goodship J: Congenital heart disease, in: Rimoin DL, Connor JM and Pyeritz RE (eds): *Emery and Rimoin's Principles and Practices of Medical Genetics.* Edinburg, Churchill Livingston, 1997, p. 790.

Cuneo BF, Driscoll DA, Gidding SS, Langman CB: Evolution of latent hypoparathyroidism in familial 22q11 deletion syndrome. *Am J Med Genet* 69:50, 1997.

Davidson HR: A large family with patent ductus arteriosus and unusual face. *J Med Genet* 30:503, 1992.

Digilio MC, Marino B, Toscano A, et al: Atrioventricular canal defect without Down syndrome: A heterogeneous malformation. *Am J Med Genet* 85:140, 1999.

Ferencz C, Boughman JA, Neill CA, et al: Congenital cardiovascular malformations: Questions on inheritance. Baltimore-Washington infant study group. *J Am Coll Cardiol* 14:756, 1989.

Gerboni S, Sabation G, Mingarelli R, Dallapiccola B: Coarctation of the aorta, interrupted aortic arch and hypoplastic left heart syndrome in three generations. *J Med Genet* 30:328, 1993.

Goldmuntz E, Clark BJ, Mitchell LA, et al: Frequency of 22q11 deletions in patients with conotruncal defects. *J Am Coll Cardiol* 32:492, 1998.

Goldmuntz E, Driscoll D, Budarf ML, et al: Microdeletions of chromosomal 22q11 in patients with congenital conotruncal cardiac defects. *J Med Genet* 30:807, 1993.

Gotzsche CO, Krag-Olsen B, Nielsen J, et al: Prevalence of cardiovascular malformations and associations with karyotypes in Turner's syndrome. *Arch Dis Child* 71:433, 1994.

Hofbeck M, Leipold G, Rauch A, et al: Clinical relevance of monosomy 22q11.2 in children with pulmonary atresia and ventricular septal defect. *Eur J Pediatr* 158:302, 1999.

Hoffman JI: Congenital heart disease: Incidence and inheritance. *Pediatr Clin North Am* 37:25, 1990.

Lin AE, Lippe B, Rosenfeld RG: Further delineation of aortic dilation, dissection, and rupture in patients with Turner syndrome. *Pediatrics* 102:1, 1998.

Lopez-Rangel E, Maurice M, Mcgillivray B, Friedman JM: William syndrome in adults. *Am J Med Genet* 44:720, 1992.

Lu JH, Chung My, Hwang B, Chien HP: Prevalence and parental origin in tetralogy of Fallot associated with chromosome 22q11 microdeletion. *Pediatrics* 104:87, 1999.

McIntosh N, Chitayat D, Bardanis M, Fouron JC: Ebstein anomaly: Report of a familial occurrence and prenatal diagnosis. *Am J Med Genet* 47:307, 1992.

Megabane A, Stephan E, Kassab R, et al: Autosomal dominant secundum atrial septal defect with various cardiac and noncardiac defects: A new midline disorder. *Am J Med Genet* 83:193, 1999.

Momma K, Matsuoka R, Takao A: Aortic arch anomalies associated with chromosome 22q11 deletion (CATCH 22). *Pediatr Cardiol* 20:97, 1999.

Nora JJ: Multifactorial inheritance hypothesis for the etiology of congenital heart diseases. *Circulation* 38:604, 1968.

Nora JJ and Nora AH: Genetic epidemiology of congenital heart diseases. *Prog Med Genet* 5:91, 1983.

Nora JJ, Nora AH and Berg K: *Cardiovascular Diseases. Genetics, Epidemiology and Prevention.* Oxford, Oxford University Press, 1991.

Swillen A, Devriendt K, Legius E, et al: Intelligence and psychosocial adjustment in velocardiofacial syndrome: A study of 37 children and adolescents with VCFS. *J Med Genet* 34:453, 1997.

Udwadia AD, Khambadkone S, Bharucha BA: Familial congenital valvar pulmonary stenosis: Autosomal dominant inheritance. *Pediatr Cardiol* 17:407, 1996.

Zetterquist PA: Clinical and genetic study of congenital heart defects. MD thesis, Institute of Medical Genetics, University of Uppsala, 1972.

INDEX

Note: Page numbers followed by *f* indicate figures; page numbers followed by *t* indicate tables.